Marine Glycobiology, Glycomics and Lectins

Marine Glycobiology, Glycomics and Lectins

Special Issue Editor

Yasuhiro Ozeki

MDPI • Basel • Beijing • Wuhan • Barcelona • Belgrade

MDPI

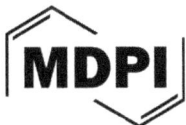

Special Issue Editor
Yasuhiro Ozeki
School of Sciences,
Yokohama City University
Japan

Editorial Office
MDPI
St. Alban-Anlage 66
4052 Basel, Switzerland

This is a reprint of articles from the Special Issue published online in the open access journal *Marine Drugs* (ISSN 1660-3397) from 2018 to 2019 (available at: https://www.mdpi.com/journal/marinedrugs/special_issues/marineglycobiology).

For citation purposes, cite each article independently as indicated on the article page online and as indicated below:

LastName, A.A.; LastName, B.B.; LastName, C.C. Article Title. *Journal Name* **Year**, *Article Number*, Page Range.

ISBN 978-3-03921-820-2 (Pbk)
ISBN 978-3-03921-821-9 (PDF)

Contents

About the Special Issue Editor

Yasuhiro Ozeki (1961–) is a Japanese lectinologist and glycobiologist. He graduated from Meijo University (known for its two Nobel laureates for blue diodes (2014) and lithium-ion batteries (2019)), School of Agriculture, Nagoya, Japan, in 1984. He started his research career in protein chemistry at the Division of Biomedical Polymer Science at the Institute of Comprehensive Medical Sciences, Fujita Health University, Toyoake Aichi, Japan. He was awarded his Ph.D. at Fujita Health University in 1992 under the supervision of Prof Koiti Titani. He conducted postdoctoral research as an NIH Fellow at The Biomembrane Institute (Otsuka Co., Ltd. President Prof Sen-itiroh Hakomori) and the University of Washington, Seattle, WA (1994–1995) on glycobiology. He has held a tenure position at Yokohama City University, Japan, since 1995. Currently, he is Scientific Advisor of Yokohama Science Frontier High School (since 2009); a Steering Committee Member, Misaki Marine Biological Station, Graduate School of Sciences, The University of Tokyo (since 2013); a Board Member of Yokohama Ocean Association (since 2016); an Editorial Board Member of the both journals Marine Drugs and Molecules of the publisher MDPI (since 2019). Dr. Ozeki has published 7 articles in MDPI journals (2012–2019) and edited this Special Issue. He has determined the representative primary structures of lectin families such as SUEL/rhamnose-binding lectin (UniProtKB P22031 1991), mytilectin (MytiLec: UniProtKB B3EWR1 2012), C1q/TNF (OXYL: GenBank MK434202.1, 2019), R-type (SeviL: GenBank MK434191, 2019) and supervised 5 Ph.D. students, 1 JSPS Postdoctoral Fellow, and 1 JSPS Invitation Fellowship scientist from Japan and Bangladesh since 2005.

Preface to "Marine Glycobiology, Glycomics and Lectins"

Glycans (carbohydrate chains) of marine creatures are rich and diverse in polysaccharides, glycoproteins, and glycolipids. The chains that are metabolized by glycan-related enzymes (glycosyltransferases and glycosidases) are recognized by glycan-binding proteins (lectins), which regulate cellular processes such as growth, differentiation, and death. Marine glycomics that involves the genome and transcriptome accelerates our understanding of the evolution of glycans, glycan-related enzymes, and lectins.

From 2017 to 2019, the Special Issue, "Marine Glycobiology, Glycomics and Lectins" of the journal Marine Drugs published scientific articles and reviews on the background of "glycobiology"—that is, glycan-based biosciences. The aim was to promote the discovery of novel biomolecules that contribute to drug development and clinical studies. This has great potential for establishing connections between the fields of both human health and marine life sciences.

This book contains 11 scientific papers representing current topics in comprehensive glycosciences related to therapeutic agents from marine natural products, as outlined.

Part 1. Marine Glycobiology (Articles No. 1–6):

- The prominent pharmacological and therapeutic effects of fucoidan, the sulfated fucose-containing polysaccharides in brown algae (phylum Ochrophyta) are introduced. A range of valuable bioactivities are represented, including the epigenetic modification and differentiation induction of malignant glioma cells, in addition to the implications for use in age-related macular degeneration.

- Polysialoglycan chains in nematocysts of hydra (phylum Cnidaria) that also rich in human tumor cells were investigated for binding to lectins. These finds have implications for future nanomedical devices and their application in cancer diagnostics and therapies.

- Glycosaminoglycans extracted from the clubs (phylum Arthropoda) inhibited β-secretase associated with Alzheimer's disease. On the other hand, another glycan with anticoagulant activity found in sea cucumber (phylum Echinodermata) was investigated with respect to structure–function relationships. The findings are certain to facilitate increased focus on the newly characterized pharmacological activities of glycosaminoglycans.

Part 2. Marine Glycomics (Articles No. 7 and 8):

- A heat-stable β-1,3-galactosidase derived from the genome of bacteria (genus Marinomonas) found in the Arctic Ocean was biotechnologically expressed in the competent cells. This can be applied to the production of sufficient galactooligosaccharides, leading to an increased number of bifidobacteria in the digestive tract, which is effective in improving immunity to prevent cancer.

- The analysis of the oyster genome (phylum Mollusca) was conducted to elucidate the evolutionary mechanisms behind the molecular diversification of C1q-domain-containing proteins, known to act as lectin-like molecules in the innate immune response of bivalves. This information is expected to lead to the discovery of new drugs with valuable immunological properties and different modes of action.

Part 3. Marine Lectins (Articles No. 9–11):

- Various lectin genes derived from horseshoe crabs (phylum Arthropoda) and abalones (phylum Mollusca) were encoded in oncolytic virus genes, where they displayed various anticancer effects.

- A β-trefoil folding lectin in mussels (phylum Mollusca) showed regulation of cancer-related genes transcription when cancer cells were killed by the lectin in vivo. The functional diversity of lectins seen here will be utilized in future biotechnology.

Yasuhiro Ozeki
Special Issue Editor

marine drugs

MDPI

Article

Effects of Crude *Fucus distichus* Subspecies *evanescens* Fucoidan Extract on Retinal Pigment Epithelium Cells—Implications for Use in Age-Related Macular Degeneration

Kevin Rohwer [1], Sandesh Neupane [2], Kaya Saskia Bittkau [2], Mayra Galarza Pérez [2], Philipp Dörschmann [1], Johann Roider [1], Susanne Alban [2] and Alexa Klettner [1,*]

[1]   Department of Ophthalmology, University Medical Center, University of Kiel, 24105 Kiel, Germany;
      k.rohwer@live.de (K.R.); Philipp.Doerschmann@uksh.de (P.D.); Johann.Roider@uksh.de (J.R.)
[2]   Department of Pharmaceutical Biology, Pharmaceutical Institute, University of Kiel, 24105 Kiel, Germany;
      sneupane@pharmazie.uni-kiel.de (S.N.); kbittkau@pharmazie.uni-kiel.de (K.S.B.);
      mperez@pharmazie.uni-kiel.de (M.G.P.); salban@pharmazie.uni-kiel.de (S.A.)
*   Correspondence: AlexaKarina.Klettner@uksh.de; Tel.: +49-431-500-24283

check for updates

Received: 14 August 2019; Accepted: 10 September 2019; Published: 16 September 2019

Abstract: Fucoidan extracts may have beneficial effects in age-related macular degeneration (AMD). Over-the-counter fucoidan preparations are generally undefined, crude extracts. In this study, we investigated the effect of a crude fucoidan extract from *Fucus distichus* subspecies *evanescens* (Fe) on the retinal pigment epithelium (RPE). Fe extract was investigated for chemical composition and molar mass. It was tested in primary RPE and RPE cell line ARPE19. Oxidative stress was induced with *tert*-butyl hydroperoxide, cell viability evaluated with MTT assay, VEGF secretion assessed in ELISA. Phagocytosis was evaluated in a fluorescence microscopic assay. Wound healing ability was tested in a scratch assay. Additionally, the inhibition of elastase and complement system by Fe extract was studied. The Fe extract contained about 61.9% fucose and high amounts of uronic acids (26.2%). The sulfate content was not as high as expected (6.9%). It was not toxic and not protective against oxidative stress. However, Fe extract was able to reduce VEGF secretion in ARPE19. Phagocytosis was also reduced. Concerning wound healing, a delay could be observed in higher concentrations. While some beneficial effects could be found, it seems to interfere with RPE function, which may reduce its beneficial effects in AMD treatment.

Keywords: *Fucus distichus* subsp. *evanescens*; fucoidan; retinal pigment epithelium; VEGF; oxidative stress; phagocytosis

1. Introduction

Fucoidans are sulfated polysaccharides derived from brown seaweed, consisting mainly of sulfated fucose. Many different biological activities have been described for fucoidan, but fucoidans are heterogeneous, varying strongly between different species [1].

Among the biological activities described for fucoidans are those interesting for potential treatment of age-related macular degeneration (AMD) [2]. AMD is the main cause for blindness and visual impairment in the elderly. Its pathogenesis is complex and multifactorial yet accepted as a major factor in the development of AMD is oxidative stress [3–5]. The retina is exposed to high degrees of oxidative stress through constant exposure to high-energetic sun light, due to a high activity of mitochondria in photoreceptors and retinal pigment epithelial cells (RPE), and due to the presence of oxidized fatty acids. The retinal pigment epithelium, a monolayer between the photoreceptors and the choroid, protects the retina from oxidative stress [6] but may succumb to the accumulating damage and degenerate later in life, leading to secondary degeneration of the photoreceptors [4,7,8]. In a subset of AMD, the exudative or wet form, choroidal vessels may grow into the retina, trying to compensate for hypoxia that may be present in the retina due to poor oxygen supply. These vessels are highly immature and leak fluids into the subretinal space, destroying RPE cells and photoreceptors. The most important factor for this neovascularization is vascular endothelial growth factor (VEGF) and VEGF inhibition is the current treatment for exudative AMD [3,9].

Fucoidans have been shown to be protective against oxidative stress in various cell assays [10–13], and we have shown such a protective, anti-oxidative stress effect of fucoidan from *Fucus vesiculosus* in ocular cells as well [14]. Furthermore, a variety of fucoidans have been shown to inhibit VEGF and VEGF-mediated angiogenesis [15–17], including in our study on fucoidan of *Fucus vesiculosus* tested on endothelial cells stimulated with RPE supernatant [18]. However, the pro- or anti-angiogenic effect as well as its influence on VEGF are highly dependent on the origin, structure, and molecular weight of the fucoidan [19] and may exert different effects in different experimental systems [14].

Most studies have been carried out with commercially available fucoidan from *Fucus vesiculosus*. In this study, we have investigated a fucoidan extract from *Fucus distichus* subspecies *evanescens*. Previous studies on fucoidans from *Fucus evanescens* mainly focused on immunomodulating effects [20–22], while there have been only limited studies in the context of potential use for AMD [23].

Several studies have reported different structure and composition of fucoidan extracted from *F. evanescens* [20,24–27]. They described fucose as the main monosaccharide with a low amount of other sugars like mannose, glucose, galactose, and xylose. The diversity in their composition can be dependent on harvest time, place, and the applied extraction method [28].

In our study, we have used a crude extract from *Fucus distichus* subsp. *evanescens* harvested in the Kiel Fjord. The extract was chemically characterized, and some additional basic activities were determined to enable an estimation of its potencies compared to purified fucoidans and was investigated regarding its potential to protect against oxidative stress-induced cell death and to inhibit VEGF secretion. Furthermore, as a functional RPE is a prerogative for functional photoreceptors and needs to be protected to avoid the development of AMD, we additionally tested the effects of the extract on parameters of RPE functions, such as toxicity, phagocytosis, and wound healing.

2. Results

2.1. Chemical Characterization of Fe Extract

We determined the basic structural composition of Fe extract (Table 1). Its content of neutral monosaccharides showed to be very low (7.54%), whereas the uronic acid content was quite high (26.1%). The neutral monosaccharides were composed of fucose (61.9%), xylose (10.1%), mannose (24.1%) and glucose (3.9%). Additionally, the molecular weight (Mw) (88.6 ± 1.0 kDa), sulfate content (SO_3Na; 6.9%), protein content (2.8%), and total phenolic content (TPC; 14.4 ± 0.7 µg GAE/mg) were determined (Table 1).

Table 1. Structural composition of extract from *Fucus distichus* subsp. *evanescens* (Fe).

Monosaccharide Composition (mol %)				Uronic Acid (%)	Mw (kDa)	SO$_3$Na (%)	Protein (%)	TPC (µg GAE/mg)
Fuc	Xyl	Man	Glc					
61.9	10.1	24.1	3.9	26.1 ± 0.2	88.60 ± 1.0	6.9	2. 8	14.4 ± 0.7

2.2. Activity Assays

Testing of the concentration-dependent inhibitory potency of Fe on elastase and complement system activation revealed half-maximal inhibitory concentrations (IC$_{50}$) of 1.48 ± 0.08 µg/mL (elastase) and 5.73 ± 1.11 µg/mL (complement system) (Table 2). The antioxidant capacity (AOC) of Fe extract

(500 µg/mL) amounted to 4.65 ± 1.80%. However, compared to the reference compound Trolox, the effect was about 500 times weaker.

Table 2. Activities of Fe extract.

Elastase Inhibition IC$_{50}$ (µg/mL)	Complement System Inhibition IC$_{50}$ (µg/mL)	DPPH AOC (%) of 500 µg/mL
1.48 ± 0.08	5.73 ± 1.11	4.65 ± 1.80

2.3. Toxicity of Fe

We have tested a potential toxic effect of Fe extract on ARPE19 and primary RPE cells. For ARPE19, no influence of Fe extract in the tested concentrations (1 µg/mL, 10 µg/mL, 100 µg/mL and 250 µg/mL) was found after one day and three days of incubation. After seven days, a slight decrease of cell viability could be noted at a concentration of 100 µg/mL (95.60 ± 3.43%), which reached statistical significance (Figure 1a–c). In primary RPE cells, no influence could be found after 1, 3 or 7 days (Figure 1d–f). In addition, even after four weeks of incubation or after use of 500 µg/mL Fe extract at any tested time point, no loss of cell viability could be seen (data not shown). Consequently, Fe extract does not impair the viability of RPE cells.

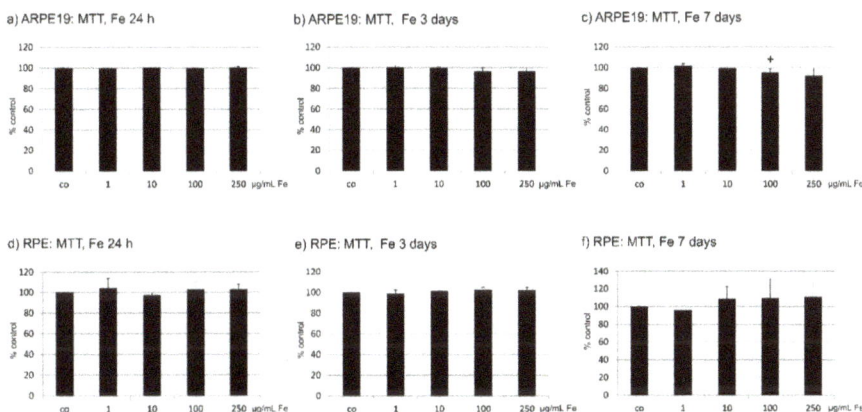

Figure 1. Cell viability tests after incubation with *Fucus distichus* subsp. *evanescens* fucoidan extract for 24 h, three days or seven days. Cell viability was determined by MTT assay. In ARPE19 cells, no influence was found on cells after 24 h (**a**) or three days (**b**). After seven days, a slight but significant reduction of cell viability was seen at a concentration of 100 µg/mL, but not at higher concentrations (**c**). In primary RPE cells, no influence on cell viability was seen after 24 h (**d**), three days (**e**), or seven days (**f**). Significance was evaluated with student's *t*-test, + $p < 0.05$, co = untreated control, Fe = crude fucoidan from *Fucus distichus* subsp. *evanescens*, h = hour.

2.4. Oxidative Stress Protection

Oxidative stress protection has been attributed to fucoidan and to polyphenols, found in crude fucoidan extracts. We tested the protective effect of Fe extract on ARPE19 cells treated with 500, 750, and 1000 µM *tert*-butyl hydroperoxide (TBHP). All three concentrations of TBHP significantly reduced cell viability in ARPE19 cells. When treated with Fe extract (1 µg/mL, 10 µg/mL, 100 µg/mL, and 250 µg/mL), no increase in cell viability was found for any TBHP or Fe extract concentration tested (Figure 2a–c). Clearly, this extract does not provide protection against oxidative stress.

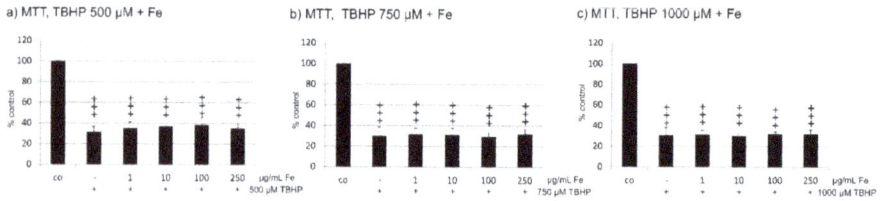

Figure 2. Cell viability after the induction of oxidative stress by *tert*-butylhydroperoxid (TBHP). Cell viability was determined by MTT assay. ARPE19 cells were incubated for 24 h with 500 μM (**a**), 750 μM (**b**), or 1000 μM (**c**) TBHP and the protective effect of Fe extract was measured for 1, 10, 100, and 250 μM. No increase of cell viability was found for any concentration of Fe extract at any oxidative stimulus tested. Significance was evaluated with student's *t*-test, $^{+++}$ $p < 0.001$ against untreated control, co = untreated control, Fe = crude fucoidan from *Fucus distichus* subsp. *evanescens*.

2.5. VEGF Secretion

VEGF secretion was detected in ARPE19 cells after incubation with the different concentrations of Fe extract (1 μg/mL, 10 μg/mL, 100 μg/mL and 250 μg/mL) after 24 h, three days or seven days (Figure 3). At all time points, Fe extract reduced the VEGF concentration in the supernatants compared to untreated control, with the most profound effect after 24 h, which reached statistical significance at concentrations of 100 and 250 μg/mL Fe extract (100 μg/mL: 54.87 ± 7.12%, $p < 0.001$; 250 μg/mL 28.87 ± 18.50%, $p < 0.001$) (Figure 3a). After three days, a significant reduction could be found at a concentration of 100 μg/mL (81.23 ± 13.48%, $p < 0.05$). Of note, 1 and 10 μg/mL resulted in a slight but significant increase of VEGF (1 μg/mL 113.61 ± 9.91%, $p < 0.05$; 10 μg/mL 113.97 ± 9.00%, $p < 0.05$) (Figure 3b). After seven days, a significant decrease of the VEGF content could be found for 250 μg/mL (67.00 ± 12.32, $p < 0.01$) (Figure 3c).

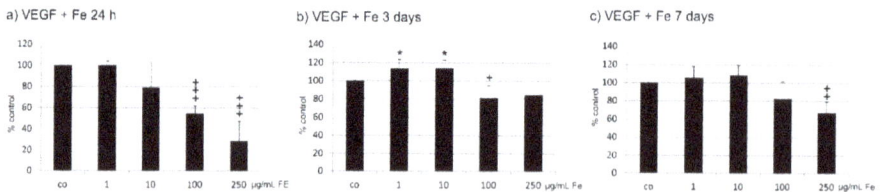

Figure 3. Effect of Fe extract on VEGF secretion of ARPE19 cells. VEGF content in the cell supernatant was investigated with a commercial ELISA. *Fucus distichus* subsp. *evanescens* fucoidan extract was tested in various concentrations (1 μg/mL, 10 μg/mL, 100 μg/mL, 250 μg/mL) for 24 h (**a**), three days (**b**), or seven days (**c**) on ARPE19 cells. After 24 h (**a**), a significant reduction of VEGF could be found for 100 and 250 μg/mL. After three days (**b**), 100 μg/mL was still significantly effective. Of note, a slight but significant increase of VEGF secretion could be found for 1 and 10 μg/mL after three days. After seven days (**c**), 250 μg/mL significantly reduced VEGF content. Significance was evaluated with student's *t*-test against untreated control, $^{+}$ $p < 0.05$, $^{++}$ $p < 0.01$, $^{+++}$ $p < 0.001$, reduction against untreated control, * $p < 0.05$, increase against untreated control, co = untreated control, Fe = crude fucoidan from *Fucus distichus* subsp. *evanescens*, h = hour.

2.6. Phagocytosis

Phagocytosis of shed photoreceptor outer segments is an important task of RPE cells. After incubation with Fe extract for 24 h, 1 μg/mL Fe extract significantly enhanced phagocytic activity (1 μg/mL 139.92 ± 68.32%, $p < 0.05$), while 100 and 250 μg/mL significantly decreased it compared to untreated control (100 μg/mL 41.00 ± 30.75%, $p < 0.001$; 250 μg/mL 24.77 ± 19.94%, $p < 0.001$) (Figure 4a). After three days, all concentrations tested significantly decreased phagocytic activity compared to untreated control (1 μg/mL 56.42 ± 40.34%; 10 μg/mL 45.29 ± 24.05%; 100 μg/mL

16.07 ± 9.39%; 250 µg/mL 21.56 ± 20.02%; all $p < 0.001$) (Figure 4b). After seven days of Fe extract incubation, a significant reduction of phagocytosis compared to untreated cells was seen at 100 µg/mL (33.97 ± 17.35%; $p < 0.001$) and 250 µg/mL (40.82 ± 34.74%; $p < 0.001$) (Figure 4c).

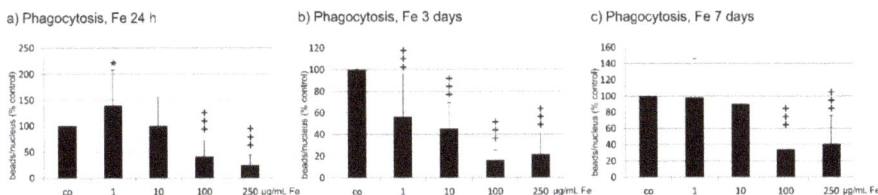

Figure 4. Phagocytic activity of RPE cells after incubation with *Fucus distichus* subsp. *evanescens* fucoidan extract. Phagocytic activity was investigated with a phagocytosis assay using photoreceptor outer segment-treated fluorescent latex beads. RPE cells were treated for 24 h (**a**), three days (**b**), or seven days (**c**) with different concentrations of Fe extract (1 µg/mL, 10 µg/mL, 100 µg/mL, 250 µg/mL). After 24 h, 1 µg/mL induced a significant increase in phagocytic activity, while 100 and 250 µg/mL significantly reduced phagocytosis. After three days, all tested concentrations significantly reduced phagocytosis. After seven days, phagocytosis was significantly reduced by 100 and 250 µg/mL. Significance was evaluated with student's *t*-test against untreated control, [+++] $p < 0.001$, reduction against untreated control, [*] $p < 0.05$, increase against untreated control. co = untreated control, Fe = crude fucoidan from *Fucus distichus* subsp. *evanescens*, h = hour.

2.7. Wound Healing

In the scratch assay, the wound area was analyzed 24 and 48 h post scratch of a confluent cell layer of RPE after treatment for 24 h, four days, or seven days with Fe extract. Incubation with Fe extract for 24 h significantly slowed down wound healing measured 24 h after scratch at 100 and 250 µg/mL Fe extract (control: 71.17 ± 7.16%; 100 µg/mL 80.31 ± 3.67%; 250 µg/mL 83.62 ± 3.18%; (both $p < 0.001$). At 48 h after scratch, also 10 µg/mL as well as 100 µg/mL and 250 µg/mL significantly delayed wound healing (co 58.89 ± 11.54%, 10 µg/mL 67.41 ± 4.30, $p < 0.01$; 100 µg/mL 68.12 ± 4.49, $p < 0.01$; 250 µg/mL 70.81 ± 6.24%, $p < 0.001$) (Figure 5a). After four days of incubation with Fe, wound healing 24 h post scratch was significantly delayed at concentrations of 10 µg/mL (co 65.01 ± 13.34%; 10 µg/mL 80.74 ± 12.42%, $p < 0.01$), 100 µg/mL (79.70 ± 9.03%; $p < 0.001$), and 250 µg/mL (89.05 ± 11.31%; $p < 0.001$) compared to scratched control not treated with Fe extract. But at 48 h after scratch, only 250 mg/mL displayed a significant delay of wound healing (co 61.60 ± 15.69%; 250 µg/mL 76.88 ± 20.12%, $p < 0.05$) (Figure 5b). Long-term incubation with Fe extract for seven days 24 h post-scratch showed a significant delay in wound healing again for 100 µg/mL (co 72.91 ± 9.46%; 100 µg/mL 81.94 ± 9.41%, $p < 0.01$) and 250 µg/mL (81.34 ± 9.71%, $p < 0.05$). After 48 hours, however, this effect was lost and conversely, wound healing was accelerated by 10 µg/mL Fe extract (co 69.54 ± 8.15%; 10 µg/mL 51.93 ± 16.29%, $p < 0.001$) (Figure 5c).

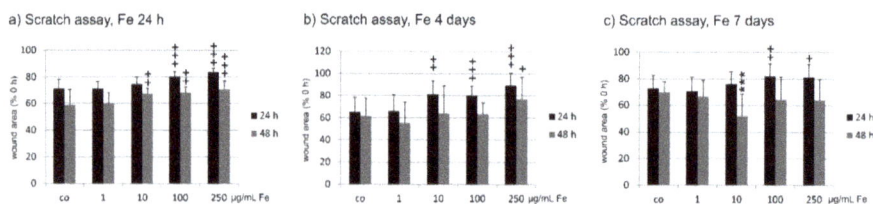

Figure 5. Wound healing of primary RPE cells after incubation with *Fucus distichus* subsp. *evanescens* fucoidan extract. A scratch was applied to a confluent RPE cell layer and the wound area was assessed 24 and 48 h after application. Cells were incubated for 24 h (**a**), four days (**b**), or seven days (**c**) with different concentrations of Fe extract (1 µg/mL, 10 µg/mL, 100 µg/mL, 250 µg/mL). (**a**) When cells were treated for 24 h with Fe extract, wound healing was significantly delayed one day after scratch at 100 and 250 µg/mL. After 48 h, wound healing was significantly delayed at 10, 100 and 250 µg/mL. When cells were treated for four days with Fe extract (**b**), wound healing was significantly delayed one day after scratch at 10, 100, and 250 µg/mL. Forty-eight hours after scratch, a significant delay could be seen at 250 µg/mL. After seven days of Fe extract incubation (**c**) and 24 h after scratch, wound healing was significantly delayed at 100 and 250 µg/mL. This effect was lost 48 h after scratch, where 10 µg/mL significantly accelerated wound healing. Significance was evaluated with student's *t*-test against untreated control, [+] $p < 0.05$, [++] $p < 0.01$, [+++] $p < 0.001$, delayed wound healing; [***] $p < 0.001$, accelerated wound healing, co = scratched control with Fe treatment, Fe = crude fucoidan from *Fucus distichus* subsp. *evanescens*, h = hour.

3. Discussion

Potential use of fucoidans in medical application has raised much interest [29]. However, the effects of fucoidans may not only differ in dependence on the algae species but also due to the used extraction methods and different degrees of purity [1]. Often, commercially available cosmetics and food supplements are declared to contain fucoidans, but these are generally poorly defined, with considerable deviation in fucoidan content. So far, much research has been done with commercially available fucoidan from *Fucus vesiculosus* [30], including our own study on *Fucus vesiculosus* fucoidan for potential use in AMD or uveal melanoma [14,18]. In the present study, we have investigated a fucoidan from another alga, *Fucus distichus* subsp. *evanescens*, which has so far not received as much attention in the literature. Recently, quite pure fucoidan from *Fucus distichus* subsp. *evanescens* (Fuc-Fe) showed to reduce the VEGF secretion in ARPE19 and displayed high affinity to VEGF but had no protective effect on ARPE19 [23]. In the current study, we used a crude extract of this alga, which can be easily produced in high amounts, elucidating its efficacy.

Despite of the high content of fucose (61%) in the Fe extract, which is the main monosaccharide of fucoidans, the low yield of neutral monosaccharides in the GLC analysis indicate that the content of fucoidan in the Fe extract is quite low. Accordingly, the sulfate content (6.9% as SO_3Na) was also quite low compared to 15–46% found in crude as well as purified fucoidans from Fucus *distichus* subsp. *evanescens* [20,25–27]. This suggests that Fe extract contains far less than 25% fucoidan, whereas the high uronic acid content (26%) indicates a high content of alginic acid, another typical cell wall compound of brown algae. This had to be expected, since methods to remove alginic acid from the extract such as a precipitation with calcium were not applied for the production of Fe extract. As previously shown, the antioxidative capacity of fucoidans is mainly due to co-extracted polyphenols [28,31]. The Fe extract exhibited only weak radical scavenging potency, which was comparable with that of Fuc-Fe and correlated with the respective total phenolic content, which turned out to be lower than that of fucoidan from *Fucus vesiculosus* (manuscript submitted). This is in line with the missing oxidative stress protection of Fe extract (see below).

Regarding a potential use of fucoidan from brown algae as a treatment option for age-related macular degeneration, we tested its effect against oxidative stress, as this comprises a general pathological pathway in AMD, and its interaction with VEGF, as this is the major pathological factor for exudative AMD.

Fe extract did not exhibit any protection against oxidative-stress induced loss of cell viability in ARPE19 cells. This is in contrast to our finding for fucoidan from *Fucus vesiculosus*, which protected the uveal melanoma from oxidative stress-induced cell death [14], and in correspondence with a paper recently published by our group, which showed a protection by Fuc-Fe of against oxidative stress in uveal melanoma cells but not in ARPE19 [23]. Obviously, different cell types react differently to oxidative stress. Uveal melanoma cell lines are rather susceptible to oxidative stress, as their superoxide dismutase (SOD) activity, which acts in oxidative stress protection, tends to be reduced [32], while RPE are highly resistant to oxidative stress, which is mainly mediated by Nrf-2 [6,33]. Fucoidan has been reported to confer its protection by activation of Nrf-2 and upregulation of SOD [12,13,34], and it is conceivable that this protective pathway may work on one cell line with reduced SOD activity (uveal melanoma) but not with a cell line with constitutive Nrf-2 activation (RPE). However, the lack of any effect concerning oxidative-stress induced cell death strongly indicates that we find no scavenging effect for this Fe extract. These data on oxidative stress protection confirm our previous findings that fucoidan from species other than *Fucus distichus* subsp. *evanescens* may be more suitable for oxidative stress protection [23] but also that the presence of additional compounds in a crude extract does not hold any beneficial effects considering oxidative stress protection.

Concerning VEGF inhibition, Fe extract turned out to reduce VEGF secretion. However, this effect was time- and concentration-dependent, showing the strongest effect after one day. Of note, however, we found an induction of VEGF secretion after three days for lower concentrations of fucoidan (1 and 10 μg/mL), which is not desirable, as the VEGF content in (exudative) AMD eyes has to be reduced. Compared with our data obtained with fucoidan from commercially available *Fucus vesiculosus* and with the purer Fuc-Fe [18,23], our data indicate that Fe extract is less suitable for VEGF secretion inhibition. As this is a crude extract, our data also suggest that no benefit can be seen from additional compounds other than fucoidan present in the extract. Furthermore, fucoidans from other species such as *Saccharina latissima* or *Fucus vesiculosus* may be more promising for further development [23].

RPE cells have a plethora of function in the retina and their functions are vital for a healthy, functioning retina [35]. Furthermore, RPE cells in AMD patients are already challenged and in danger of degeneration. Therefore, any substance to be considered for use in AMD should interfere as little with RPE function as possible. We have tested toxicity, wound healing and phagocytosis as parameters. Similar to our findings with *Fucus vesiculosus* fucoidan as well as fucoidans from five other algae [36], we did not find a relevant toxic effect. However, some minor but nevertheless significant reduction was seen after seven days, which was not observed for *Fucus vesiculosus* fucoidan [18]. Notably, both *Fucus vesiculosus* and Fe extract reduced the wound healing abilities of RPE cells. However, the data obtained 24 and 48 hours after scratch suggest that this is a transient effect and might therefore not be of further consequence for RPE cell function. More importantly, considering the function of RPE cells, Fe extract reduced phagocytic activity of the cells at all tested time points at 100 and 250 μg/mL (and additionally at 1 and 10 μg/mL after three days). A previous study testing fucoidan of *Fucus vesiculosus* at a concentration of 100 μg/mL did not exhibit a reduction of phagocytic activity [18]. In that study, phagocytosis was evaluated only after short term incubation, therefore the effect could be related to duration of fucoidan exposition. However, the effect of the Fe extract was found at every time point tested, indicating a species-dependent effect. In addition, it is possible that other components present in the extract are interfering with phagocytic activity. As a prolonged reduction of phagocytosis could possibly impair the function of the retina, which is not desirable when treating AMD, further testing is needed to elucidate the effects of purity and species of fucoidans on RPE function.

The results so far indicate some beneficial effects of this crude extract of *Fucus distichus* subsp. *evanescens* with regard to AMD, concerning VEGF inhibition. Previous investigations with the purer Fuc-Fe suggest that beneficial effects are due to the fucoidan content and not due to other compounds of the Fe extract. The reduction of phagocytic activity in RPE cells may be of concern.

There are other aspects of interest for AMD pathology that we did not test in our assays, such as lipid metabolism [37,38], which may be influenced by fucoidans [39,40], or inflammatory aspects [41], which also could be influenced by fucoidans and especially by fucoidan of *Fucus distichus* subsp. *evanescens* [22,42]. Future studies should address these issues, but for these, highly purified fucoidans should be used. In conclusion, crude extracts from *Fucus distichus* subsp. *evanescens* are of some interests in regard to potential AMD treatment considering their effect on RPE cells. However, fucoidans of other species may be of higher interest, and, importantly, further studies should be performed with highly purified fucoidans.

4. Materials and Methods

4.1. Extraction

Fucus distichus subsp. *evanescens* was cleaned from epiphytes and washed with tap water, drained and autoclaved. The material was mixed with four volumes of extraction buffer (100 mM Tris base, pH 10.0) and shredded and blended with Ultraturrax (Sigma-Aldrich, Steinheim, Germany) for 1 min at maximum speed. After centrifugation and separation of the supernatant, the algae material was two further times treated as described with one volume of extraction buffer each. Then, NaCl and citric acid were added to the combined supernatants resulting in 600 mM NaCl and pH 4.75. The extract was then mixed with ethanol (final concentration 50%) (v/v) for precipitation over night at room temperature. After centrifugation, the pellet was dissolved in 20 mM NaOH, and the precipitation procedure including the addition of NaCl and citric acid was repeated once, and was finally dissolved in pure water (pH ~6.0), frozen, and lyophilized. The yield amounted to about 4% in relation to wet algae mass and to 18.4% in dry algae mass.

4.2. Elemental Analysis

The contents of hydrogen, carbon, nitrogen, and sulfur in the crude *Fucus distichus* subsp. *evanescens* fucoidan extract (Fe) were determined by elemental analysis performed with the HEKAtech CHNS Analyser (HEKAtech, Wegberg, Germany; calibrator: sulfanil amide). After gas liquid chromatographic separation (carrier gas: helium), the respective analyte gases were detected in a thermal conductivity detector. The nitrogen content (%) was multiplied by 6.25 to estimate the protein content [43]. Based on the sulfur content (%), the content of sulfate groups (as $-SO_3Na$) was calculated.

4.3. Molecular Weight (Mw) Determination

The average molecular weight (Mw) of the fucoidan extract was examined by size exclusion chromatography (SEC) (ÄKTA Pure 25 from GE Healthcare, Munich, Germany), coupled with online multi-angle light scattering (MALS) and refractive index (RI) detection using DAWN 8+ and Optilab T-rex (Wyatt Technology Corporation, Dernbach, Germany). For the separation by hydrodynamic volume, an OHPak LB-806M 8.0 mmID X 300 mmL (ShodexTM, Munich, Germany) column was used. The mobile phase was composed of 0.15 mol/L NaCl, 0.025 mol/L NaH_2PO_4, 0.025 mol/L Na_2HPO_4 (pH 7.0) and a flow rate of 0.5 mL/min was applied. The sample was dissolved in the elution buffer to a concentration of 2.0 mg/mL, and 100 μL were injected. The elution buffer was degassed using ultrasound for 30 min. The MALS detector was calibrated by the manufacturer using toluol. The used refractive index increment (dn/dc) was 0.150 mL/g. The Mw values were calculated with ASTRA 7.1.2.5 (Wyatt Technology Corporation, Dernbach, Germany). The chromatographic system was controlled by UNICORN 7.2 GE (Healthcare, Munich, Germany).

4.4. Monosaccharide Composition by Acetylation Analysis

For the determination of neutral monosaccharide composition, the Fe extract was hydrolyzed with 2.0 mol/L trifluoroacetic acid (TFA) at 121 °C [44] and, after evaporation of TFA, converted into alditol acetate derivatives (AA) by reduction and acetylation [45]. The AA were separated by gas liquid chromatography (GLC) on an OPTIMA-225-0.25 µm fused silica capillary column (25 m × 0.25 mm i.d., film thickness 0.25 µm, Macherey-Nagel, Düren, Germany) using an GC 7890B gas chromatograph (Agilent Technologies, Waldbronn, Germanywith integrated flame ionization detector. The helium flow rate was 1.0 mL/min, the oven temperature was 180 °C for 5 min followed by an increase of 1 °C/min up to 210 °C held for 10 min, the temperatures of injector and detector were 250 °C and 240 °C, respectively. The AA were identified by their retention times. For quantitative analysis, the samples were supplemented with a defined amount of myo-inositol as an internal standard. The percentage of the respective AA was calculated by Agilent MassHunter Qualitative Analysis Workflows B.08.00, (Waldbronn, Germany).

4.5. Uronic Acid Determination

Uronic acids were quantified by reaction with 3-hydroxydiphenyl according to the method by Blumenkrantz and Asboe-Hansen modified by Filisetti-Cozzi and Carpita [46].

4.6. Total Phenolic Content

The total phenolic content (TPC) was determined by a modified Folin–Ciocalteu method in a microplate format [47] with slightly adapted volumes. Aqueous fucoidan extract (20 µL) was mixed with 0.025 N Folin–Ciocalteu reagent (200 µL; Merck Millipore, Cat. 109001) and incubated for 5 min. Then, 2 M Na_2CO_3 (30 µL) was added and absorption was measured at 660 nm (FLUOstar Omega, BMG LABTECH GmbH, Ortenberg, Germany) after 2 h. Gallic acid (Roth, Cat. 7300.1) was used as reference and TPC of sample was expressed as gallic acid equivalents (GAE) in µg per mg of the dry substance.

4.7. DPPH Scavenging Assay

The antioxidant potency of the crude *Fucus distichus* subsp. *evanescens* fucoidan extract was determined by the 2,2-diphenyl-1-picrylhydrazyl radical (DPPH; Sigma-Aldrich, Munich, Germany, Cat. D9132) scavenging microplate assay as previously described [48]. An aliquot of 100 µL of a 0.20 mmol/L DPPH-solution in ethanol 70% (V/V) was mixed with 100 µL of the sample (0.5 mg/mL in ethanol 70% (V/V)). For the control, 100 µL DPPH solution were mixed with 100 µL ethanol 70% (V/V). After incubation for 30 min at 20 °C in the dark, the absorption (A) was measured at 520 nm using the plate reader FLUOstar Omega (BMG LABTECH GmbH, Ortenberg, Germany). The radical scavenging potency of the fucoidan samples was calculated by the formula

$$\text{radical scavenging potency (\%)} = (A \text{ control} - A \text{ sample})/A \text{ control} \times 100.$$

Trolox (6-hydroxy-2,5,7,8-tetramethylchroman-2-carboxylic acid; Sigma Aldrich, Munich, Germany) dissolved in ethanol 70% (V/V) was used as reference substance. Its concentration ranged from 3 to 12 µg/mL.

4.8. Fluorigenic PMN-Elastase Activity Assay

The elastase inhibitory activity was examined by a fluorogenic microplate assay using elastase from human polymorph nuclear granulocytes (PMN, EC 3.4.21.37, Merck Millipore, Germany) and the substrate MeOSuc-Ala-Ala-Pro-Val-7-amido-4-methylcoumarin (Bachem, Bubendorf, Switzerland) as previously described [49,50]. By means of the concentration-dependent inhibition curves, the concentration of test compound for 50% inhibition of elastase activities (IC_{50} in µg/mL) was calculated.

4.9. Hemolytic Classical Complement Modulation Assay

An aliquot of 75 µL fucoidan extract in veronal buffered saline (VBS: 5,5-diethylbarbituric acid 4.94 mmol/L, NaCl 145 mmol/L, $MgCl_2$ 0.83 mmol/L, $CaCl_2$ 0.25 mmol/L, pH 7.3) was mixed with 50 µL of a hemolytic system consisting of sheep erythrocytes sensitized with rabbit antibodies (Labor

Dr. Merk & Kollegen, Ochsenhausen, Germany) in the well of a V-bottom microplate (nunc™ 249570, Thermo Fisher Scientific, Germany). Then, 25 µL of a 2.1% human pooled serum dilution in VBS were added. After incubation for 45 min at 37 °C and subsequent centrifugation for 15 min at 952× *g* at room temperature, 100 µL of the supernatant was transferred into a well of a flat bottom microplate (nunc™ 269620, Thermo Fisher Scientific, Regensburg, Germany) and diluted with 100 µL distilled water. The optical density was measured at 405 nm. For control values, VBS instead of crude Fe extract and hemolytic system were mixed with 2.1% serum dilution (100% hemolysis) and inactivated 2.1% serum dilution (0% hemolysis), respectively. By means of the concentration-dependent hemolysis curves, the IC_{50} (µg/mL) was calculated.

4.10. Cell Culture

Primary porcine RPE cells were prepared and cultivated as previously described [51] with modifications [52]. In brief, eyes were obtained from a local slaughterhouse, cleaned, the anterior segment and retina were discarded, and RPE cells harvested by trypsin digestion. Cells were used in the first passage at confluence, morphology, and confluency observed in light microscopy. Cells were maintained in HyClone DMEM (GE Healthcare, Munich, Germany, supplemented with penicillin/streptomycin (1%), HEPES (2.5%), sodium pyruvate (110 mg/mL), and 10% fetal calf serum, Linaris GmbH, Wertheim-Bettingen, Germany). The immortal RPE cell line ARPE19 was obtained from ATCC and cultivated in DMEM (Merck, Darmstadt, Germany), supplemented with penicillin/streptomycin (1%), non-essential amino acids (1%), and 10% fetal calf serum.

4.11. Treatment with Fucus distichus subsp. evanescens extract (Fe)

Fe extract was solved in Ampuwa water (Fresenius Kabi, Bad Homburg, Germany) in a concentration of 10 mg/mL and filtered through a 0.2 µm filter. Cells were treated with 1, 10, 100, and 250 µg/mL Fe extract for indicated time periods, diluted in cell culture medium. If stimulation time exceeded three days, medium (including Fe extract) was renewed twice a week.

4.12. Oxidative Stress

Oxidative stress was induced by *tert*-butyl hydroperoxide (TBHP), a stable inducer of oxidative stress in RPE cells, as previously described [33]. In this study, we used 500 µM, 750 µM, and 1000 µM TBHP for 24 h on ARPE19 cells. Cells were incubated with indicated concentration of Fe extract for 30 min, then TBHP (500 µM, 750 µM, and 1000 µM, respectively) was added. After incubation for 24 h, cell viability was tested using an MTT test as described below.

4.13. Methyl Thiazolyl Tetrazolium (MTT) Assay

MTT assay is an established viability assay [53] and was conducted as previously described [18]. In brief, cells were incubated with 0.5 mg/mL MTT (3-(4,5-dimethylthiazol-2-yl)-2,5-diphenyltetrazoliumbromid), solved in DMEM without phenol red, washed, and lysed in dimethyl sulfoxide (DMSO). Absorption was measured at 550 nm with a spectrometer (Elx800, BioTek, Bad Friedrichshall, Germany).

4.14. VEGF ELISA

ARPE19 supernatants were collected after 24 h, three days and seven days, by quick centrifugation and stored at −20 °C until assessment. VEGF content of the supernatant of ARPE19 cells were determined using a commercially available ELISA kit (R&D Systems), following the manufacturer's instructions.

4.15. Phagocytosis Assay

Phagocytosis assay was conducted as previously described [54]. In brief, photoreceptor outer segments were prepared from porcine retina and used to opsonize fluorescence-labelled latex beads. Cells were incubated with Fe extract for indicated time periods and treated with opsonized latex beads for four hours. Uptake of beads was detected by fluorescence microscopy (Apotome, Zeiss Microscopy GmbH, Jena, Germany) and evaluated in Axiovision software (Zeiss).

4.16. Wound Healing Assay (Scratch Assay)

Scratch assay was conducted as previously described [18]. In brief, a wound ("scratch") was applied to a confluent cell layer of primary RPE cells using a pipet tip. Photos were taken immediately after the wound application as well as 24 and 48 h later in light microscopy. Area of wound was assessed with Axiovision software. Wound healing is depicted as % wound area in relation to wound area at time of scratch.

4.17. Statistics

Each experiment was independently repeated at least three times. Calculation of mean, standard deviation, and significance was conducted in Microsoft Excel. Significance was assessed with student's *t*-test. A *p*-value of 0.05 or below was considered significant.

5. Conclusions

In conclusion, crude extracts from *Fucus distichus* subsp. *evanescens* are of some interests in regard to potential AMD treatment considering their VEGF reducing effect on RPE cells. However, other fucoidans have shown more promising effects. Furthermore, the tested crude extracts interfere with RPE function, such as phagocytosis, which may be a cause of concern. Taken together, fucoidans of other species may be of higher interest, and, importantly, further studies should be performed with highly purified fucoidans.

Author Contributions: Conceptualization, A.K. and S.A.; methodology, A.K., K.S.B., K.R., P.D., M.G.P., and S.A.; S.N. validation, A.K., K.S.B., K.R., S.A., and S.N.; formal analysis, A.K., K.S.B., K.R., M.G.P.; P.D., S.A., and S.N.; investigation, K.R., K.S.B., M.G.P., and S.N.; resources, A.K., J.R., and S.A.; data curation, K.S.B., K.R., and S.N.; writing—original draft preparation, A.K. and S.A.; writing—review and editing, A.K., J.R., K.R., K.S.B., P.D., S.N., and S.A.; visualization, A.K. and K.R.; supervision, A.K., J.R., and S.A.; project administration, A.K.; funding acquisition, A.K.

Funding: This study has been conducted with funding of the Baltic Blue Biotechnology Alliance (InterReg5b) and with funding of the FucoSan Health from the Sea Project, supported by EU InterReg-Deutschland-Denmark and the European Fond of Regional Development.

Acknowledgments: We especially thank Coastal Research & Management and Kiel, for the collection of the algae and Christoph Plieth, Center for Biochemistry and Molecular Biology, University of Kiel, for providing the extracts.

Conflicts of Interest: The authors declare no conflict of interest.

References

1. Li, B.; Lu, F.; Wei, X.; Zhao, R. Fucoidan: Structure and bioactivity. *Molecules* **2008**, *13*, 1671–1695. [CrossRef] [PubMed]
2. Klettner, A. Fucoidan as a potential therapeutic for major blinding dieases—A hypothesis. *Mar. Drugs* **2016**, *14*, 31. [CrossRef] [PubMed]
3. Miller, J.W. Age-related macular degeneration revisited-piecing the puzzle: The LXIX Edward Jackson memorial lecture. *Am. J. Ophthalmol.* **2013**, *155*, 1–35. [CrossRef]
4. Bellezza, I. Oxidative Stress in Age-Related Macular Degeneration: Nrf2 as Therapeutic Target. *Front. Pharmacol.* **2018**, *9*, 1280. [CrossRef] [PubMed]
5. Klettner, A. Age-related macular degeneration—Biology and treatment. *Med. Monatsschr. Pharm.* **2015**, *38*, 258–264. [PubMed]

6. Klettner, A. Oxidative stress induced cellular signaling in RPE cells. *Front. Biosci.* **2012**, *4*, 392–411. [CrossRef]
7. Datta, S.; Cano, M.; Ebrahimi, K.; Wang, L.; Handa, J.T. The impact of oxidative stress and inflammation on RPE degeneration in non-neovascular AMD. *Prog. Retin. Eye Res.* **2017**, *60*, 201–218. [CrossRef] [PubMed]
8. Nowak, J.Z. Oxidative stress, polyunsaturated fatty acids-derived oxidation products and bisretinoids as potential inducers of CNS diseases: Focus on age-related macular degeneration. *Pharmacol. Rep.* **2013**, *65*, 288–304. [CrossRef]
9. Schmidt-Erfurth, U.; Chong, V.; Loewenstein, A.; Larsen, M.; Souied, E.; Schlingemann, R.; Eldem, B.; Monés, J.; Richard, G.; Bandello, F. European Society of Retina Specialists. Guidelines for the management of neovascular age-related macular degeneration by the European Society of Retina Specialists (EURETINA). *Br. J. Ophthalmol.* **2014**, *98*, 1144–1167. [CrossRef]
10. Kim, K.J.; Yoon, K.Y.; Lee, B.Y. Low molecular weight fucoidan from the sporophyll of Undaria pinnatifida suppresses inflammation by promoting the inhibition of mitogen-activated protein kinases and oxidative stress in RAW264.7 cells. *Fitoterapia* **2012**, *83*, 1628–1635. [CrossRef]
11. Kim, E.A.; Lee, S.H.; Ko, C.I.; Cha, S.H.; Kang, M.C.; Kang, S.M.; Ko, S.C.; Lee, W.W.; Ko, J.Y.; Lee, J.H.; et al. Protective effect of fucoidan against AAPH-induced oxidative stress in zebrafish model. *Carbohydr. Polym.* **2014**, *102*, 185–191. [CrossRef] [PubMed]
12. Ryu, M.J.; Chung, H.S. Fucoidan reduces oxidative stress by regulating the gene expression of HO−1 and SOD−1 through the Nrf2/ERK signaling pathway in HaCaT cells. *Mol. Med. Rep.* **2016**, *14*, 3255–3260. [CrossRef] [PubMed]
13. Wang, Y.Q.; Wei, J.G.; Tu, M.J.; Gu, J.G.; Zhang, W. Fucoidan Alleviates Acetaminophen-Induced Hepatotoxicity via Oxidative Stress Inhibition and Nrf2 Translocation. *Int. J. Mol. Sci.* **2018**, *19*, 4050. [CrossRef] [PubMed]
14. Dithmer, M.; Kirsch, A.M.; Richert, E.; Fuchs, S.; Wang, F.; Schmidt, H.; Coupland, S.E.; Roider, J.; Klettner, A. Fucoidan does not exert anti-tumorigenic effects on uveal melanoma cell lines. *Mar. Drugs* **2017**, *15*, 193. [CrossRef] [PubMed]
15. Koyanagi, S.; Tanigawa, N.; Nakagawa, H.; Soeda, S.; Shimeno, H. Oversulfation of fucoidan enhances its anti-angiogenic and antitumor activities. *Biochem. Pharmacol.* **2003**, *65*, 173–179. [CrossRef]
16. Chen, H.; Cong, Q.; Du, Z.; Liao, W.; Zhang, L.; Yao, Y.; Ding, K. Sulfated fucoidan FP08S2 inhibits lung cancer cell growth in vivo by disrupting angiogenesis via targeting VEGFR2/VEGF and blocking VEGFR2/Erk/VEGF signaling. *Cancer Lett.* **2016**, *382*, 44–52. [CrossRef] [PubMed]
17. Rui, X.; Pan, H.F.; Shao, S.L.; Xu, X.M. Anti-tumor and anti-angiogenic effects of Fucoidan on prostate cancer: Possible JAK-STAT3 pathway. *BMC Complement. Altern. Med.* **2017**, *17*, 378. [CrossRef]
18. Dithmer, M.; Fuchs, S.; Shi, Y.; Schmidt, H.; Richert, E.; Roider, J.; Klettner, A. Fucoidan reduces secretion and expression of vascular endothelial growth factor in the retinal pigment epithelium and reduces angiogenesis in vitro. *PLoS ONE* **2014**, *9*, e89150. [CrossRef]
19. Ustyuzhanina, N.E.; Bilan, M.I.; Ushakova, N.A.; Usov, A.I.; Kiselevskiy, M.V.; Nifantiev, N.E. Fucoidans: Pro- or antiangiogenic agents? *Glycobiology* **2014**, *24*, 1265–1274. [CrossRef]
20. Anastyuk, S.D.; Shevchenko, N.M.; Ermakova, S.P.; Vishchuk, O.S.; Nazarenko, E.L.; Dmitrenok, P.S.; Zvyagintseva, T.N. Anticancer activity in vitro of a fucoidan from the brown alga Fucus evanescens and its low-molecular fragments, structurally characterized by tandem mass-spectrometry. *Carbohydr. Polym.* **2012**, *87*, 186–194. [CrossRef]
21. Kuznetsova, T.A.; Besednova, N.N.; Somova, L.M.; Plekhova, N.G. Fucoidan extracted from Fucus evanescens prevents endotoxin-induced damage in a mouse model of endotoxemia. *Mar. Drugs* **2014**, *12*, 886–898. [CrossRef]
22. Makarenkova, I.D.; Logunov, D.Y.; Tukhvatulin, A.I.; Semenova, I.B.; Besednova, N.N.; Zvyagintseva, T.N. Interactions between sulfated polysaccharides from sea brown algae and Toll-like receptors on HEK293 eukaryotic cells in vitro. *Bull. Exp. Biol. Med.* **2012**, *154*, 241–244. [CrossRef]
23. Dörschmann, P.; Bittkau, K.S.; Neupane, S.; Roider, J.; Alban, S.; Klettner, A. Effects of Fucoidans from Five Different Brown Algae on Oxidative Stress and VEGF Interference in Ocular Cells. *Mar. Drugs* **2019**, *17*, 258. [CrossRef]
24. Skriptsova, A.V.; Shevchenko, N.M.; Tarbeeva, D.V.; Zvyagintseva, T.N. Comparative study of polysaccharides from reproductive and sterile tissues of five brown seaweeds. *Mar. Biotechnol.* **2012**, *14*, 304–311. [CrossRef]

25. Vishchuk, O.S.; Ermakova, S.P.; Zvyagintseva, T.N. The fucoidans from brown algae of Far-Eastern seas: Anti-tumor activity and structure-function relationship. *Food Chem.* **2013**, *141*, 1211–1217. [CrossRef]
26. Bilan, M.I.; Grachev, A.A.; Ustuzhanina, N.E.; Shashkov, A.S.; Nifantiev, N.E.; Usov, A.I. Structure of a fucoidan from the brown seaweed Fucus evanescens C.Ag. *Carbohydr. Res.* **2002**, *337*, 719–730. [CrossRef]
27. Cumashi, A.; Ushakova, N.A.; Preobrazhenskaya, M.E.; D'Incecco, A.; Piccoli, A.; Totani, L.; Tinari, N.; Morozevich, G.E.; Berman, A.E.; Bilan, M.I.; et al. Consorzio Interuniversitario Nazionale per la Bio-Oncologia, Italy. A comparative study of the anti-inflammatory, anticoagulant, antiangiogenic, and antiadhesive activities of nine different fucoidans from brown seaweeds. *Glycobiology* **2007**, *17*, 541–552. [CrossRef]
28. Schneider, T.; Ehrig, K.; Liewert, I.; Alban, S. Interference with the CXCL12/CXCR4 axis as potential antitumor strategy: Superiority of a sulfated galactofucan from the brown alga Saccharina latissima and fucoidan over heparins. *Glycobiology* **2015**, *25*, 812–824. [CrossRef]
29. Fitton, J.H.; Stringer, D.N.; Karpiniec, S.S. Therapies from Fucoidan: An Update. *Mar. Drugs* **2015**, *13*, 5920–5946. [CrossRef]
30. Sanjeewa, K.K.A.; Lee, J.S.; Kim, W.S.; Jeon, Y.J. The potential of brown-algae polysaccharides for the development of anticancer agents: An update on anticancer effects reported for fucoidan and laminaran. *Carbohydr. Polym.* **2017**, *177*, 451–459. [CrossRef]
31. Lahrsen, E.; Liewert, I.; Alban, S. Gradual degradation of fucoidan from Fucus vesiculosus and its effect on structure, antioxidant and antiproliferative activities. *Carbohydr. Polym.* **2018**, *192*, 208–216. [CrossRef]
32. Blasi, M.A.; Maresca, V.; Roccella, M.; Roccella, F.; Sansolini, T.; Grammatico, P.; Balestrazzi, E.; Picardo, M. Antioxidant pattern in uveal melanocytes and melanoma cell cultures. *Investig. Ophthalmol. Vis. Sci.* **1999**, *40*, 3012–3016.
33. Koinzer, S.; Reinecke, K.; Herdegen, T.; Roider, J.; Klettner, A. Oxidative Stress Induces Biphasic ERK1/2 Activation in the RPE with Distinct Effects on Cell Survival at Early and Late Activation. *Curr. Eye Res.* **2015**, *40*, 853–857. [CrossRef]
34. Kim, H.; Ahn, J.H.; Song, M.; Kim, D.W.; Lee, T.K.; Lee, J.C.; Kim, Y.M.; Kim, J.D.; Cho, J.H.; Hwang, I.K.; et al. Pretreated fucoidan confers neuroprotection against transient global cerebral ischemic injury in the gerbil hippocampal CA1 area via reducing of glial cell activation and oxidative stress. *Biomed. Pharmacother.* **2019**, *109*, 1718–1727. [CrossRef]
35. Strauss, O. The retinal pigment epithelium in visual function. *Physiol. Rev.* **2005**, *85*, 845–881. [CrossRef]
36. Bittkau, K.S.; Dörschmann, P.; Blümel, M.; Tasdemir, D.; Roider, J.; Klettner, A.; Alban, S. Comparison of the Effects of Fucoidans on the Cell Viability of Tumor and Non-Tumor Cell Lines. *Mar. Drugs* **2019**, *17*, 441. [CrossRef]
37. Handa, J.T.; Cano, M.; Wang, L.; Datta, S.; Liu, T. Lipids, oxidized lipids, oxidation-specific epitopes, and Age-related Macular Degeneration. *Biochim. Biophys. Acta Mol. Cell Biol. Lipids* **2017**, *1862*, 430–440. [CrossRef]
38. Van Leeuwen, E.M.; Emri, E.; Merle, B.M.J.; Colijn, J.M.; Kersten, E.; Cougnard-Gregoire, A.; Dammeier, S.; Meester-Smoor, M.; Pool, F.M.; de Jong, E.K.; et al. A new perspective on lipid research in age-related macular degeneration. *Prog. Retin. Eye Res.* **2018**, *67*, 56–86. [CrossRef]
39. Yokota, T.; Nomura, K.; Nagashima, M.; Kamimura, N. Fucoidan alleviates high-fat diet-induced dyslipidemia and atherosclerosis in ApoE(shl) mice deficient in apolipoprotein E expression. *J. Nutr. Biochem.* **2016**, *32*, 46–54. [CrossRef]
40. Park, M.K.; Jung, U.; Roh, C. Fucoidan from marine brown algae inhibits lipid accumulation. *Mar. Drugs* **2011**, *9*, 1359–1367. [CrossRef]
41. Copland, D.A.; Theodoropoulou, S.; Liu, J.; Dick, A.D. A Perspective of AMD Through the Eyes of Immunology. *Investig. Ophthalmol. Vis. Sci.* **2018**, *59*, AMD83–AMD92. [CrossRef]
42. Li, C.; Gao, Y.; Xing, Y.; Zhu, H.; Shen, J.; Tian, J. Fucoidan, a sulfated polysaccharide from brown algae, against myocardial ischemia-reperfusion injury in rats via regulating the inflammation response. *Food Chem. Toxicol.* **2011**, *49*, 2090–2095. [CrossRef]
43. Mariotti, F.; Tomé, D.; Mirand, P.P. Converting nitrogen into protein–beyond 6.25 and Jones' factors. *Crit. Rev. Food Sci. Nutr.* **2008**, *48*, 177–184. [CrossRef]
44. Albersheim, P.; Nevins, D.J.; English, P.D.; Karr, A. A method for the analysis of sugars in plant cell-wall polysaccharides by gas-liquid chromatography. *Carbohydr. Res.* **1967**, *5*, 340–345. [CrossRef]

45. Blakeney, A.B.; Harris, P.J.; Henry, R.J.; Stone, B.A. A simple and rapid preparation of alditol acetates for monosaccharide analysis. *Carbohydr. Res.* **1983**, *113*, 291–299. [CrossRef]
46. Filisetti-Cozzi, T.M.; Carpita, N.C. Measurement of uronic acids without interference from neutral sugars. *Anal. Biochem.* **1991**, *197*, 157–162. [CrossRef]
47. Sánchez-Rangel, J.C.; Benavides, J.; Heredia, J.B.; Cisneros-Zevallos, L.; Jacobo-Velázquez, D.A. The Folin–Ciocalteu assay revisited. Improvement of its specificity for total phenolic content determination. *Anal. Methods* **2013**, *5*, 5990. [CrossRef]
48. Gerhäuser, C.; Klimo, K.; Heiss, E.; Neumann, I.; Gamal-Eldeen, A.; Knauft, J.; Frank, N. Mechanism-based in vitro screening of potential cancer chemopreventive agents. *Mutat. Res.* **2003**, *523*, 163–172. [CrossRef]
49. Groth, I.; Alban, S. Elastase inhibition assay with peptide substrates—An example for the limited comparability of in vitro results. *Planta Med.* **2008**, *74*, 852–858. [CrossRef]
50. Becker, M.; Franz, G.; Alban, S. Inhibition of PMN-elastase activity by semisynthetic glucan sulfates. *Thromb. Haemost.* **2003**, *89*, 915–925. [CrossRef]
51. Wiencke, A.K.; Kiilgaard, J.F.; Nicolini, J.; Bundgaard, M.; Röpke, C.; La Cour, M. Growth of cultured porcine retinal pigment epithelial cells. *Acta Ophthalmol. Scand.* **2003**, *81*, 170–176. [CrossRef]
52. Klettner, A.; Roider, J. Comparison of bevacizumab, ranibizumab, and pegaptanib in citro: Efficiency and possible additional pathways. *Investig. Ophthalmol. Vis. Sci.* **2008**, *49*, 4523–4527. [CrossRef]
53. Riss, T.L.; Moravec, R.A.; Niles, A.L.; Duellman, S.; Benink, H.A.; Worzella, T.J.; Minor, L. *Assay Guidance Manual [Internet]*; Eli Lilly & Company and the National Center for Advancing Translational Sciences: Bethesda, MD, USA, 2004; 1 May 2013 [updated 1 July 2016]; Available online: https://www.ncbi.nlm.nih.gov/books/NBK144065/ (accessed on 12 September 2019).
54. Klettner, A.; Möhle, F.; Lucius, R.; Roider, J. Quantifying FITC-labeled latex beads opsonized with photoreceptor outer segment fragments: An easy and inexpensive method of investigating phagocytosis in retinal pigment epithelium cells. *Ophthalmic Res.* **2011**, *46*, 88–91. [CrossRef]

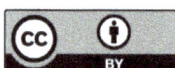

marine drugs

MDPI

Article

Epigenetic Modification and Differentiation Induction of Malignant Glioma Cells by Oligo-Fucoidan

Chien-Huang Liao [1,†], I-Chun Lai [2,†], Hui-Ching Kuo [1], Shuang-En Chuang [3], Hsin-Lun Lee [4], Jacqueline Whang-Peng [1,5,6], Chih-Jung Yao [1,7,*] and Gi-Ming Lai [1,3,5,6,7,*]

[1]   Cancer Center, Wan Fang Hospital, Taipei Medical University, Taipei 11696, Taiwan
[2]   Division of Radiation Oncology, Department of Oncology, Taipei Veterans General Hospital, Taipei 11217, Taiwan
[3]   National Institute of Cancer Research, National Health Research Institutes, Miaoli 35053, Taiwan
[4]   Department of Radiation Oncology, Taipei Medical University Hospital, Taipei Medical University, Taipei 11031, Taiwan
[5]   Taipei Cancer Center, Taipei Medical University, Taipei 11031, Taiwan
[6]   Division of Hematology and Medical Oncology, Department of Internal Medicine, Wan Fang Hospital, Taipei Medical University, Taipei 11696, Taiwan
[7]   Department of Internal Medicine, School of Medicine, College of Medicine, Taipei Medical University, Taipei 11031, Taiwan
*   Correspondence: yao0928@tmu.edu.tw (C.-J.Y.); gminlai@nhri.org.tw (G.-M.L.);
    Tel.: +886-2-2930-7930 (ext. 8130) (G.-M.L.); Fax: +886-2-8663-6454 (G.-M.L.)
†   These authors contributed equally to this work.

Received: 30 July 2019; Accepted: 3 September 2019; Published: 8 September 2019

check for updates

Abstract: Malignant glioma (MG) is a poor prognostic brain tumor with inevitable recurrence after multimodality treatment. Searching for more effective treatment is urgently needed. Differentiation induction via epigenetic modification has been proposed as a potential anticancer strategy. Natural products are known as fruitful sources of epigenetic modifiers with wide safety margins. We thus explored the effects of oligo-fucoidan (OF) from brown seaweed on this notion in MG cells including Grade III U87MG cells and Grade IV glioblastoma multiforme (GBM)8401 cells and compared to the immortalized astrocyte SVGp12 cells. The results showed that OF markedly suppress the proliferation of MG cells and only slightly affected that of SVGp12 cells. OF inhibited the protein expressions of DNA methyltransferases 1, 3A and 3B (DNMT1, 3A and 3B) accompanied with obvious mRNA induction of differentiation markers (*MBP*, *OLIG2*, *S100β*, *GFAP*, *NeuN* and *MAP2*) both in U87MG and GBM8401 cells. Accordingly, the methylation of *p21*, a DNMT3B target gene, was decreased by OF. In combination with the clinical DNMT inhibitor decitabine, OF could synergize the growth inhibition and *MBP* induction in U87MG cells. Appropriated clinical trials are warranted to evaluate this potential complementary approach for MG therapy after confirmation of the effects in vivo.

Keywords: malignant glioma; oligo-fucoidan; differentiation induction; epigenetic modification; DNA methyltransferases

1. Introduction

Cancer is widely considered as a developmental disease, caused by the dysregulation of cellular proliferation and differentiation [1,2]. Cancer cells generally belong to incomplete cell differentiation mainly in profound impairment of terminal differentiation. Substantial evidence has revealed that this highly de-differentiated and plastic state reflects acquisition of genetic events that actively promote stemness [3]. Tumors thus originate from cells with stem cell characteristics that have acquired aberrant gene expression patterns, mostly due to mutations and epimutations. These aberrant gene expression patterns lead to a block in differentiation and trigger uncontrolled proliferation. Loss of differentiation is thus an important characteristic of tumor cells and represents a defining feature of human cancers. As a consequence, differentiation therapy has been developed into an important approach for the treatment of cancers, particularly hematologic malignancy [4,5].

Malignant glioma (MG) is the most common primary adult brain tumor. According to the 2007 World Health Organization (WHO) classification, gliomas are graded according to the extent of anaplasia ("de-differentiation") status, with less aggressive designated as WHO grade II, more aggressive forms designated as WHO grade III and the most aggressive one as glioblastoma multiforme (GBM, WHO grade IV). The prognosis of MG remains poor despite a great deal of advances in surgery, radiation and chemotherapy, with a median overall survival of 12–15 months [6–8]. The cell origin of MG remains a matter of argument, with evidence indicating it originates from neural stem cells (NSCs), oligodendrocyte precursors (OPCs), or de-differentiated neurons and astrocytes [9–11]. Therefore, MG is a developmental disease with incomplete differentiation. Recent studies have demonstrated that substances such as BMPs (bone morphogenetic proteins), Znf179 (a RING (Really Interesting New Gene) finger protein) and CG500354 (a small molecule targeting for cAMP-specific 3′,5′-cyclic phosphodiesterase 4D) are able to reprogram malignant GBM cells to a more-differentiated, less-oncogenic phenotype, which could extend the probability of manipulating the GBM cells toward less-aggressive circumstances [12–14]. In addition to hematologic malignancy, MG may also be effectively treated by differentiation therapy. Searching for appropriate effective differentiation inducers is of great importance for this approach.

Drugs that modulate epigenetic processes in human cancer cells represent an important aspect in the development of differentiation therapy for cancer. All-trans-retinoic acid (ATRA), a well-known differentiation-inducing compound, was among the first substances used for differentiation therapy of acute promyelocytic leukemia [4]. The influential finding that the differentiation-inducing cytosine analogue 2′-deoxy-5-azacytidine (decitabine) acts as an effective inhibitor of DNA methyltransferases provided an important link between cellular differentiation and epigenetic regulation [15,16]. Decitabine is widely used in myelodysplastic syndrome [17]. It also has been evaluated in clinical trials for the treatments of acute myeloid leukemia in recent years [18]. However, many challenges remain in using these epigenetic drugs for the differentiation therapy in solid tumors such as MG. The development of alternative appropriate agents to effectively induce differentiation of MG is needed.

Fucoidan is a natural sulfated polysaccharide found in the cell wall matrix of brown seaweed. Structurally, fucoidan is a heparin-like molecule with a substantial percentage of L-fucose, sulfated ester groups, as well as small proportions of D-xylose, D-galactose, D-mannose and glucuronic acid [19]. Various biological activities of fucoidan, such as antioxidant, anti-inflammatory, antiproliferative and proapoptotic activities have been reported [20,21]. It induces apoptosis in human lymphoma cells by activation of caspase-3 [22], in A549 (human lung adenocarcinoma) cells by activation of caspase-9 [23] and in MCF-7 (human breast cancer) cells by activation of caspases-8 [24], respectively. In addition, fucoidan inhibits invasion and angiogenesis in human fibrosarcoma cells via repression of the activities of matrix metalloproteinases 2 and 9 [25]. Of note, several studies have shown the ability of fucoidan to induce osteoblast differentiation in human osteoblast [26] and adipose-derived stem cells [27]. Furthermore, fucoidan was also reported to stimulate osteoblast differentiation via c-Jun N-terminal kinase (JNK)- and extracellular signal-related kinase (ERK)-dependent bone morphogenetic protein 2 (BMP2)-Smad 1/5/8 signaling in human mesenchymal stem cells [28]. These studies suggest the potential of fucoidan in the differentiation induction of tumor cells, especially MG cells.

The oligo-fucoidan (OF) used in this study is a low-molecular-weight (<667 Da) fucoidan, which was derived from the glycolytic cleavage product of original fucoidan from brown seaweed *Laminaria japonica* [29]. Various anticancer effects of OF have been reported over the last decade. For examples, the effects of OF against breast and lung cancers via ubiquitin proteasome pathway (UPP)-mediated transforming growth factor β receptor (TGFR) degradation have been demonstrated in animal models by Hsu et al. [30,31]. Our previous study showed that OF regulates miR-29b-DNMT3B-MTSS1 axis and inhibits epithelial–mesenchymal transition (EMT) and invasion in hepatocellular carcinoma cells [32]. In the present study, we explored the effects of OF on the differentiation induction in MG cells and studied the underlying molecular mechanism in the aspect of epigenetic modification. In addition, its combination effects with decitabine, a clinically available demethylating epigenetic agent, in MG cells were also investigated.

2. Results

2.1. Oligo-Fucoidan Inhibits Proliferation and Clonogenicity, and Arrests Cell Cycle in Human Malignant Glioma Cells

The effect of OF on the proliferation of human MG cells (GBM8401 and U87MG) determined by sulforhodamine (SRB) assay is shown in Figure 1. Varying degrees of growth inhibition were observed after 72 h exposure to OF. At a concentration of 400 μg/mL, the cell growth of GBM8401 and U87MG cells were inhibited to 40% and 46% of the control, respectively (Figure 1A). In contrast, OF only had a slight inhibitory effect on the growth of immortalized astrocyte SVGp12 cells at the same concentration, suggesting the preferential suppression of cancer cells by OF. At concentration of 200 μg/mL, OF significantly decreased the colony formation of GBM8401 and U87MG cells to 14% and 32%, respectively (Figure 1B,C). The 50% inhibitory concentration (IC_{50}) of OF in clonogenicity of GBM8401 and U87MG cells upon 12-day treatment was 62 ± 8 and 92 ± 13 μg/mL, respectively (Figure 1B,C). A higher grade of MG cells seemed to be more sensitive to OF.

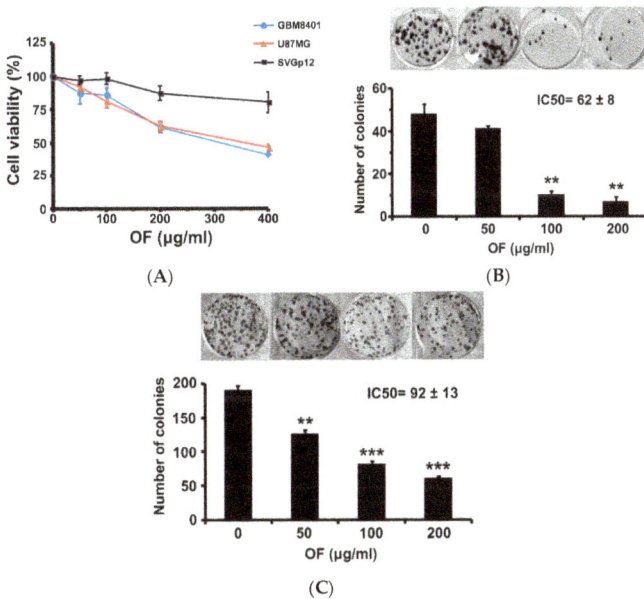

Figure 1. Inhibitory effects of oligo-fucodian (OF) on cell viability and colony formation of human malignant glioma cells. (**A**) Two malignant glioma (MG) cell lines (GBM8401 and U87MG) and immortalized astrocyte SVGp12 cells were treated with various concentrations of OF for 72 h. The cell proliferation was measured by sulforhodamine (SRB) assay. Values are expressed as the mean ± standard error of triplicate wells. (**B**) Effects of OF on the clonogenicity of GBM8401, and (**C**) U87MG cells. Each experiment was performed in triplicate, and the representative examples are shown (column, mean, bar, standard error; ** $p < 0.01$; *** $p < 0.001$). The IC_{50} indicates the 50% inhibitory concentration (μg/mL) of OF in the 12-day clonogenicity assay of GBM8401 and U87MG cells, respectively. Data are expressed as mean ± standard error.

Figure 2A,B show the cell-cycle distribution of GBM8401 and U87MG cells after treatment with OF at concentrations of 200 and 400 μg/mL for 72 h. OF arrested the cell cycle of GBM8401 cells by increasing the proportion of G1 phase from 58% (control) to 69% and 71%, respectively (Figure 2A). In U87MG cells, OF concentration dependently increased the S phase from 7% (control) to 10% and 14%, respectively (Figure 2B). The results indicate that in different types of MG cells, OF could inhibit proliferation via arresting the cell cycle at either the G1 or S phase.

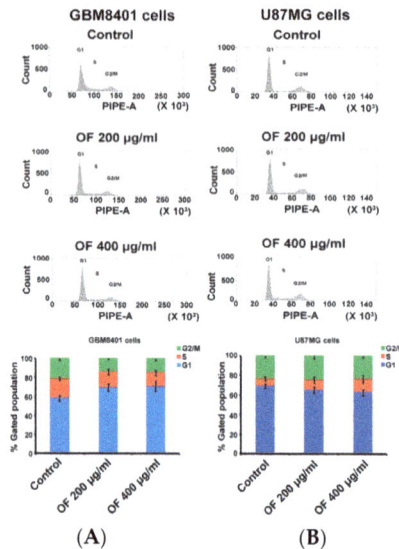

Figure 2. Analysis of cell-cycle distribution in malignant glioma cells after treatment with oligo-fucoidan (OF). After 72 h treatment, the effects of OF on cell-cycle distributions of GBM8401 (**A**) and U87MG (**B**) cells were analyzed by flow cytometry. The quantitative measurement of G1, S and G2/M phases of GBM8401 and U87MG cells after treating with OF.

2.2. Oligo-Fucoidan Induces Differentiation of Malignant Glioma Cells

As shown in Figure 2, apoptosis induction was not observed in OF-treated MG cells. Nonetheless, marked changes of cellular shape to the morphologies of neural, oligodendrocyte or glial cells were displayed after treatment with OF. This suggests that OF-mediated inhibition of MG cells might attribute to differentiation induction rather than cytotoxic effect. To confirm this assumption, a panel of early (astrocyte (GFAP), oligodendrocyte (Olig2) and neuron (MAP2 and Tuj1)) and terminal (astrocyte (S-100β), oligodendrocytes (myelin basic protein, MBP) and neuron (NeuN)) differentiation markers were measured in OF-treated MG cells by quantitative PCR assay. As shown in Figure 3A, neural and oligodendrocyte-like cellular shapes were observed in OF-treated GBM8401 cells. In support of this, early differentiation markers of oligodendrocytes (*Olig2*) and neurons (*MAP2*) were markedly elevated in these GBM8401 cells (Figure 3A). In OF (400 μg/mL)-treated U87MG cells, more oligodendrocyte-like and less glial-like cellular shapes were observed (Figure 3B). In accordance, a dramatic elevation of terminal oligodendrocyte differentiation marker *MBP* and significant increase of astrocyte markers (*GFAP* and *S100B*) were detected in these U87MG cells (Figure 3B). Together, OF might induce re-differentiation of MG cells, which were driven to malignant transformation by the de-differentiation events described in Section 1.

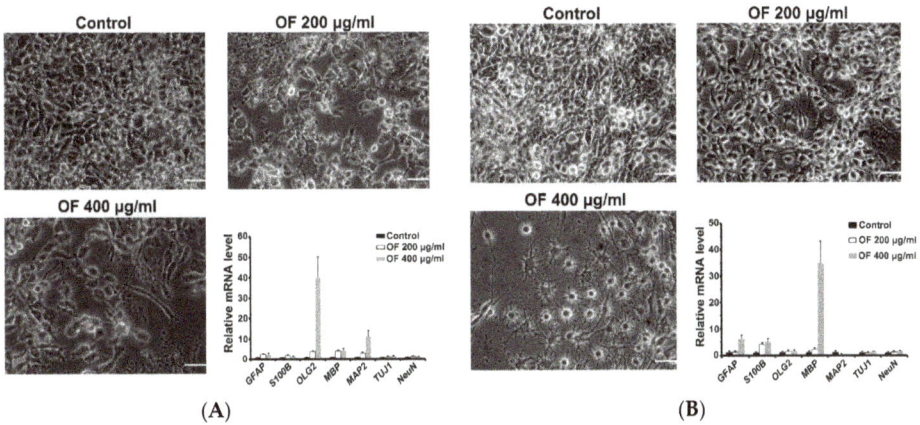

Figure 3. Differentiation induction of human MG cells after treatment with oligo-fucodian (OF). (A) GBM8401 and (B) U87MG cells were treated with OF for seven days. Morphology of the MG cells was examined by inverted phase contrast microscopy. Scale bar is 50 μm. Expression of differentiation marker genes was analyzed by quantitative PCR. Astrocyte markers: *GFAP* and *S100B*; oligodentrocyte markers: *Olig2* and *MBP*; neuron markers: *MAP2*, *TUJ1* and *NeuN*. Data were expressed as mean ± standard error.

2.3. Oligo-Fucoidan Inhibits DNA Methyltransferases (DNMTs) in Human Malignant Glioma Cells

Next, we investigated the molecular mechanism underlying the differentiation of OF-treated MG cells. Epigenetic modulation involving DNA demethylation was known to play a crucial role in the differentiation of MG cells [33]. Our previous study found that OF is able to induce miR-29b [32], which suppresses DNMTs (DNMT1, 3A and 3B) in cancer cells [34]. We thus determined if the DNMTs of MG cells were inhibited during differentiation induction by OF. As expected, OF repressed the protein levels of DNMTs in both GBM8401 (Figure 4A) and U87MG (Figure 4B) cells. Epigenetic mechanism involving DNA demethylation might play a crucial role in the differentiation induction by OF.

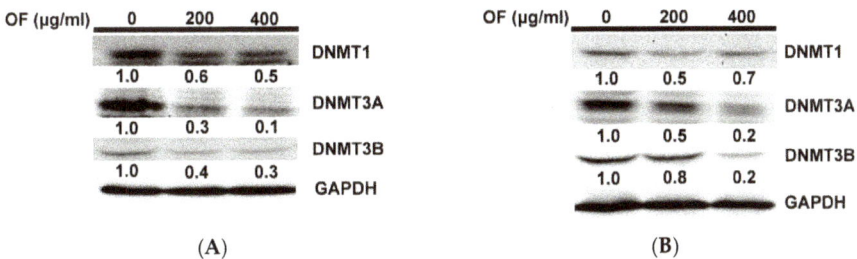

Figure 4. Oligo-fucodian (OF) represses protein levels of DNA methyltransferases (DNMTs) in human MG cells. After treatment with OF for 72 h, the protein levels of DNMT1, DNMT3A and 3B in GBM8401 (A) and U87MG (B) cells were analyzed by Western blot analysis. Glyceraldehyde-3-phosphate dehydrogenase (GAPDH) was used as the loading control for Western blot analysis. The fold changes of these protein levels were indicated below the band.

2.4. Oligo-Fucoidan Decreases the Methylation of p21 Gene Accompanied with Induction of Its Expression in Human Malignant Glioma Cells

The expression of *p21* (*CDKN1A*, cyclin dependent kinase inhibitor 1A) is known to be repressed by DNMT3B through methylating the CpG islands in its promoter region [35]. Regarding the substantial inhibition of DNMT3B protein level by OF in U87MG cells, it may decrease the methylation of *p21* gene and restore its expression. In agreement, OF induced the mRNA (Figure 5A) and protein (Figure 5B) levels of p21 in U87MG cells in a concentration-dependent manner. Through further examination of the methylation status of *p21* gene by methyl-specific PCR, we found that OF increased the proportion of unmethylated (U) p21 promoter and decreased the methylated (M) (Figure 5C). The U/M ratio in control U84MG cells was 0.89 and increased to 1.28 and 1.51 by OF at concentrations of 200 and 400 μg/mL, respectively (Figure 5C). The known demethylating agent decitabine (5-aza-2′-deoxycytidine) was used as a positive control, which increased the U/M ratio of *p21* gene from 0.89 to 1.18 at concentration of 5 μM (Figure 5C). As *p21* is a tumor suppressor and cyclin-dependent kinases (CDK) inhibitor, epigenetic induction of its expression would play a crucial role in OF-mediated growth inhibition in MG cells. It is considered that the repressed differentiation marker genes might be epigenetically induced by OF through the similar mechanism of action in demethylation.

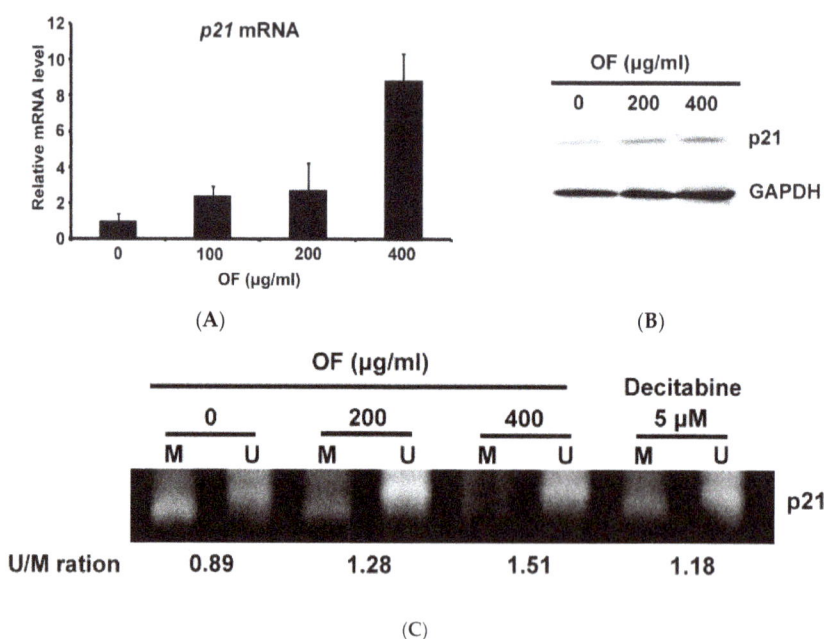

Figure 5. Oligo-fucodian (OF) increases p21 expression and decreases *p21* gene methylation in human MG cells. The *p21* mRNA (**A**) and p21 protein (**B**) levels of U87MG cells were increased after treatment with OF for seven days. The mRNA and protein levels were analyzed by quantitative PCR and Western blot analysis, respectively. (**C**) Analysis of *p21* gene methylation by methylation-specific PCR. PCR products amplified with methylated (M) and unmethylated (U) sequence-specific primers were shown. The quantitative U/M ratios are indicated below each pair of bands. Decitabine was used as positive control.

2.5. Combination with Oligo-Fucoidan (OF) Enhances Decitabine-Mediated Growth Inhibition and Differentiation Induction in MG Cells

Aberrant methylation of DNA has been proposed as a target for novel cancer treatment [36]. However, substantial hurdles (low efficacy and high toxicity) limit the extension of this proposal to solid tumors [36]. Considering the substantial demethylating effect of OF shown in Figure 5C, its combination with decitabine might be an alternative way for the epigenetic therapy of MG via demethylation. As shown in Figure 6A,B, decitabine only slightly inhibited the growth of GBM8401 and U87MG cells to 64% and 70% of the control, respectively, even at the maximum concentration of 10 µM. When combined with OF (400 µg/mL), decitabine decreased the growth of GBM8401 and U87MG cells to less than 40% of the control (Figure 6A,B). In contrast, the immortalized astrocyte SVGp12 cells were much less sensitive to the combination effect of decitabine and OF (Figure 6C), suggesting the selectivity of this combination against MG cells. The combination effect was further examined by the so-called combination index (CI), which quantitatively depicts synergism (CI < 1), additive effect (CI = 1) and antagonism (CI > 1) [37]. As shown in Figure 6D,E, the CI values in both GBM8401 and U87MG cells were all below 1, indicating synergisms of this combination against the proliferation of MG cells. By contrast, the CI values of decitabine combined with OF in SVGp12 cells were above 1 (Figure 6F), suggesting an antagonism effect on cell proliferation.

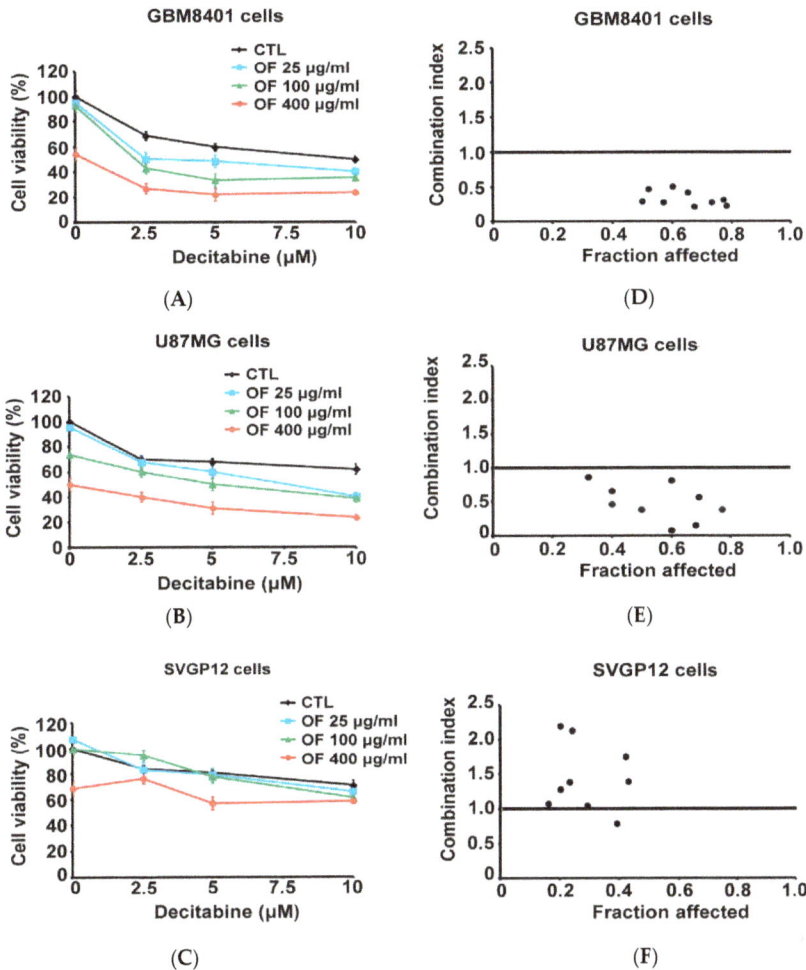

Figure 6. Combination effects of oligo-fucoidan (OF) and decitabine on the proliferation of MG cells. (**A–C**) GBM8401, U87MG and immortalized human astroglia (SVGp12) cells were treated with various concentrations of decitabine in combination of OF as indicated for 72 h. The proliferation of cells was measured by sulforhodamine (SRB) assay. Values are expressed as the mean ± standard error of triplicate wells. (**D–F**) Combination index values of decitabine–OF combinations vs. the inhibition (fraction affected) of cell proliferation. Values lower than 1 show synergistic effects, whereas those equal or close to 1 are additive and those higher than 1 are antagonistic.

In line with the combination effect on growth inhibition, the differentiation induction of U87MG cells by decitabine at 2.5 µM was also markedly enhanced by OF at 100 µg/mL. As shown in Figure 7A, the display of oligodendrocyte-like morphology induced by OF or decitabine in U87MG cells was markedly enhanced in the combination-treated group. In support of this, OF or decitabine alone induced the mRNA expression of terminal differentiation marker *MBP* to 7 and 180 folds of the control, respectively (Figure 7B). In combination-treated U87MG cells, the expression of *MBP* was markedly enhanced to 357 folds of the control (Figure 7B). Thus, consistent with that observed in morphologic changes, combining OF and decitabine has an obvious synergistic effect on not only the inhibition of cell proliferation, but also the differentiation induction in MG cells.

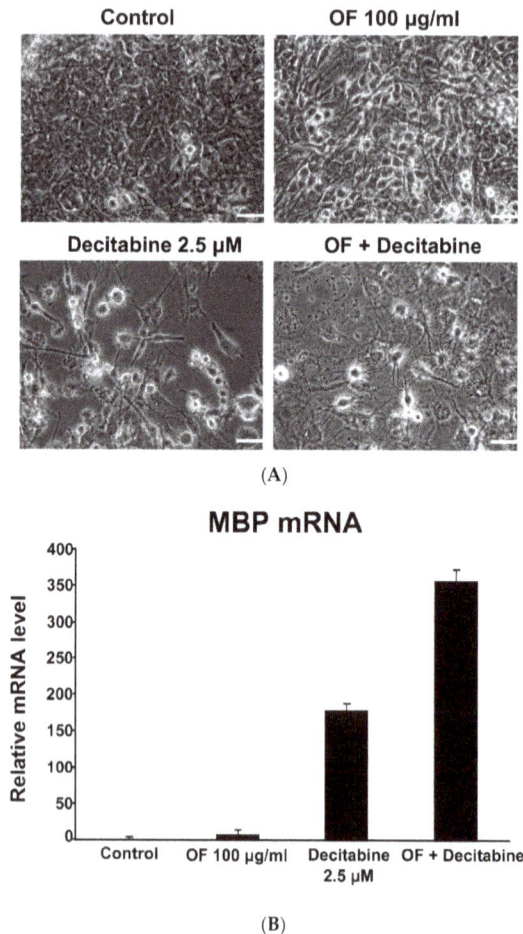

(A)

(B)

Figure 7. Combination effects of oligo-fucoidan (OF) and decitabine on the differentiation induction of MG cells. (**A**) U87MG cells were treated with OF (100 µg/mL), decitabine (2.5 µM) or a combination of each other for seven days. Morphology of the MG cells was examined by inverted phase contrast microscopy. Scale bar is 50 µm. (**B**) U87MG cells were treated with OF (100 µg/mL), decitabine (2.5 µM) or a combination of each other as indicated for seven days. The gene induction of differentiation marker *MBP* was analyzed by quantitative PCR.

3. Discussion

Fucoidan is a botanical sulfated polysaccharide extracted from brown seaweed. Its widespread bioactivity has gained significant research attention. Previous studies have reported that the in vitro anticancer activity of low-molecular-weight fucoidan (<5000 Da) was significantly higher than that of native fucoidan (>30 kDa) from sporophyll of *Undaria pinnatifida* [38,39]. However, the sulfate contents in both fucoidans are similar [38], suggesting that the anticancer activity of fucoidan could be considerably improved by lowering the molecular weight. As such, we chose the low-molecular weight (<667 Da) oligo-fucoidan (OF) [29] as the research material in this study.

Numerous researches have reported various anticancer effects of OF in many different types of tumor cells, including hepatoma, breast cancer and lung adenocarcinoma cells [30–32]. However, as far as we know, no literature has shown the effects of OF on MG cells. In this study, we demonstrated the growth arrest of MG cells by OF, accompanied with induction of differentiation marker genes expression. Current treatments of MG remain focused on achieving maximal surgical resection followed by concurrent radiation therapy with temozolomide. Conventional treatment offers patients with GBM additional survival time with generally acceptable quality of life, but a cure is never achieved [40]. In addition to killing cancer cells by conventional chemotherapy or radiotherapy, reactivation of their endogenous differentiation program to resume the maturation process and abolish tumor phenotypes has been proposed [41]. However, its application in MG treatment is hampered by the toxicity and limited efficacy of current clinically-used differentiation agents such as ATRA, azacitidine and decitabine in solid tumors [42,43]. Hopefully, our results in this study might help to shed light on the approach of MG differentiation therapy.

In response to previous reports showing the effects of fucoidan to stimulate osteogenic differentiation of adipose-derived stem cells [27] and mesenchymal stem cells [28], we demonstrated the effects of OF on differentiation induction in MG cells, accompanied with simultaneous DNMTs inhibition. It has been hypothesized that in glioma hypermethylator phenotype tumors, the extensive DNA methylation maintains MG cells in a de-differentiated state [33]. In support of this, differentiation induction and growth inhibition in IDH1 (isocitrate dehydrogenase 1) mutant MG cells by the DNMT inhibitor decitabine has been demonstrated [33]. Therefore, the down-regulation of DNMTs in OF-treated MG cells suggests the epigenetic mechanisms involving DNA demethylation for this OF-mediated differentiation induction. Moreover, it has been reported that DNMT1 and DNMT3B are overexpressed in gliomas and inhibiting DNMTs by 5-azacytidine (azacytidine, DNMT inhibitor) enhances expression of tumor suppressor genes such as p21 [44]. Accordingly, we found the induction of *p21* accompanied the decrease of its methylated promotor region in OF-treated U87 MG cells. Our previous work showed the inhibition of DNMT3B by OF via miR-29b induction [32]. As miR-29b has been shown to directly target DNMT3A and 3B and indirectly down-regulate DNMT1 by targeting Sp1 [34], miR-29b induction might participate in OF-mediated inhibition of DNMTs in MG cells. The epigenetic modification activities of OF make it an attractive option for the complementary management of MG.

There is evidence that epigenetic regulation plays a crucial role not only in cell differentiation and embryonic development, but also in the self-renewal of cancer stem cells [45]. Exploring the manipulation of epigenetic networks may provide new insights for differentiation therapy in solid tumors [45]. In contrast to genomic mutations, epigenetic changes remain reversible and have been targeted by agents such as DNA methylation inhibitor decitabine (5-Aza-2′-deoxycytidine) and histone deacetylase inhibitor suberoylanilide hydroxamic acid (SAHA; vorinostat) in cancer clinical trials [46]. In brain cancers, many loci exhibit epigenetic alterations and therapies to reverse these changes are thus being pursued [46]. As there are a lack of effective DNA demethylating agents with low toxicity and ease of delivery to the brain, clinical trials for epigenetic therapies of MG are currently limited to SAHA [46].

To promote clinical trials in brain tumors, combining inhibitors of DNA methylation and histone deacetylation has been proposed to reduce toxicity and increase efficacy through their synergistic effects at lower doses [46]. In line, OF combined with chidamide, a histone deacetylase inhibitor, could synergistically inhibit growth of MG cells (Supplementary Data 1). Moreover, synergistic induction of oligodendrocyte terminal differentiation marker MBP in U87MG cells was achieved by combination of decitabine and OF. Consistently, OF also synergized the effect of decitabine against the proliferation of GBM8401 and U87MG but not the immortalized astrocyte SVGp12 cells. It is expected that epigenetic therapies for MG will be established in the near future [45]. Our results suggest the potential of combining OF and currently-used epigenetic drugs as the complementary approach for this goal.

As mentioned above, epigenetic regulation also plays a crucial role in the self-renewal of cancer stem cells [45], which are more resistant to conventional chemotherapy and radiotherapy than more differentiated tumor cells [47]. In agreement of this, we found that OF could reduce the elevated stem markers in the cancer stem-like U87 sphere cells, resulting in the diminishment of sphere number and size, and the reduction of cancer stem-like side population percentage (Supplementary Data 2). Triggering the differentiation of cancer stem cells has been proposed to restore their sensitivities to regular chemotherapy and radiotherapy [47]. Regarding the epigenetic- and differentiation-inducing effects of OF shown in this study, it might be able to enhance the efficacy of chemotherapy and radiotherapy for MG and warrants further investigation. In parallel, previous studies have shown the enhancing effects of fucoidan on the activities of chemotherapeutic agents, such as tamoxifen, cisplatin and paclitaxel against cancer cells [48,49]. In glioblastoma, it has been proposed that targeting the cancer stem cells rather than the bulk tumor mass would be more effective [47]. Combination with OF might be an alternative way to enhance the chemotherapeutic effects against MG stem cells and is worthy of further investigation.

On the other hand, whether OF can pass the blood-brain barrier (BBB) is critical for its application in differentiation therapy of MG. The BBB is constituted from cerebrovascular endothelial cells through forming complex tight junctions, which obstruct the passing of chemical agents to enter the brain. The tissue distribution of naïve fucoidan after intragastric administration to rats had been studied by Pozharitskaya et al. [50]. In their study, the average molecular mass of the naïve fucoidan was estimated to be 735 kDa [50], which is much higher than the upper limit (400 Da) [51] for efficient permeability through the BBB. Pozharitskaya et al. did not analyze the brain distribution of the fucoidan they used [50]. As aforementioned, the OF used in the present study is a low-molecular-weight (<667 Da) fucoidan, which was derived from the glycolytic cleavage product of original fucoidan from brown seaweed *Laminaria japonica* [29]. The molecular weight of OF is much smaller than that of the naïve fucoidan (735 kDa) [50] and is near the upper limit (400 Da) [51] for efficient permeability through the BBB. Moreover, in brain tumors, the increased permeability of the BBB by disrupting endothelial tight junction proteins via vascular endothelical growth factor (VEGF) in GBM [52] and the fenestration and vesicles in the capillary endothelium of pilocytic astrocytomas [53] have been found. These abnormalities in the BBB of MG suggest the possibility for OF to pass through. Ultimately, an appropriate animal study is warranted to further confirm the OF-mediated differentiation of MG in vivo.

In summary, our results demonstrate the induction of OF-mediated DNMTs inhibition and differentiation markers in MG cells (Scheme 1). Its synergistic combination effects with decitabine against MG cells suggest a potential complementary approach for the epigenetic differentiation therapy of MG. After confirmation of the effects in vivo, an appropriated clinical trial is warranted to evaluate its clinical benefit for MG.

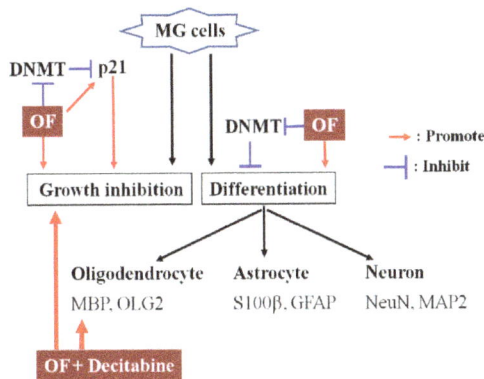

Scheme 1. Schematic diagram displays the proposed mechanisms of action of OF (oligo-fucoidan) in MG (malignant glioma) cells.

4. Materials and Methods

4.1. Reagents

The fucoidan powder from *Laminaria japonica*, a commercial product named Hi-Q Oligo-fucoidan®, was provided by Hi-Q Marine Biotech International Ltd. (New Taipei City, Taiwan). Briefly, the crude extract of *Laminaria japonica* was eluted with a NaCl gradient on a DEAE (Diethylaminoethyl)-Sephadex A-25 column. The fucose- and sulfate-enriched fraction eluted at a higher concentration of NaCl was collected and then hydrolyzed with glycolytic enzyme preparation to obtain our oligo-fucoidan (OF) sample [54]. The characteristics of oligo-fucoidan (OF) were as follows: average molecular weight of <667 Da with a 85.9% fucose content (127.2 ± 1.3 µmol/g), sulfate content 28.4% ± 2.1% (*w/w*), protein content 4.3% ± 0.3% (*w/w*), fat content 0.6% ± 0.1% (*w/w*), ash 4.1% ± 0.1% (*w/w*) and moisture content 3.9% ± 0.8% (*w/w*) [29]. It was dissolved in double-distilled H_2O and stirred at 25 °C for 30 min. The dissolved solution was filtered using 0.22 µm sterile filters (Millipore, Billerica, MA, USA). Decitabine (5-aza-2'-deoxycytidine, Cat #A3656, Sigma-Aldrich, St Louis, MO, USA) was used as a demethylating agent. Stock solutions of decitabine (20 mM) were dissolved in dimethyl sulfoxide (Cat #D2650, Sigma-Aldrich).

4.2. Cell Culture

The human glioblastoma multiforme cell line GBM8401 (BCRC 60163) was purchased from the BCRC (Bioresource Collection and Research Center, Hsin Chu, Taiwan). Human glioblastoma cell line U87MG was obtained from American Type Culture Collection (Manassas, VA, USA). GBM8401 cells were maintained as monolayers in Dulbecco's modification Eagle's medium (DMEM, Gibco, CA, USA) and U87MG cells were maintained in Roswell Park Memorial Institute (RPMI) 1640 (Gibco). These culture mediums supplemented with 10% fetal bovine serum (Gibco) and 1× penicillin-streptomycin-glutamine (PSG, Gibco). Cells were cultured at 37 °C in a water jacketed 5% CO_2 incubator.

4.3. Cellular Viability

Cells were seeded in 96-well plates at a density of 2000 cells per well and treated with various concentrations of oligo-fucoidan (OF) for 3 days. At harvest, the cell numbers were determined by sulforhodamine (SRB) that measured the cellular protein content. Briefly, cells were fixed in 10% trichloroacetic acid and stained with 0.4% SRB (Sigma-Aldrich). After incubation and washing, bound SRB was dissolved in 100 µL of 10 mM unbuffered Tris base and optical density was measured at 570 nm using a microtiter plate reader (ELx800; BioTek, Winooski, VT, USA). At least three independent measurements were performed for each experiment.

4.4. Clonogenicity

Cells were plated at a density of 200 cells/well in 6-well plate. After seeding for 24 h, cells were treated with indicated agents for 12 days. At the end, cells were stained with crystal violet (Sigma-Aldrich), photographed and the colonies that expanded to >50 cells were counted.

4.5. Photograph of the Cells

The phase contrast images of cells were photographed using a digital microscope camera (PAXcam2+, Villa Park, IL, USA) adapted to an inverted microscope (CKX31; Olympus, Tokyo, Japan) at 40× objective lens magnification.

4.6. Cell-Cycle Distribution Analysis

Cells were seeded in 6-cm dishes at a density of 4×10^5 per dish. After treatment with OF at indicated concentrations for 72 h, cells were trypsinized, washed twice by PBS, fixed in ice-cold 70% ethanol and stored at 4 °C. The cells were then washed twice with ice-cold phosphate-buffered saline and then incubated with RNase and DNA intercalating dye propidium iodide (50 µg/mL) at room temperature for 20 min. The cell-cycle distributions were then analyzed using a CytoFLEX flow cytometer (Beckman Coulter). A minimum of 10,000 events were collected and analyzed.

4.7. Quantitative RT-PCR

Total RNA was extracted from untreated or oligo-fucoidan (OF)-treated malignant glioma cells, using an RNeasy Mini Kit, and treated with an RNase-free DNase I set (Qiagen, Hilden, Germany) according to the manufacturer's protocol. Total RNA (1 µg) was reverse-transcribed using oligo $(dT)_{15}$ primers and a reverse transcription system (Promega, Madison, WI, USA). Reactions were carried out using Fast SYBR® Green PCR Master Mix (Applied Biosystems, Warrington, UK) on the Step One Plus Real-Time PCR System (Applied Biosystems, Foster City, CA, USA) by denaturation at 95 °C for 10 min, followed by 40 cycles at 95 °C for 15 s and 60 °C for 40 s. Melting curve analyses were performed to verify the amplification specificity. Relative quantification of gene expression was performed according to the ∆∆-CT (threshold cycle) method using StepOne Software 2.0 (Applied Biosystems). The sequences of qPCR primers used to probe differentiation marker genes of astrocyte, oligodendrocytes and neurons are listed in Table S1. Glyceraldehyde-3-phosphate dehydrogenase (GAPDH) was used as an internal control.

4.8. Western Blotting

Cell extracts were prepared from cells that were suspended in Radio-Immunoprecipitation Assay (RIPA) lysis buffer with protease inhibitor (Roche, Pleasanton, CA, USA). After centrifugation, supernatants were dissolved in the Laemmli sample buffer (Bio-Rad, Hercules, CA, USA) for sodium dodecyl sulfate-polyacrylamide gel electrophoresis (SDS-PAGE). Approximately 50 µg of protein were separated in SDS-PAGE and electrotransferred onto a Polyvinylidene Fluoride (PVDF) membrane. The membrane was blocked with 5% skim milk and then probed with the following primary antibodies: anti-DNMT1 (ab13537, Abcam MA, USA), anti-DNMT3A (GTX129125, Gene Tex, Irvine, CA, USA), anti-DNMT3B (GTX129127, Gene Tex), anti-GAPDH (ab8245, Abcam) and anti-p21 (ab109199, Abcam) at 4 °C for overnight. After incubation with horseradish peroxidase-conjugated secondary antibody (Jackson Immunoresearch, West Grove, PA, USA), the membrane was then visualized using Immobilon Western Chemiluminescent HRP Substrate (Millipore, Burlington, MA, USA). The Western blotting results were quantified with Image J software (NIH, Bethesda, MD, USA).

4.9. DNA Isolation and Sodium Bisulfite Conversion

Genomic DNA was isolated from malignant glioma cells after treatment with oligo-fucoidan (OF) using the QIAquick kit (Qiagen, Germantown, MD, USA). Bisulfite conversion of genomic DNA was performed using EZ DNAMethylation-Gold™ kit (Zymo Research, Irvine, CA, USA) following the manufacturer's instruction. After bisulfite treatment, unmethylated cytosines were converted to uracil (which was amplified as thymidine in subsequent PCR assays), whereas methylated cytosine remained unaltered.

4.10. Methylation Specific PCR (MSP)

The methylation status of *p21* genes was assessed by using conventional methylation specific PCR. Appropriate primer pairs (*p21* methylation forward primer, 5'-TACGCGAGGTTTCGGGATC-3'; reverse primer, 5'-CCCTAATATACAACCGCCCCG-3'; *p21* unmethylation forward primer, 5'-GGA TTGGTTGGTTTGTTGGAATTT-3'; reverse primer, 5'-ACAACCCTAATATACAACCA CCCCA-3') were employed. The presence of methylated cytosine residues was indicated by an amplification product using the primer pair specific for methylated DNA. The reaction mixture was preheated at 95 °C for 5 min, followed by 40 cycles at 95 °C for 30 s, 60 °C for 45 s, 72 °C for 30 s and the final step at 72 °C for 5 min.

4.11. Synergistic Combination Effect

The synergism between OF and decitabine on the growth inhibition of cancer cells was analyzed by the combination index (CI) derived from the median effect principle of Chou and Talalay [55], using the CalcuSyn software (version 1.1.1; Biosoft, Cambridge, UK). The value of CI < 1 points to a synergism effect, whereas the value of CI = 1 points to an additive effect and CI > 1 indicates an antagonism effect.

4.12. Statistical Analysis

Differences between the clonogenicity data of control and treated groups were evaluated by one-way ANOVA followed by Dunnett's *t*-test. Probability value of $p < 0.05$ was considered statistically significant. Single asterisk (*) indicates $p < 0.05$; double asterisks (**) indicate $p < 0.01$; triple asterisks (***) indicate $p < 0.001$.

Supplementary Materials: The following are available online at http://www.mdpi.com/1660-3397/17/9/525/s1, Figure S1: Combination effects of Oligo-Fucoidan (OF) and Chidamide on the proliferation of MG cells, Figure S2: Effects of OF on the cancer stemness of U87MG cells, Table S1: Primers used in Real-Time PCR analyses, Experimental Procedures: Sphere formation assay and Side Population Analysis.

Author Contributions: C.-H.L., I.-C.L., C.-J.Y. and G.-M.L. contributed to the study design and writing of the manuscript. C.-H.L. drafted the manuscript and worked with H.-C.K. to carry out the experiments and analyze the data. S.-E.C., H.-L.L. and J.W.-P. provided important suggestions for data processing and manuscript editing. C.-H.L. and I.-C.L. equally contributed to the paper.

Funding: This work was supported by the joint grant of Wan Fang Hospital, Taipei Medical University and Hi-Q Marine Biotech International Ltd., New Taipei City, Taiwan (Grant W330-1), Health and Welfare Surcharge of Tobacco Products (MOHW108-TDU-B-212-124020) and Ministry of Science and Technology, Taiwan (MOST107-2314-B-038-080-MY2).

Acknowledgments: The authors would like to thank Hi-Q Marine Biotech International Ltd. (New Taipei City, Taiwan) for providing the OF (oligo-fucoidan) powder from *Laminaria japonica*.

Conflicts of Interest: The authors declare that this study received funding from Hi-Q Marine Biotech International Ltd., New Taipei City, Taiwan.

References

1. Von Wangenheim, K.H.; Peterson, H.P. The role of cell differentiation in controlling cell multiplication and cancer. *J. Cancer Res. Clin. Oncol.* **2008**, *134*, 725–741. [CrossRef]
2. Capp, J.P. Stochastic gene expression, disruption of tissue averaging effects and cancer as a disease of development. *Bioessays* **2005**, *27*, 1277–1285. [CrossRef] [PubMed]
3. Takebe, N.; Harris, P.J.; Warren, R.Q.; Ivy, S.P. Targeting cancer stem cells by inhibiting Wnt, Notch, and Hedgehog pathways. *Nat. Rev. Clin. Oncol.* **2011**, *8*, 97–106. [CrossRef] [PubMed]

4.   Sell, S. Stem cell origin of cancer and differentiation therapy. *Crit. Rev. Oncol. Hematol.* **2004**, *51*, 1–28. [CrossRef] [PubMed]
5.   Degos, L. Differentiating agents in the treatment of leukemia. *Leuk. Res.* **1990**, *14*, 717–719. [CrossRef]
6.   Stupp, R.; Mason, W.P.; van den Bent, M.J.; Weller, M.; Fisher, B.; Taphoorn, M.J.B.; Belanger, K.; Brandes, A.A.; Marosi, C.; Bogdahn, U.; et al. Radiotherapy plus concomitant and adjuvant temozolomide for glioblastoma. *N. Engl. J. Med.* **2005**, *352*, 987–996. [CrossRef]
7.   Schwartzbaum, J.A.; Fisher, J.L.; Aldape, K.D.; Wrensch, M. Epidemiology and molecular pathology of glioma. *Nat. Clin. Pract. Neurol.* **2006**, *2*, 494–503. [CrossRef]
8.   Wen, P.Y.; Kesari, S. Malignant gliomas in adults. *N. Engl. J. Med.* **2008**, *359*, 492–507. [CrossRef]
9.   Alderton, G.K. Tumorigenesis: The origins of glioma. *Nat. Rev. Cancer* **2011**, *11*, 627.
10. Friedmann-Morvinski, D.; et al. Dedifferentiation of neurons and astrocytes by oncogenes can induce gliomas in mice. *Science* **2012**, *338*, 1080–1084. [CrossRef]
11. Lee, D.Y.; Gianino, S.M.; Gutmann, D.H. Innate neural stem cell heterogeneity determines the patterning of glioma formation in children. *Cancer Cell* **2012**, *22*, 131–138. [CrossRef] [PubMed]
12. Piccirillo, S.G.; Reynolds, B.A.; Zanetti, N.; Lamorte, G.; Binda, E.; Broggi, G.; Brem, H.; Olivi, A.; Dimeco, F.; Vescovi, A.L. Bone morphogenetic proteins inhibit the tumorigenic potential of human brain tumour-initiating cells. *Nature* **2006**, *444*, 761–765. [CrossRef] [PubMed]
13. Lee, K.H.; Chen, C.L.; Lee, Y.C.; Kao, T.J.; Chen, K.Y.; Fang, C.Y.; Chang, W.C.; Chiang, Y.H.; Huang, C.C. Znf179 induces differentiation and growth arrest of human primary glioblastoma multiforme in a p53-dependent cell cycle pathway. *Sci. Rep.* **2017**, *7*, 4787. [CrossRef] [PubMed]
14. Kang, T.W.; Choi, S.W.; Yang, S.R.; Shin, T.H.; Kim, H.S.; Yu, K.R.; Hong, I.S.; Ro, S.; Cho, J.M.; Kang, K.S. Growth arrest and forced differentiation of human primary glioblastoma multiforme by a novel small molecule. *Sci. Rep.* **2014**, *4*, 5546. [CrossRef] [PubMed]
15. Alcazar, O.; Achberger, S.; Aldrich, W.; Hu, Z.; Negrotto, S.; Saunthararajah, Y.; Triozzi, P. Epigenetic regulation by decitabine of melanoma differentiation in vitro and in vivo. *Int. J. Cancer* **2012**. *Int. J. Cancer* **2012**, *131*, 18–29. [CrossRef]
16. Jones, P.A.; Taylor, M.S. Cellular differentiation, cytidine analogs and DNA methylation. *Cell* **1980**, *20*, 85–93. [CrossRef]
17. Steensma, D.P. Myelodysplastic syndromes current treatment algorithm 2018. *Blood Cancer J.* **2018**, *8*, 47. [CrossRef]
18. Bohl, S.R.; Bullinger, L.; Rucker, F.G. Epigenetic therapy: Azacytidine and decitabine in acute myeloid leukemia. *Expert. Rev. Hematol.* **2018**, *11*, 361–371. [CrossRef]
19. Senthilkumar, K.; Manivasagan, P.; Venkatesan, J.; Kim, S.K. Brown seaweed fucoidan: Biological activity and apoptosis, growth signaling mechanism in cancer. *Int. J. Biol. Macromol.* **2013**, *60*, 366–374. [CrossRef]
20. Atashrazm, F.; Lowenthal, R.M.; Woods, G.M.; Holloway, A.F.; Dickinson, J.L. Fucoidan and cancer: A multifunctional molecule with anti-tumor potential. *Mar. Drugs* **2015**, *13*, 2327–2346. [CrossRef]
21. Kwak, J.Y. Fucoidan as a marine anticancer agent in preclinical development. *Mar. Drugs* **2014**, *12*, 851–870. [CrossRef] [PubMed]
22. Aisa, Y.; Miyakawa, Y.; Nakazato, T.; Shibata, H.; Saito, K.; Ikeda, Y.; Kizaki, M. Fucoidan induces apoptosis of human HS-sultan cells accompanied by activation of caspase-3 and down-regulation of ERK pathways. *Am. J. Hematol.* **2005**, *78*, 7–14. [CrossRef] [PubMed]
23. Boo, H.J.; Hyun, J.H.; Kim, S.C.; Kang, J.I.; Kim, M.K.; Kim, S.Y.; Cho, H.; Yoo, E.S.; Kang, H.K. Fucoidan from Undaria pinnatifida induces apoptosis in A549 human lung carcinoma cells. *Phytother. Res.* **2011**, *25*, 1082–1086. [CrossRef] [PubMed]
24. Yamasaki-Miyamoto, Y.; Yamasaki, M.; Tachibana, H.; Yamada, K. Fucoidan induces apoptosis through activation of caspase-8 on human breast cancer MCF-7 cells. *J. Agric. Food Chem.* **2009**, *57*, 8677–8682. [CrossRef] [PubMed]
25. Ye, J.; Li, Y.; Teruya, K.; Katakura, Y.; Ichikawa, A.; Eto, H.; Hosoi, M.; Hosoi, M.; Nishimoto, S.; Shirahata, S. Enzyme-digested Fucoidan Extracts Derived from Seaweed Mozuku of Cladosiphon novae-caledoniae kylin Inhibit Invasion and Angiogenesis of Tumor Cells. *Cytotechnology* **2005**, *47*, 117–126. [CrossRef] [PubMed]
26. Jang, H.O.; Park, Y.S.; Lee, J.H.; Seo, J.B.; Koo, K.I.; Jeong, S.C.; Jin, S.D.; Lee, Y.H.; Eom, H.S.; Yun, I. Effect of extracts from safflower seeds on osteoblast differentiation and intracellular calcium ion concentration in MC3T3-E1 cells. *Nat. Prod. Res.* **2007**, *21*, 787–797. [CrossRef] [PubMed]

27. Park, S.J.; Lee, K.W.; Lim, D.S.; Lee, S. The sulfated polysaccharide fucoidan stimulates osteogenic differentiation of human adipose-derived stem cells. *Stem. Cells Dev.* **2012**, *21*, 2204–2211. [CrossRef]

28. Kim, B.S.; Kang, H.J.; Park, J.Y.; Lee., J. Fucoidan promotes osteoblast differentiation via JNK- and ERK-dependent BMP2-Smad 1/5/8 signaling in human mesenchymal stem cells. *Exp. Mol. Med.* **2015**, *47*, e128. [CrossRef]

29. Hwang, P.A.; Yan, M.D.; Lin, H.T.; Li, K.L.; Lin, Y.C. Toxicological Evaluation of Low Molecular Weight Fucoidan in Vitro and in Vivo. *Mar. Drugs* **2016**, *14*, 121. [CrossRef]

30. Hsu, H.Y.; Lin, T.Y.; Hwang, P.A.; Tseng, L.M.; Chen, R.H.; Tsao, S.M.; Hsu, J. Fucoidan induces changes in the epithelial to mesenchymal transition and decreases metastasis by enhancing ubiquitin-dependent TGFbeta receptor degradation in breast cancer. *Carcinogenesis* **2013**, *34*, 874–884. [CrossRef]

31. Hsu, H.Y.; Lin, T.Y.; Wu, Y.C.; Tsao, S.M.; Hwang, P.A.; Shih, Y.W.; Hsu, J. Fucoidan inhibition of lung cancer in vivo and in vitro: Role of the Smurf2-dependent ubiquitin proteasome pathway in TGFbeta receptor degradation. *Oncotarget* **2014**, *5*, 7870–7885. [CrossRef] [PubMed]

32. Yan, M.D.; Yao, C.; Chow, J.M.; Chang, C.L.; Hwang, P.A.; Chuang, S.E.; Whang-Peng, J.; Lai, G.M. Fucoidan Elevates MicroRNA-29b to Regulate DNMT3B-MTSS1 Axis and Inhibit EMT in Human Hepatocellular Carcinoma Cells. *Mar. Drugs* **2015**, *13*, 6099–6116. [CrossRef] [PubMed]

33. Turcan, S.; Fabius, A.W.; Borodovsky, A.; Pedraza, A.; Brennan, C.; Huse, J.; Viale, A.; Riggins, G.J.; Chan, T.A. Efficient induction of differentiation and growth inhibition in IDH1 mutant glioma cells by the DNMT Inhibitor Decitabine. *Oncotarget* **2013**, *4*, 1729–1736. [CrossRef] [PubMed]

34. Garzon, R.; Liu, S.; Fabbri, M.; Liu, Z.; Heaphy, C.E.; Callegari, E.; Schwind, S.; Pang, J.; Yu, J.; Muthusamy, N.; et al. MicroRNA-29b induces global DNA hypomethylation and tumor suppressor gene reexpression in acute myeloid leukemia by targeting directly DNMT3A and 3B and indirectly DNMT1. *Blood* **2009**, *113*, 6411–6418. [CrossRef] [PubMed]

35. Blanc, R.S.; Vogel, G.; Chen, T.; Crist, C.; Richard, S. PRMT7 Preserves Satellite Cell Regenerative Capacity. *Cell Rep.* **2016**, *14*, 1528–1539. [CrossRef] [PubMed]

36. Issa, J.P.; Kantarjian, H.M. Targeting DNA methylation. *Clin. Cancer Res.* **2009**, *15*, 3938–3946. [CrossRef]

37. Chou, T.-C. The combination index (CI1) as the definition of synergism and of synergy claims. *Synergy* **2018**, *7*, 49. [CrossRef]

38. Cho, M.L.; Lee, B.Y.; You, G.S. Relationship between oversulfation and conformation of low and high molecular weight fucoidans and evaluation of their in vitro anticancer activity. *Molecules* **2010**, *16*, 291–297. [CrossRef]

39. Yang, C.; Chung, D.; Shin, I.S.; Lee, H.; Kim, J.; Lee, Y.; You, S. Effects of molecular weight and hydrolysis conditions on anticancer activity of fucoidans from sporophyll of Undaria pinnatifida. *Int. J. Biol. Macromol.* **2008**, *43*, 433–437. [CrossRef]

40. Das, S.; Srikanth, M.; Kessler, J.A. Cancer stem cells and glioma. *Nat. Clin. Pract. Neurol.* **2008**, *4*, 427–435. [CrossRef]

41. Yan, M.; Liu, Q. Differentiation therapy: A promising strategy for cancer treatment. *Chin. J. Cancer* **2016**, *35*, 3. [CrossRef] [PubMed]

42. Yang, D.; Luo, W.; Wang, J.; Zheng, M.; Liao, X.H.; Zhang, N.; Lu, W.; Wang, L.; Chen, A.Z.; Wu, W.G.; et al. A novel controlled release formulation of the Pin1 inhibitor ATRA to improve liver cancer therapy by simultaneously blocking multiple cancer pathways. *J. Control. Release* **2018**, *269*, 405–422. [CrossRef] [PubMed]

43. Nervi, C.; De Marinis, E.; Codacci-Pisanelli, G. Epigenetic treatment of solid tumours: A review of clinical trials. *Clin. Epigenetics* **2015**, *7*, 127. [CrossRef] [PubMed]

44. Rajendran, G.; Shanmuganandam, K.; Bendre, A.; Muzumdar, D.; Goel, A.; Shiras, A. Epigenetic regulation of DNA methyltransferases: DNMT1 and DNMT3B in gliomas. *J. Neurooncol.* **2011**, *104*, 483–494. [CrossRef] [PubMed]

45. Kawamura, Y.; Takouda, J.; Yoshimoto, K.; Nakashima, K. New aspects of glioblastoma multiforme revealed by similarities between neural and glioblastoma stem cells. *Cell Biol. Toxicol.* **2018**, *34*, 425–440. [CrossRef] [PubMed]

46. Fouse, S.D.; Costello, J.F. Epigenetics of neurological cancers. *Future Oncol.* **2009**, *5*, 1615–1629. [CrossRef] [PubMed]

47. Santamaria, S.; Delgado, M.; Kremer, L.; Garcia-Sanz, J.A. Will a mAb-Based Immunotherapy Directed against Cancer Stem Cells Be Feasible? *Front. Immunol.* **2017**, *8*, 1509. [CrossRef] [PubMed]
48. Zhang, Z.; Teruya, K.; Yoshida, T.; Eto, H.; Shirahata, S. Fucoidan extract enhances the anti-cancer activity of chemotherapeutic agents in MDA-MB-231 and MCF-7 breast cancer cells. *Mar. Drugs* **2013**, *11*, 81–98. [CrossRef]
49. Hsu, H.Y.; Lin, T.Y.; Hu, C.H.; Shu, D.T.F.; Lu, M.K. Fucoidan upregulates TLR4/CHOP-mediated caspase-3 and PARP activation to enhance cisplatin-induced cytotoxicity in human lung cancer cells. *Cancer Lett.* **2018**, *432*, 112–120. [CrossRef]
50. Pozharitskaya, O.N.; Shikov, A.N.; Faustova, N.M.; Obluchinskaya, E.D.; Kosman, V.M.; Vuorela, H.; Makarov, V.G. Pharmacokinetic and Tissue Distribution of Fucoidan from Fucus vesiculosus after Oral Administration to Rats. *Mar. Drugs* **2018**, *16*, 132. [CrossRef]
51. Pardridge, W.M. Drug transport across the blood-brain barrier. *J. Cereb. Blood Flow Metab.* **2012**, *32*, 1959–1972. [CrossRef] [PubMed]
52. Wen, L.; Tan, Y.; Dai, S.; Zhu, Y.; Meng, T.; Yang, X.; Liu, Y.; Liu, X.; Yuan, H.; Hu, F. VEGF-mediated tight junctions pathological fenestration enhances doxorubicin-loaded glycolipid-like nanoparticles traversing BBB for glioblastoma-targeting therapy. *Drug Deliv.* **2017**, *24*, 1843–1855. [CrossRef] [PubMed]
53. Takeuchi, H.; Kubota, T.; Sato, K.; Arishima, H. Ultrastructure of capillary endothelium in pilocytic astrocytomas. *Brain Tumor Pathol.* **2004**, *21*, 23–26. [CrossRef] [PubMed]
54. Hwang, P.A.; Lin, H.V.; Lin, H.Y.; Lo, S.K. Dietary Supplementation with Low-Molecular-Weight Fucoidan Enhances Innate and Adaptive Immune Responses and Protects against Mycoplasma pneumoniae Antigen Stimulation. *Mar. Drugs* **2019**, *17*, 175. [CrossRef] [PubMed]
55. Chou, T.C. Drug combination studies and their synergy quantification using the Chou-Talalay method. *Cancer Res.* **2010**, *70*, 440–446. [CrossRef] [PubMed]

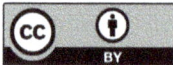

marine drugs

MDPI

Review

Therapeutic Effects of Fucoidan: A Review on Recent Studies

Sibusiso Luthuli †, Siya Wu †, Yang Cheng, Xiaoli Zheng, Mingjiang Wu * and Haibin Tong *

College of Life and Environmental Science, Wenzhou University, Wenzhou 325035, China
* Correspondence: wmj@wzu.edu.cn (M.W.); tonghb@wzu.edu.cn (H.T.); Tel.: +86-577-86689078 (M.W. & H.T.)
† Contributed equally to this work.

Received: 29 June 2019; Accepted: 19 August 2019; Published: 21 August 2019

check for
updates

Abstract: Fucoidan is a polysaccharide largely made up of L-fucose and sulfate groups. Fucoidan is favorable worldwide, especially amongst the food and pharmaceutical industry as a consequence of its promising therapeutic effects. Its applaudable biological functions are ascribed to its unique biological structure. Classical bioactivities associated with fucoidan include anti-oxidant, anti-tumor, anti-coagulant, anti-thrombotic, immunoregulatory, anti-viral and anti-inflammatory effects. More recently, a variety of in vitro and in vivo studies have been carried out to further highlight its therapeutic potentials. This review focuses on the progress towards understanding fucoidan and its biological activities, which may be beneficial as a future therapy. Hence, we have summarized in vitro and in vivo studies that were done within the current decade. We expect this review and a variety of others can contribute as a theoretical basis for understanding and inspire further product development of fucoidan.

Keywords: fucoidan; therapeutic effects; bioactivity; anti-viral

1. Introduction

The marine environment is renowned as a rich source of chemical and biological diversity. This type of diversity has been regarded as a unique source of chemical compounds for cosmetics, dietary supplementation, agrochemicals and pharmaceuticals [1]. Seaweeds, such as green algae, red algae and brown algae, are able to produce various metabolites characterized by a broad spectrum of biological activities [2]. A number of studies have been conducted towards their nutraceutical and pharmaceutical properties [3–5].

For about a period of 2000 years, brown algae, such as *Sargassum* spp., has been put to use as traditional Chinese medicine (TCM) towards treating various diseases, including thyroid diseases such as goiters [6]. In addition, it has also been used traditionally to treat scrofula, tumors, edema, testicular pain, swelling, cardiovascular diseases, arteriosclerosis, ulcer, renal issues, eczema, scabies, psoriasis and asthma [6]. Their therapeutic effects have been scientifically approved and may, therefore, be explained by means of in vivo and in vitro pharmacological activities, such as producing anti-cancer, anti-inflammatory, anti-bacterial, anti-viral, neuroprotective and anti-HIV activities.

Several studies and reviews have been done in the past on the bioactivity of fucoidan e.g., by producing anti-oxidant, anti-tumor, immunoregulation, anti-viral and anti-coagulant activities [7]. Our aim is to cover a variety of angles on the contributing factors behind the bioactivities of fucoidan, such as their source, molecular weight (Mw), sulfate group and extraction methods. In addition, we did a follow up on some studies done by certain groups with the aim to observe and compare progress based on their previous studies.

2. Summary of The Literature

It seems evident that fucoidan is gaining interest as a potential therapy, which is part of the highlight of this literature. Though this may be the case, a lot of ground still needs to be covered, first by understanding the concept, origin and source of fucoidan (Sections 3 and 4). One of the most important points in this review is the structure and pharmacokinetics of fucoidan, which sort of gives us a general idea on how the mechanism of bioactivity gets executed by fucoidan, especially when it comes to its structure and pharmacokinetics (Sections 5 and 6). Since fucoidan is identified as possessing pro-apoptotic abilities, we summarized studies that were stimulated by fucoidan—for instance in cancers. We also reflected upon different mechanisms within the process of apoptosis e.g., cell-cycle arrest, intrinsic and extrinsic pathways (Section 7). Sections 8–11 provides a summary of the anti-viral activities of fucoidan, including anti-influenza virus, anti-hepatitis B, anti-HIV and anti-canine distemper virus (CDV). In the past, a variety of studies have shown fucoidan's potential as possessing anti-diabetic capabilities. Some in vitro studies have characterized fucoidan's ability to reverse the classical symptoms of diabetes and related metabolic syndromes, and we have provided a summary of these characterizations in Section 12. Plants of marine origin, such as fucoidan, based on previous literature are also regarded as an anti-coagulant, hence it was suitable to include such a summary in Section 13. Therefore, the aim was to use an all-round approach into the health benefits (e.g., anti-cancer, anti-viral, anti-coagulant, anti-diabetic) that are generally mentioned by authors who focus their studies of fucoidan, while looking into the structure and characteristics of fucoidan.

3. Fucoidan

The first extraction of fucoidan was in 1913 from a species of brown algae [8], such as *Laminaria digitata*, *Ascophyllum nodosum* and *Fucus vesiculosus*. Fucoidan is a negatively charged and highly hygroscopic polysaccharide [9]. A high content of fucoidan is mainly found in the leaves of *L. digitata*, *A. nodosum*, *Macrocystis pyrifera* and *F. vesiculosus*. Fucoidan is soluble in both water and acid solutions. After the first publication took place in 1913, the number of published articles (studies) on fucoidan has increased significantly, especially in the modern era. The reason behind the increase in studies is that fucoidan has anti-tumor, anti-coagulant and anti-oxidant activities, as well as the importance in terms of regulating the metabolism of glucose and cholesterol [10]. Also, there has been an interest in fucoidan because of its potential to provide protection against liver damage and urinary system failures. It is evident that research on fucoidan is gradually flourishing, as these activities are carried out, and more of its bio-activities and health-related benefits are being discovered as studies continue to accumulate.

4. Sources of Fucoidan

Fucoidan is a sulfated polysaccharide which can be found amongst a number of marine sources, including sea cucumbers [11] or brown algae [12]. A great number of algae and invertebrates have been ascertained for their fucoidan contents inclusive of *Fucus vesiculosus*, *Sargassum stenophyllum*, *Chorda filum*, *Ascophyllum nodosum*, *Dictyota menstrualis*, *Fucus evanescens*, *Fucus serratus*, *Fucus distichus*, *Caulerpa racemosa*, *Hizikia fusiforme*, *Padina gymnospora*, *Kjellmaniella crassifolia*, *Analipus japonicus* and *Laminaria hyperborea* exhibited in Figure 1. In these sources, different types of fucoidan can be obtained and the methods of extraction employed are different, especially when they are reported in different studies.

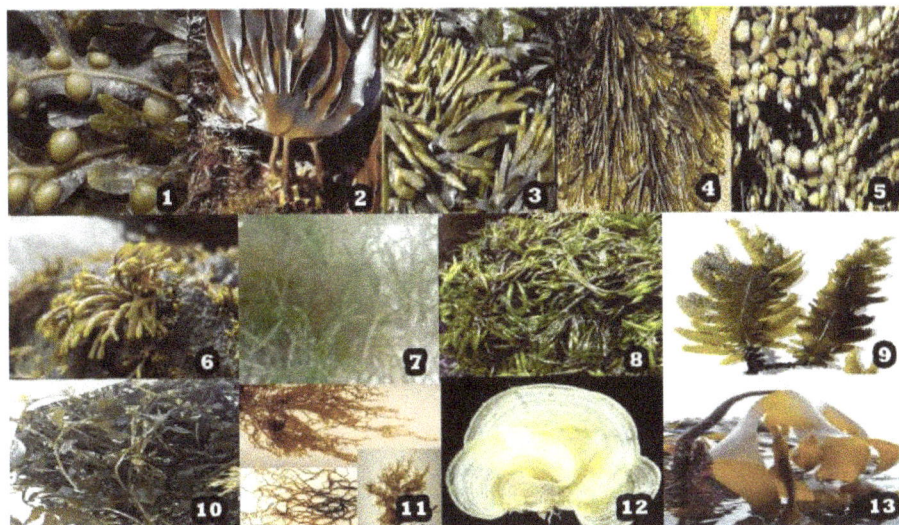

Figure 1. Sources of fucoidan. 1. *Fucus vesiculosus*, 2. *Laminaria digitata*, 3. *Fucus evanescens*, 4. *Fucus serratus*, 5. *Ascophyllum nodosum*, 6. *Pelvetia canaliculata*, 7. *Cladosiphon okamuranus*, 8. *Sargassum fusiforme*, 9. *Laminaria japonica*, 10. *Sargassum horneri*, 11. *Nemacystus decipiens*, 12. *Padina gymnospora*, 13. *Laminaria hyperborea*.

5. Structure of Fucoidan

Fucoidan is known as a fucose-enriched and sulfated polysaccharide that is mainly sourced from the extracellular matrix of brown algae. Fucoidan is made up of L-fucose, sulfate groups and one or more small proportions of xylose, mannose, galactose, rhamnose, arabinose, glucose, glucuronic acid and acetyl groups in a variety of brown algae [13–15]. In a number of studies, researchers have also used galactofucan to represent a kind of fucoidan. Galactofucan is known as a monosaccharide, and the composition of the monosaccharide is galactose accompanied by fucose, similar to rhamnofucan (rhamnose and fucose) and rhamnogalactofucan (rhamnose, galactose and fucose). In addition to the structure of fucoidan, there is also a variation amongst different seaweed types. Nevertheless, fucoidan normally has two types of homofucose (Figure 2). One type (I) encompasses repeated (1→3)-L-fucopyranose, and the other type (II) encompasses alternating and repeated (1→3)- and (1→4)-L-fucopyranose [16].

Reports based on structures of fucoidan, sourced from different species of brown algae, brought about an improved categorization in terms of structures. By a way of illustration, most of the fucoidans sourced from species belonging to the *Fucales* have an alternating linkage of (1→3)-α-L-fucose and (1→4)-α-L-fucose [17–21]. Structures of *Ascophyllum nodosum* fucoidan [22] and *F. vesiculosus* fucoidan show a resemblance of one another, the difference is only significant based on sulfate patterns and the presence of glucuronic acid. A number of *Fucales* species, such as *Fucus serratus*, *Fucus distichus* and *Pelvetia canaliculate*, present similar fucoidan backbone, but show more diversity in the branching and the presence of different monosaccharides [20,21,23]. However, exceptions do exist, for instance, fucoidans from the *Bifurcaria bifucardia* and *Himanthalia elongate* do not follow or ascribe to such a structural feature [24]. Hence, identifying the structure of fucoidan based on the species they belong to presents a challenge.

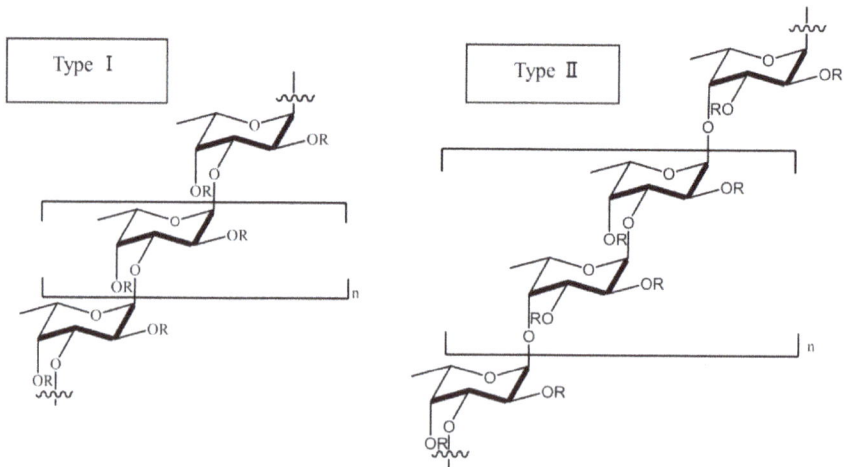

Figure 2. Type I and type II of common backbone chains in brown seaweed fucoidan. R can be fucopyranose, glucuronic acid and sulfate groups, while the location of galactose, mannose, xylose, rhamnose, arabinose and glucose in several kinds of seaweed species remains unknown.

Another important fact that deserves mentioning is that the structure of fucoidan is also highly dependent on the harvest season. This is based on the *Undaria pinnafida* fucoidan, which exhibited distinct characteristics and bioactivity, especially when harvested during different seasons [25,26]. In addition, it should be indicated that the purification method also plays a critical role in the structure of fucoidan. To such an extent that new purification methods have led to the revelation that the fucoidan structure is comprised of multiple fractions [27]. An investigation reported that the structure of crude fucoidan sourced from *A. nodosum* showed a predominant repetition of [→(3)-α-L-Fuc(2SO$_3^-$) − (1→4)-α-Fuc(2,3diSO$_3^-$)-(1)]n [28]. However, from the same species, a purified fraction comprised of primarily α-(1→3)-fucosyl residues with a sparse linkage of α-(1→4) and was found to be highly branched [29]. Therefore, the employment of different extraction methods results in distinct structures. For example, a report states that one species produced two distinct fucoidan structures, particularly galactofuctans and uronofucoidans [30]. Hence, it should be emphasized that purification techniques are one of the determining factors towards the structure and the associated bioactivities.

6. Pharmacokinetics Research of Fucoidan

It can be mentioned that quite a few experimental activities have been undertaken to address the so-called ADME i.e., absorption, distribution, metabolism and excretion of fucoidan. The confirmation of fucoidan absorption was determined using ELISA with fucoidan-specific antibody [31–33]. An absorption study was performed on rats using *F. vesiculosus* fucoidan (737 kDa), while 4 h after administration, a maximum concentration of fucoidan in serum was reached, which then resulted in the accumulation of the absorbed fucoidan in the kidneys. The fucoidan accumulation in organs has also been confirmed by the absorption of *C. okamuranus* fucoidan in rats [34]. In addition, authors' observation from healthy volunteers who either orally ingested or were administered with fucoidan showed that some portion of fucoidan was absorbed by means of endocytosis, and was detected both in their serum and urine [35]. It could be mentioned that LMWF (low molecular weight fucoidan) may be further developed to be used for clinical purposes. This is in relation to a comparative investigation (i.e., LMWF and MMWF (middle molecular weight fucoidan) from *S. japonica*), the outcome was that LMWF presented with a better absorption rate and bioavailability, hence supporting its biological potential [36]. However, fucoidan may still present with favorable pharmacokinetics in relation to toxicity; the information on its biodistribution in human is still insufficient. Animal models indicate its bioavailability, sparking interest toward the LWMF as a potential solution. The latest study by Kadena et al. [37] pursued a slightly different approach when investigating the absorption of fucoidan based on oral administration. They concluded that "the habit of eating mozuku was speculated to be a factor in the absorption of fucoidan". A total of 396 volunteers were investigated after they ingested 3 g of mozuku fucoidan, fucoidan was detected in the urine specimens of the 385 participants out of the 396. Hence, in addition to the conclusion, participants residing in the location of Okinawa presented with increased urinary excretion of fucoidan, because the locals of the Okinawa region generally consumed greater amounts of mozuku than those outside the region. Although further studies on absorption across the intestinal tract should be performed, it is rather interesting to have scientists pursuing different angles towards fucoidan absorption. Hence, future developments of fucoidan as a drug will be based on well-informed choices, due to a wide range of information that is gradually accumulating.

To date, two clinical trials are underway, such trials are focused on the biodistribution and tolerance of fucoidan. Healthy individuals or volunteers are engaged in tests that involve the biodistribution, safety and dosimetry of a labeled fucoidan (ClinicalTrials.gov, Identifier: NCT03422055). In another trial, patients with stage III-IV non-small cell lung cancer (NSCLC) are being studied (in a placebo-controlled trial), whereby fucoidan is added to their chemotherapy treatment to determine the impact it would present on their quality of life (ClinicalTrials.gov, Identifier: NCT03130829). The results of these studies (clinical trials) will play an important role in gaining insight in ADME and toxicity of fucoidan in human beings.

7. Anti-Cancer Capacity

Apoptosis is a physiological process that is known as programmed cell death and is essential for embryonic development and homeostasis in organisms, but it can also participate in pathological processes, e.g., cancer [38]. Therefore, this section follows up on how malignant or cancer cells undergo apoptosis after the administration or stimulation by fucoidan, in different manners, i.e., caspases, cell cycle arrest, intrinsic and extrinsic pathways. *C. okamuranus* fucoidan (average Mw 75.0 kDa), which consists of 5.01 mg/mL of L-fucose, 2.02 mg/mL of uronic acids and 1.65 ppm of sulfate, has revealed that at the concentration of 1.0 mg/mL, the G0/G1-phase population in Huh7 hepatocarcinoma cell was increased, accompanied by a decrease in the S phase, highly suggesting that fucoidan may cause the cell cycle arrest at the G0/G1 phase [39]. In a recent study by Zhang et al. [40], it was reported that a high Mw fucoidan HMWF had been extracted from *Cladosiphon navae*. It was then digested with glysidases to acquire LMWF. LMWF was comprised of a digested low-molecular-weight fraction (72%, <500 kDa) and a non-digested fraction that consisted of less than 28% (800 kDa). LMWF consisted mainly of fucose (73%), xylose (12%) and mannose (7%). Their results showed that the LMWF enabled an induction of apoptosis in MDA-MB-231 breast cancer cells, showing a decreased trend in cell viability at the concentrations between 82 and 1640 µg/mL, followed by nuclear shrinkage and fragmentation on further analysis, which was an indication that the cytotoxic effect of LMWF was mediated through apoptotic induction. Kasai et al. [41] performed comparative studies involving apoptosis, where they discovered that type II fucoidan isolated from *F. vesiculosus* (600 kDa), exhibited similar apoptosis-inducing activities through the activation of caspase-8 and -9 in MCF-7 and HeLa cells at concentrations between 10–1000 µg/mL when compared to the low-molecular-weight of a type I fucoidan derivative.

Fucoidan has also been identified as a possible or potential counteracting agent to melanoma. Though therapeutic strategies exist in a form of a single agent or combined therapies, the efficacy depends on a number of factors which include the overall health of the patient, stage of cancer or metastasis and location of melanoma [42]. However, the efficacy of such treatments can somewhat be decreased due to the development of diverse resistance mechanisms. Hence, new therapeutic targets have been urgently needed for melanoma. For instance, *F. vesiculosus* fucoidan (purchased from Sigma) exhibited significant inhibitory effects on the cell proliferation and induction of apoptosis on

B16 melanoma cells at 550 µg/mL for 48 h [43]. Such evidence was well executed, which indeed was evidently shown by a strong contention on the side of fucoidan to possess therapeutic potentials.

The efficiency of fucoidan to inhibit cancer cells through activating apoptosis indicates a promising potential as a therapeutic agent. It is also encouraging to note that a couple of clinical studies have been undertaken to develop fucoidan as an anti-cancer therapy by means of combining it with other anti-cancer agents, and the little amount of data accumulated so far seems to be leaning in a positive direction. However, serious considerations in terms of further anti-cancer studies are still required, especially the discrepancy of results between the animal experiments and clinical trials in human. This may be under the influence of how the body absorbs and processes fucoidan, including the way in which fucoidan affects the body. In most cases, such processes are similar across species if not the same, occasionally they can be so different in that a substance may be benign in one species but invalid to the other. Therefore, some sort of a multidisciplinary approach can be considered, with an aim to produce credible results and avoid the discrepancy between animal studies and clinical trials as much as possible. With that being mentioned, a lot of ground still needs to be uncovered, hence it is proper to term fucoidan a 'potential therapy' rather than a cure for cancer at this stage until further updates are available.

8. Therapeutic Potential against Influenza A Virus

Among viral infections, the flu, with its seasonal outbreaks, has been one of the most problematic viruses worldwide, while medicine and science are in pursuit of amicable solutions. For example, influenza A virus (IAV) has been a formidable pathogen, which has been involved in at least three pandemics since the last century. One of its featured pandemics, which was regarded to be severe, claimed at least 40 million lives worldwide 1918–1919 [44]. In late April of 2009, an influenza A virus i.e., H1N1 [45], was in the limelight causing major awareness and surveillance in countries around the world. Though its prevalence was only for a brief period, its negative impact was rather great [46]. Therefore, scientists have been seeking solutions to eradicate or at least control over IAV. The scientific activities have extended as far as exploring marine sources such as fucoidan.

Recently, a study from Wang et al. [47] was undertaken to inhibit IAV infection by *Kjellmaniella crassifolia* fucoidan (536 kDa, sulfate content 30.1%) targeting the viral neuraminidase and cellular EGFR pathway. The selection of this type of fucoidan was based on one of the other requirements—that the development of anti-IAV drugs must have a high efficacy and minimal or no toxicity [46], hence the study on fucoidan was rather favorable as a consequence that most studies mention that fucoidan has less or no toxicity and is cost-effective compared to possible alternatives. The results revealed that *K. crassifolia* fucoidan blocked IAV infection in vitro with low toxicity, it also exhibited a broad spectrum against IAV and showed a low tendency in the induction of viral resistance, outperforming the regular anti-IAV drug amantadine. *K. crassifolia* fucoidan was able to inactivate virus particles before infection and some stages after adsorption. This was because it could also bind to viral neuraminidase (NA) and inhibit the activity of NA to block the release of IAV. In addition, intranasal administration of *K. crassifolia* fucoidan significantly improved survival and showed a decreased in the viral titers in IAV-infected mice. Sun et al. [48] obtained two *L. japonica* LMWF fractions LF1 and LF2 by degradation, which contained fucose of 42.0% and 30.5%; galactose content of 19.8% and 23.9%; uronic acid content of 5.3% and 3.7%; and sulfate content of 30.7% and 32.5%, respectively. They found a weight-average Mw and number-average Mw to be 7600 and 7300 for LF1 and 3900 and 3700 for LF2, respectively. LF1 and LF2 presented remarkable anti-viral activity in vitro especially in middle and high doses (0.15, 0.3, 0.6, 1.2 and 2.4 mg/mL). In vivo results also indicated that LF1 and LF2 were able to prolong the survival time of virus-infected mice, in addition, it presented an ability to significantly improve the quality of immune organs, immune cell phagocytosis and humoral immunity after intravenous administration of LMWFs (2.5, 5, 10 and 15 mg/kg; a period of 14 days). While such fucoidans present broad-spectrum anti-viral activity, the structure–activity relationship still remains unclear.

Despite the success of the currently available drugs, drug resistance, toxicity and cost still remain unresolved issues in the fight against IAV infection. Hence, the development of novel anti-IAV agents that could be used alone or in conjunction with existing anti-viral drugs is of critical importance. It may be possible that this kind of fucoidan from *K. crassifolia* may be developed further against highly pathogenic strains such as H5N1 or H7N9. In some way, fucoidan also has the potential of being a novel nasal drop or spray for influenza therapy and could serve as prophylaxis in the near future [49].

9. The Role of Fucoidan as A Potential Anti-Hepatitis B Virus Treatment

Another virus that presents detrimental effects is the hepatitis B virus (HBV). HBV infects more than 300 million people worldwide and is one of the leading causes of liver disease and liver cancer. The current challenge associated with HBV is the lack of knowledge in terms of predicting the outcome and progression of the HBV infection and an unfulfilled need in understanding the molecular, cellular, immunological and genetic basis of various disease manifestations allied with HBV infection [50]. A number of efforts have been made to improve the immunogenicity of HBV vaccines. There was a study conducted with an aim to investigate on *Fucus evanescens* fucoidan towards HBV vaccination, due to the fact that fucoidan was used as an adjuvant as reported previously. This study found that *Fucus evanescens* fucoidan (130–400 kDa) indeed acted as adjuvants by stimulating the formation of specific antibodies towards the surface of HBV, such as HBs-AG in mice [51]. The mice were immunized with compositions of vaccines contained HBs-AG and fucoidan samples, causing the increase of cytokines (TNF-a, IFN-g and IL-2) in the serum. An increase in the production of such cytokines was detected in the culture of splenocytes stimulated in vitro by fucoidan. A comparison was made that the adjuvant effect of fucoidan and its derivatives was similar to aluminum hydroxide, a traditional licensed adjuvant. Based on a structural analysis, this sample possesses the glycosidic linkage and structural features as follows: 3)-a-L-Fucp (2.4-SO_3)-(1→4)-a-L-Fucp (2-SO_3)-(1n. Another investigation showed that *F. vesiculosus* fucoidan was able to inhibit the replication of HBV both in vivo and in vitro [52]. Fucoidan suppressed the HBV replication by the activation of the EKR signal pathway and also enhanced the production of type I interferon via the activation of the host immune system. This newly discovered mechanism suggested another approach, which can be effectively employed to inhibit HBV replication. It was further mentioned that fucoidan alone and/or synergistically can be used to serve as a new therapeutic drug against HBV. The investigation determined that fucoidan significantly inhibited HBV replication in a mouse model in vivo (100 mg of fucoidan at 0, 1, 3, 5 and 7 days post-infection) and in HepG2.2.15 cells in vitro (at the concentration of <200 µg/mL). The results indicated *F. vesiculosus* fucoidan could activate MAPK-ERK1/2 pathway and subsequently promote the expression of IFN-α, causing a decrease in the production of HBV DNA and related proteins. This may suggest the possibility of using fucoidan as an alternative therapeutic strategy against HBV infection. Without a doubt, the consideration of safety and other related mechanisms of fucoidan still require further investigation prior to clinical application.

10. Therapeutic Potential as Veterinary Medicine against Canine Distemper Virus (CDV)

Viral infection does not only limit its impact on humans, but also affects wild and domestic animals as well. Though, not a lot of data are available, there are viruses that tend to be lethal to domestic animals e.g., canines [53]. The disadvantage is that therapies or medications suitable for such animals are rather limited and not well documented. This leads to such domestic pets succumbing to certain viruses, especially at their infancy due to a low immune system. For example, canine distemper virus (CDV), a morbillivirus genus member, is a virus that infects quite a range of terrestrial and aquatic carnivores [54]. This infection is characterized by presentations of respiratory and gastrointestinal disorders, followed by immunosuppression and neurological complications in infected hosts [54].

A study was performed to assess the fucoidan's anti-viral activity against CDV, since this type of virus is quite difficult to treat among canines. However, fucoidan may be part of the solution among the strategies and developments that are currently being undertaken, since the cure is still not available. Trejo-Avila et al. [55] reported that fucoidan extracted from *C. okamuranus* was able to inhibit CDV replication. This extraction contained 90.4% fucoidan and its mean molecular weight was 92.1 kDa, with fucose (38.6%), sulfate (15.9%) and other sugars (23%). It did not only show a reduction in the number of plaques but reduced the size of them as well. This fucoidan enabled an inhibition of CDV replication in Vero cells at an amount of 50% inhibitory concentration (IC50) of 0.1 µg/mL. The selectivity index (SI50) derived was >20,000. This showed that the fucoidan possesses an ability to inhibit the viral infection by interfering in the early steps and also by inhibiting CDV-mediated cell fusion. Therefore, fucoidan may be useful for the development of pharmacological strategies to treat and control CDV infection. Results such as these and many others to follow could be a stepping stone towards inventing the medication or cure against this deadly disease among canines.

11. Therapeutic Potential against HIV

A search for a cure towards HIV has been one of the focal points by a number of scientists worldwide. Though, a breakthrough has been noted in terms of the currently available treatment (in the form of anti-retrovirals) to tame the virus. However, a need still exists to eradicate it completely. The challenge with current treatment is related to side effects, especially during the initial introduction. Current treatments can also be cost-prohibitive, though certain countries subsidize affected individuals. This, in turn, places some constraints on governments in terms of exorbitant expenditures in an aim to sustain the lives of the people. Taking this into consideration, research for novel compounds to overcome such limitations is desperately needed.

Their anti-viral activity is dependent on the physical and chemical properties of fucoidan. An investigation found various fucoidans could suppress the infection of Jurkat cells utilizing pseudo-HIV-1 particles which contain envelope proteins of HIV-1 [56]. Therefore, based on the data obtained, the fucoidans (*Saccharina cichorioides* (1.3-α-ʟ-fucan) and *S. japonica* (galactofucan) presented a significant inhibitory effect. This was demonstrated by the efficiency against the lentiviral transduction of fucoidan at rather low concentrations of 0.001–0.05 µg/mL. Another potential anti-HIV agent was *S. swartzii* fucoidan [57]. Bioactive fucoidan fractions (CFF: Crude Fucoidan Fraction; FF1: Fucoidan Fraction 1; FF2: Fucoidan Fraction 2) were isolated from *S. swartzii*. The fucoidan fractions were placed under investigation for anti-HIV-1 properties. Fraction FF2 significantly exhibited anti-HIV-1 activity at concentrations of 1.56 and 6.25 µg/mL which was observed by >50% reduction in HIV-1 p24 antigen levels and reverse transcriptase activity. These fractions were mainly composed of sugars, sulfate and uronic acid, and the total sugar content in the FF1 and FF2 was 61.8% and 65.9%; the sulfate content—19.2% and 24.5%, uronic acid—17.6% and 13.4%, Mw—45 and 30 kDa, respectively. In addition, Thanh et al. [58] concluded that fucoidans derived from the three brown seaweeds, *S. mcclurei* (F_{SM}), *S. polycystum* (F_{SP}) and *Turbinara ornate* (F_{TO}), also displayed similar anti-HIV activities with a mean IC50 ranging from 0.33 to 0.7 g/mL. While the highest sulfate content was found in F_{SM} when compared to the other two fucoidans, and their anti-viral activities were not significantly different, suggesting that sulfate content is not the essential factor for anti-HIV activities of fucoidan. Those fucoidans inhibited HIV-1 infection when they were pre-incubated with the virus but not with the cells, and not after infection, showing that they were able to block the early steps of HIV entry into target cells. Hence, such studies are an indication that fucoidans with a naturally high molecular weight are possibly effective as anti-HIV agents regardless of their backbone. Though, the above results may present a rather positive outlook towards fucoidan as an anti-HIV treatment, more in vitro and in vivo studies are still necessary before proceeding to clinical trials.

12. Diabetic and Metabolic Syndrome Control

In recent years, fucoidan has received some intense interest as an agent for treating diabetes and other types of metabolic syndromes (MetS). Fucoidan extracted from *F. vesiculosus* has been known as an α-glucosidase inhibitor that is able to treat diabetes [59]. Among other studies, fucoidan was mentioned to have an ability to attenuate diabetic retinopathy through inhibiting VEGF signaling [60].

Additionally, a report of a low Mw fucoidan was noted to provide protection against diabetic associated symptoms in Goto-Kakizaki rats [61]. Fucoidan also improves glucose tolerance by modulating AMPK signaling and GLUT4 activity [62]. Some studies mention that Fuc-Pg (fucoidan from the sea cucumber *Pearsonothuria graeffei*) with an Mw of 310 kDa can be used as a form of functional food to treat MetS [63]. Fuc-Pg enabled weight reduction in high fat diet-fed mice, it also reduced hyperlipidemia, and protected the liver from steatosis. Concurrently, Fuc-Pg reduced the serum inflammatory cytokines combined with reduced macrophage infiltration into adipose tissue. Furthermore, it was declared that the treatment effect for MetS was primarily related to the 4-O-sulfated structure of fucoidan, since it was identified as a tetrasaccharide repeating unit with a backbone of [→3Fuc (2S, 4S) α1→3Fucα1→3Fuc(4S) α1→3Fucα1→]n.

With the rapid development of investigations related to intestinal microbes, in some cases, fucoidan is recognized as a prebiotic to regulate the intestinal ecosystem or microbiome [64]. It promotes the growth of beneficial bacteria which represents a mechanism inhibiting the development of MetS [65]. A report by Parnell et al. [66] showed that prebiotics containing fucoidan can regulate blood glucose and metabolism by providing a beneficial environment for the growth stimulation of probiotics. Cheng et al. [67] also demonstrated that *S. fusiforme* fucoidan (SFF) could modify gut microbiota during the alleviation of streptozotocin-induced hyperglycemia in mice. The yield of SFF was 6.02%., with sulfate content up to 14.55% and the average Mw of 205.8 kDa. This study was done with diabetic mice where after a 6-week administration, SFF impressively decreased the fasting blood glucose, diet and water intake. Additionally, SFF attenuated the pathological changes in the heart and liver tissues, hence, improving liver function. Also, SFF suppressed oxidative stress in STZ-induced diabetic mice which are manifestations associated with MetS. Concurrently, SFF significantly altered the gut microbiota in diabetic mice, what was noted is SFF decreased the relative abundances of the diabetes-related intestinal bacteria, which might be the potential mechanism for relieving the symptoms of diabetes [67].

Though the results indicated in this section seem significant in favor of reversing diabetes and MetS, it should be mentioned that related research is still in progress worldwide. The reason is based on the fact that scientists are still in pursuit of the mechanism which affords fucoidan the ability to reverse diabetes or MetS. Other factors to be considered are short-chain fatty acids (SCFAs), which are known to play a role in providing a conducive environment in the intestine after the oral intake of fucoidan since fucoidan cannot be digested by gastrointestinal enzymes, although their fermentation is regarded to be ideal for gut microbiota to produce SCFAs. Therefore, depending on interest, others would study fucoidan through the disciplines of physiology or pathophysiology in the intestine, some may explore the liver and/or pancreas as they play an integral role in digestion especially in the intestine, some may examine the microbiological context, while also looking into the exact mechanism of fucoidan. The reality is that before fucoidan can be considered as medication or future therapy towards MetS and diabetes, the studies that are still in their early stages would need to be completed. Perhaps a solid future project and/or direction needs to be well established while using a specific type of fucoidan.

13. Anti-Coagulant Function

Vascular related disease, such as ischemic heart disease, atherosclerosis and deep vein thrombosis, are still among the leading causes of death worldwide. As reported by the World Health Organization, complications associated with these diseases account for over one-quarter of death throughout the world [68]. In most cases, thrombotic related episodes are usually managed by using anti-coagulant and anti-thrombotic medications, such as heparin, a sulfated glycan belonging to the family of glycosaminoglycans (CAGs) [69]. As it would be anticipated, such therapies tend to present with undesirable and come with severe to moderate side effects that are unavoidable [70]. The side effects linked to heparin include thrombocytopenia [71] and hemorrhagic episodes [72], hence this can limit, defeat or hinder its pharmacological applications.

According to evidence from available studies, it is mentioned that the anti-coagulant activity of fucoidan is dependent on its Mw, sulfate group/total sugar ratio, sulfate position, sulfate degree, and glycoside branching [73]. Chandria et al. [74] discovered that, by preparing *Lessonia vadosa* LMWF using free-radical depolymerization, a better anti-coagulant activity is then exhibited than the naïve fucoidan in a dose-dependent-manner. Jin et al. [75] discovered that fucoidan's Mw and content of galactose, presented anti-coagulant activity. Documentation based on previous studies indicates that fucoidans with an Mw of 5–100 kDa present as potential anti-coagulants, while fractions greater than 850 kDa are lack of anti-coagulant activity [76]. The fucoidans with an Mw ranging from 10–300 kDa, are regarded as having by far the strongest anti-coagulant activity. In a previous study [77], the authors performed a comparative study of anti-thrombotic and anti-platelet activities of different fucoidans from *L. japonica*, where their results showed that the fucoidan of Mw 27–32 kDa exhibited a much better anti-coagulant and anti-thrombin activity than low molecular weight fucoidans (3.7–7.2 kDa) through intravenous administration. A recent study [78] reported that two dry *Fucus* extracts, DFE-1 and DFE-2, prepared using ultrasound technique, were investigated for their anti-coagulant activity compared to the reference agent heparin. An in vivo experiment on Wistar rats was conducted based on anti-coagulant activities whereby increased blood clotting time was studied—measured by activated partial thromboplastin time (APTT) and prothrombin time (PT). The results indicated that DFE-2 was analogous to the anti-coagulatory effect produced by the reference agent heparin, while DFE-1 showed a weak effect compared to DFE-2 or heparin. The distinct anti-coagulant effect between DFE-1 and DFE-2 might be due to their different physiochemical properties, including fucoidan content, monosaccharide composition and the differences in the contents of polyphenols and sulfate groups. This was indicative that the chemical composition plays an essential role in the anti-coagulant activities of fucoidan.

14. Methods

An electronic search was conducted with an aim to identify articles relevant for this literature, from the online database Web of Science from 2000 until 2019. The search included 'structure of fucoidan', 'pharmacokinetics', 'fucoidan', 'seaweed', 'apoptosis' and 'anti-viral'. The citation lists were searched manually for other related articles. The strategy used to search is explained in Appendix A.

15. Conclusions and Future Perspectives

Fucoidan continues to be promising towards a wide range of potential applications. Since the modern era, reviews and research articles based on the therapeutic applications of fucoidan are on the rise. Therefore, support has been growing in terms of the role that fucoidan could play as a form of therapy. This stems from the fact that brown algae has been used for many years to treat certain ailments in TCM, hence there is a bit of history to be considered. It remains significant or essential that each type of fucoidan necessitates screening and validation for a particular therapeutic activity. A serious consideration on pharmacokinetics, uptake and biodistribution still requires further assessment. Despite the numerous studies done on fucoidan so far, there are still few clinical trials planned and completed. This may be due to a lack of comparative studies, on a specific fucoidan for instance. In most cases, studies are examining different types of fucoidan on different cell lines or animal models. Hence, this makes it difficult to establish a general mechanism that is for a specific type of fucoidan. In addition, there is relatively little information available with regards to the absorption, distribution and excretion of fucoidan. With that being mentioned, the structure of fucoidans still requires attention, since they present a complex structure, even their refined structures are not yet clear or fully understood. The biological activities presented by fucoidan are attractive. However, because most of these studies are carried out by using a relatively crude fucoidan, it is quite difficult to determine the relationships between structure and activity. Future studies based on the clear conformation of fucoidan should assist in establishing a better understanding of their biological properties. This might soon be practically possible, as a consequence of the gradual increase in the availability of detection and measurement techniques. The key element in developing successful therapeutic products is based on the understanding of the chemistry and structural variability of each type of fucoidan. It should be appreciated that some studies indicated in this review are currently undertaking further studies, following up on what they have done previously. Additionally, they also indicate that future studies are currently underway, and will be available soon that is based on the past and present work. This paves the way for what will be known as a 'tried and tested' regimen, should it one day be used as therapy.

Author Contributions: Conceptualization, S.L. and H.T.; resources, S.L., X.Z. and Y.C.; writing—original draft preparation, S.L. and S.W.; writing—review and editing, M.W. and H.T.; visualization, S.W.; supervision, H.T.; funding acquisition, M.W.

Funding: This work was financially supported by the National Natural Science Foundation of China (41876197, 31470430 and 81872952), the Natural Science Foundation of Zhejiang Province (LY18C020006), the Science and Technology Program of Wenzhou (Y20180210).

Acknowledgments: We thank Alan K Chang (Wenzhou University) for helpful discussion and for revising the language of the manuscript. We thank the Department of Higher Education and Training (DHET) of South Africa for their financial contribution and general support. We thank the China Scholarship Council (CSC) for the support. We also thank A. Luthuli of Majesty Graphic Designs (MGD) for the helpful advice and work on graphics.

Conflicts of Interest: The authors declare no conflict of interest.

Appendix A

Appendix A.1 Search Strategy

Web of Science:

- TOPIC: (fucoidan)
- TOPIC: (fucoidan) AND TOPIC: (structure)
- TOPIC: (sulfated polysaccharides) AND TOPIC:(structure)
- TOPIC: (sulfated polysaccharides) AND TOPIC:(pharmacokinetics)
- TOPIC: (sulfated polysaccharides) AND TOPIC:(absorption)
- TOPIC: (fucoidan) AND TOPIC: (absorption)
- TOPIC: (fucoidan) AND TOPIC:(pharmacokinetics)
- TOPIC: (fucoidan) AND TOPIC: (preparation)
- TOPIC: (fucoidan) AND TOPIC: (sulfate)
- TOPIC: (fucoidan) AND TOPIC: (species)
- TOPIC: (fucoidan) AND TOPIC: (Fucus vesiculosus)
- TOPIC: (fucoidan) AND TOPIC: (cladosiphon okamuranus)
- TOPIC: (fucoidan) AND TOPIC: (ascophyllum nodosum)
- TOPIC: (fucoidan) AND TOPIC: (fucales)
- TOPIC: (fucoidan) AND TOPIC: (brown algae)
- TOPIC: (fucoidan) AND TOPIC: (cancer)
- TOPIC: (fucoidan) AND TOPIC: (antiviral)
- TOPIC: (fucoidan) AND TOPIC: (synergy)
- TOPIC: (fucoidan) AND TOPIC: (anti-influenza)
- TOPIC: (fucoidan) AND TOPIC: (diabetes)
- TOPIC: (fucoidan) AND TOPIC: (metabolic syndrome)
- TOPIC: (fucoidan) AND TOPIC: (anti-coagulant)
- TOPIC: (fucoidan) AND TOPIC: (anti-canine distemper)
- TOPIC: (Low molecular weight fucoidan)
- TOPIC: (fucoidan) AND TOPIC: (apoptosis)
- TOPIC: (fucoidan) AND TOPIC: (caspase)

- TOPIC: (fucoidan) AND TOPIC: (caspase pathway)
- TOPIC: (fucoidan) AND TOPIC: (intrinsic & extrinsic apoptosis)

Appendix A.2 Criteria for Considering Studies for This Review

We considered all the subject-related studies for this literature, experimental articles published around 2000–2019 (mainly the summary of the experimental data portrayed, excluding background information covered before year 2000) to have provoked our interest. In addition, relevant articles from the bibliography of articles we found with above-mentioned search terms were selected for this review.

References

1. Blunt, J.W.; Copp, B.R.; Hu, W.P.; Munro, M.H.G.; Northcote, P.T.; Prinsep, M.R. Marine natural products. *Nat. Prod. Rep.* **2007**, *24*, 31–86. [CrossRef]
2. Rajasulochana, P.; Dhamotharan, R.; Krishnamoorthy, P.; Murugesan, S. Antibacterial activity of the extracts of marine red and brown algae. *J. Am. Sci.* **2009**, *5*, 20–25.
3. Liu, X.; Du, P.; Liu, X.; Cao, S.; Qin, L.; He, M.; He, X.; Mao, W. Anticoagulant properties of a green algal phamnan-type sulfated polysaccharide and its low-molecular-weight fragments prepared by mild acid degradation. *Mar. Drugs* **2018**, *16*, 445. [CrossRef] [PubMed]
4. Chandini, S.K.; Ganesan, P.; Bhaskar, N. In vitro antioxidant activities of three selected brown seaweeds of India. *Food Chem.* **2008**, *107*, 707–713. [CrossRef]
5. Gomes, D.L.; Melo, K.R.T.; Queiroz, M.F.; Batista, L.A.N.C.; Santos, P.C.; Costa, M.S.S.P.; Almeida-Lima, J.; Camara, R.B.G.; Costa, L.S.; Rocha, H.A.O. In vitro studies reveal antiurolithic effect of antioxidant sulfated polysaccharides from the green seaweed *Caulerpa cupressoides var* flabellata. *Mar. Drugs* **2019**, *17*, 326. [CrossRef] [PubMed]
6. Liu, L.; Heinrich, M.; Myres, S.; Dworjanyn, S.A. Towards a better understanding of medicinal uses of the brown seaweed *Sargassum* in traditional Chinese medicine: A phytochemical and pharmacological review. *J. Ethnopharmacol.* **2012**, *142*, 591–619. [CrossRef] [PubMed]
7. Yoo, H.J.; You, D.J.; Lee, K.W. Characterization and immunomodulatory effects of high molecular weight fucoidan fraction from the *Sporophyll* of *Undaria pinnatifida* in cyclophosphamide-induced immunosuppressed mice. *Mar. Drugs.* **2019**, *17*, 447. [CrossRef]
8. McDowell, P.E. 15—Algal polysaccharides. In *Methods in Plant Biochemistry*, 1st ed.; Elsever: Amsterdam, The Netherlands, 1990; Volume 2, pp. 523–547.
9. Cui, K.; Tai, W.; Shan, X.; Hao, J.; Li, G.; Yu, G. Structural characterization and anti-thrombotic properties of fucoidan from *Nemacystus decipiens*. *Int. J. Biol. Macromol.* **2018**, *120*, 1817–1822. [CrossRef] [PubMed]
10. Yokota, T.; Nomura, K.; Nagashima, M.; Kamimura, N. Fucoidan alleviates high-fat diet-induced dyslipidemia and atherosclerosis in ApoE^{shl} mice deficient in apolipoprotein E expression. *J. Nutr. Biochem.* **2016**, *32*, 46–54. [CrossRef]
11. Mansour, M.B.; Balti, R.; Yacoubi, L.; Ollivier, V.; Chaubet, F.; Maaroufi, R.M. Primary structure and anticoagulant activity of fucoidan from the sea cucumber *Holothuria polii*. *Int. J. Biol. Macromol.* **2019**, *121*, 1145–1153. [CrossRef]
12. Zhao, Y.; Zheng, Y.; Wang, J.; Ma, S.; Yu, Y.; White, W.L.; Yang, S.; Yang, F.; Lu, J. Fucoidan extracted from *Undaria pinnatifida*: Source for nutraceuticals/functional foods. *Mar Drugs* **2018**, *16*, 321. [CrossRef] [PubMed]
13. Koh, H.S.A.; Lu, J.; Zhou, W. Structure characterization and antioxidant activity of fucoidan isolated from *Undaria pinnatifida* grown in New Zealand. *Carbohydr. Polym.* **2019**, *212*, 178–185. [CrossRef] [PubMed]
14. Jin, W.; Wu, W.; Tang, H.; Wei, B.; Wang, H.; Sun, J.; Zhang, W.; Zhong, W. Structure analysis and anti-tumor and anti-angiogenic activities of sulfated galactofucan extracted from *Sargassum thunbergii*. *Mar. Drugs* **2019**, *17*, 52. [CrossRef] [PubMed]
15. Usoltseva, R.V.; Anastyuk, S.D.; Surits, V.V.; Shevchenko, N.M.; Thinh, P.D.; Zadorozhny, P.A.; Ermakova, S.P. Comparison of structure and in vitro anticancer activity of native and modified fucoidans from *Sargassum feldmannii* and *S. duplicatum*. *Int. J. Biol. Macromol.* **2019**, *124*, 220–228. [CrossRef] [PubMed]
16. Usoltseva, R.V.; Shevchenko, N.M.; Malyarenko, O.S.; Anastyuk, S.D.; Kasprik, A.E.; Zvyagintsev, N.V.; Ermakova, S.P. Fucoidans from brown algae *Laminaria longipes* and *Saccharina cichorioides*: Structural

characteristics, anticancer and radio-sensitizing activity in vitro. *Carbohydr. Polym.* **2019**, *221*, 157–165. [CrossRef] [PubMed]

17. Lahrsen, E.; Liewert, I.; Alban, S. Gradual degradation of fucoidan from *Fucus vesiculosus* and its effect on structure, antioxidant and antiproliferative activities. *Carbohydr. Polym.* **2018**, *192*, 208–216. [CrossRef]

18. Zhang, Z.; Till, S.; Jiang, C.; Knappe, S.; Reutterer, S.; Scheiflinger, F.; Szabo, C.M.; Dockal, M. Structure-activity relationship of the pro- and anticoagulant effects of *Fucus vesiculosus* fucoidan. *Thromb. Haemost.* **2014**, *111*, 429–437.

19. Bilan, M.I.; Grachev, A.A.; Ustuzhanina, N.E.; Shashkov, A.S.; Nifantiev, N.E.; Usov, A.I. Structure of a fucoidan from the brown seaweed *Fucus evanescens* C. Ag. *Carbohydr. Res.* **2002**, *337*, 719–730. [CrossRef]

20. Bilan, M.I.; Grachev, A.A.; Ustuzhanina, N.E.; Shashkov, A.S.; Nifantiev, N.E.; Usov, A.I. A highly regular fraction of a fucoidan from the brown seaweed *Fucus distichus* L. *Carbohydr. Res.* **2004**, *339*, 511–517. [CrossRef]

21. Bilan, M.I.; Grachev, A.A.; Shashkov, A.S.; Nifantiev, N.E.; Usov, A.I. Structure of a fucoidan from the brown seaweed *Fucus serratus* L. *Carbohydr. Res.* **2006**, *341*, 238–245. [CrossRef]

22. Foley, S.A.; Szegezdi, E.; Mulloy, B.; Samali, A.; Tuohy, M.G. An unfractionated fucoidan from *Ascophyllum nodosum*: Extraction, characterization, and apoptotic effects in vitro. *J. Nat. Prod.* **2012**, *75*, 1674. [CrossRef]

23. Descamps, V.; Colin, S.; Lahaye, M.; Jam, M.; Richard, C.; Potin, P.; Barbeyron, T.; Yvin, J.C.; Kloareg, B. Isolation and culture of a marine bacterium degrading the sulfated fucans from marine brown algae. *Mar. Biotechnol.* **2006**, *8*, 27–39. [CrossRef] [PubMed]

24. Jabbar Mian, A.; Percival, E. Carbohydrates of the brown seaweeds *Himanthalia lorea* and *Bifurcaria bifurcata*: Part II. structural studies of the "fucans". *Carbohydr. Res.* **1973**, *26*, 147–161. [CrossRef]

25. Mak, W.; Hamid, N.; Liu, T.; Lu, J.; White, W.L. Fucoidan from New Zealand *Undaria pinnatifida*: Monthly variations and determination of antioxidant activities. *Carbohydr. Polym.* **2013**, *95*, 606–614. [CrossRef] [PubMed]

26. Fletcher, H.R.; Biller, P.; Ross, A.B.; Adams, J.M.M. The seasonal variation of fucoidan within three species of brown macroalgae. *Algal Res.* **2017**, *22*, 79–86. [CrossRef]

27. Garcia-Vaquero, M.; Rajauria, G.; O'Doherty, J.V.; Sweeney, T. Polysaccharides from macroalgae: Recent advances, innovative technologies and challenges in extraction and purification. *Food Res. Int.* **2017**, *99*, 1011–1020. [CrossRef] [PubMed]

28. Chevolot, L.; Foucault, A.; Chaubet, F.; Kervarec, N.; Sinquin, C.; Fisher, A.M.; Boisson-Vidal, C. Further data on the structure of brown seaweed fucans: Relationships with anticoagulant activity. *Carbohydr. Res.* **1999**, *319*, 154–165. [CrossRef]

29. Marais, M.F.; Joseleau, J.P. A fucoidan fraction from *Ascophyllum nodosum*. *Carbohydr. Res.* **2001**, *336*, 155–159. [CrossRef]

30. Ponce, N.M.A.; Pujol, C.A.; Damonte, E.B.; Flores, M.L.; Stortz, C.A. Fucoidans from the brown seaweed *Adenocystis utricularis*: Extraction methods, antiviral activity and structural studies. *Carbohydr. Res.* **2003**, *338*, 153–165. [CrossRef]

31. Irhimeh, M.R.; Fitton, J.H.; Lowenthal, R.M.; Kongtawelert, P. A quantitative method to detect fucoidan in human plasma using a novel antibody. *Methods Find. Exp. Clin. Pharmacol.* **2005**, *27*, 705–710. [CrossRef]

32. Pozharitskaya, O.N.; Shikov, A.N.; Faustova, N.M.; Obluchinskaya, E.D.; Kosman, V.M.; Vuorela, H.; Makarov, V.G. Pharmacokinetic and tissue distribution of fucoidan from *Fucus vesiculosus* after oral administration to rats. *Mar. Drugs* **2018**, *16*, 132. [CrossRef] [PubMed]

33. Torode, T.A.; Marcus, S.E.; Jam, M.; Tonon, T.; Blackburn, R.S.; Hervé, C.; Knox, J.P. Monoclonal antibodies directed to fucoidan preparations from brown algae. *PLoS ONE* **2015**, *10*, e0118366. [CrossRef] [PubMed]

34. Nagamine, T.; Nakazato, K.; Tomioka, S.; Iha, M.; Nakajima, K. Intestinal absorption of fucoidan extracted from the brown seaweed, *Cladosiphon okamuranus*. *Mar. Drugs* **2015**, *13*, 48–64. [CrossRef] [PubMed]

35. Tokita, Y.; Nakajima, K.; Mochida, H.; Iha, M.; Nagamine, T. Development of a fucoidan-specific antibody and measurement of fucoidan in serum and urine by sandwich ELISA. *Biosci. Biotechnol. Biochem.* **2010**, *74*, 350–357. [CrossRef]

36. Matsubara, K.; Xue, C.; Zhao, X.; Mori, M.; Sugawara, T.; Hirata, T. Effects of middle molecular weight fucoidans on in vitro and ex vivo angiogenesis of endothelial cells. *Int. J. Mol. Med.* **2005**, *15*, 695–699. [CrossRef] [PubMed]

37. Kadena, K.; Tomori, M.; Iha, M.; Nagamine, T. Absorption study of mozuku fucoidan in Japanese volunteers. *Mar. Drugs* **2018**, *16*, 254. [CrossRef] [PubMed]

38. Burz, C.; Berindan-Neagoe, I.; Balacescu, O.; Irimie, A. Apoptosis in cancer: Key molecular signaling pathways and therapy targets. *Acta Oncol.* **2009**, *48*, 811–821. [CrossRef] [PubMed]

39. Nagamine, T.; Hayakawa, K.; Kusakabe, T.; Takada, H.; Nakazato, K.; Hisanaga, E.; Iha, M. Inhibitory effect of fucoidan on Huh7 hepatoma cells through downregulation of CXCL12. *Nutr. Cancer* **2009**, *61*, 340–347. [CrossRef]

40. Zhang, Z.; Teruya, K.; Hiroshi Eto, H.; Shirahata, S. Induction of apoptosis by low-molecular-weight fucoidan through calcium- and caspase-dependent mitochondrial pathways in MDA-MB-231 breast cancer cells. *Biosci. Biotechnol. Biochem.* **2013**, *77*, 235–242. [CrossRef]

41. Kasai, A.; Arafuka, S.; Koshiba, N.; Takahashi, D.; Toshima, K. Systematic synthesis of low-molecular weight fucoidan derivatives and their effect on cancer cells. *Org. Biomol. Chem.* **2015**, *13*, 10556–10568. [CrossRef]

42. Domingues, B.; Lopes, J.M.; Soares, P.; Pópulo, H. Melanoma treatment in review. *Immunotargets Ther.* **2018**, *7*, 35–49. [CrossRef] [PubMed]

43. Wang, Z.J.; Xu, W.; Liang, J.W.; Wang, C.S.; Kang, Y. Effect of fucoidan on B16 murine melanoma cell melanin formation and apoptosis. *Afr. J. Tradit. Complement. Altern. Med.* **2017**, *14*, 149–155. [CrossRef] [PubMed]

44. Peltier, M. The influenza epidemic that occurred in New Caledonia in 1921. *Bull. de l'Office Int. d'Hygiene Publique* **1922**, *6*, 677–685.

45. Schoch-Spana, M.; Bouri, N.; Rambhia, K.J.; Norwood, A. Stigma, health disparities, and the 2009 H1N1 influenza pandemic: How to protect Latino farmworkers in future health emergencies. *Biosecur. Bioterror.* **2010**, *8*, 243–254. [CrossRef] [PubMed]

46. Tognotti, E. Lessons from the history of quarantine, from plague to influenza A. *Emerg. Infect. Dis.* **2013**, *19*, 254–259. [CrossRef] [PubMed]

47. Wang, W.; Wu, J.; Zhang, X.; Hao, C.; Zhao, X.; Jiao, G.; Shan, X.; Tai, W.; Yu, G. Inhibition of influenza A virus infection by fucoidan targeting viral neuraminidase and cellular EGFR pathway. *Sci. Rep.* **2017**, *7*, 40760. [CrossRef]

48. Sun, T.; Zhang, X.; Miao, Y.; Zhou, Y.; Shi, J.; Yan, M.; Chen, A. Studies on antiviral and immuno-regulation activity of low molecular weight fucoidan from *Laminaria japonica*. *J. Ocean Univ. China* **2018**, *3*, 705–711. [CrossRef]

49. Moscona, A. Global transmission of oseltamivir-resistant influenza. *N. Engl. J. Med.* **2009**, *360*, 953–956. [CrossRef]

50. Liang, T.J. Hepatitis B: The virus and disease. *Hepatology* **2009**, *49*, 13–21. [CrossRef]

51. Kuznetsova, T.; Ivanushko, L.; Persiyanova, E.V.; Shutikova, A.L.; Ermakova, S.P.; Khotimchenko, M.Y.; Besednova, N.N. Evaluation of adjuvant effects of fucoidane from brown seaweed *Fucus evanescens* and its structural analogues for the strengthening vaccines effectiveness. *Biomed. Khim.* **2017**, *63*, 553–558. [CrossRef]

52. Li, H.F.; Li, J.; Tang, Y.; Lin, L.; Xie, Z. Fucoidan from *Fucus vesiculosus* suppresses hepatitis B virus replication by enhancing extracellular signal-regulated kinase activation. *Virol. J.* **2017**, *14*, 178. [CrossRef] [PubMed]

53. Williams, E.S.; Barker, I.K. Canine distemper. *Infect. Dis. Wild Mamm.* **2001**, *3*, 50–59.

54. Beineke, A.; Puff, C.; Seehusen, F.; Baumgärtner, W. Pathogenesis and immunopathology of systemic and nervous canine distemper. *Vet. Immunol. Immunopathol.* **2009**, *127*, 1–18. [CrossRef] [PubMed]

55. Trejo-Avila, L.M.; Morales-Martínez, M.E.; Ricque-Marie, D.; Cruz-Suarez, L.E.; Zapata-Benavides, P.; Morán-Santibañez, K.; Rodríguez-Padillan, C. In-vitro anti-canine distemper virus activity of fucoidan extracted from the brown alga *Cladosiphon okamuranus*. *Virus Dis.* **2014**, *25*, 474–480. [CrossRef] [PubMed]

56. Prokofjeva, M.M.; Imbs, T.I.; Shevchenko, N.M.; Spirin, P.V.; Horn, S.; Fehse, B.; Zvyagintseva, T.N.; Prassolov, V.S. Fucoidans as potential inhibitors of HIV-1. *Mar. Drugs* **2013**, *11*, 3000–3014. [CrossRef] [PubMed]

57. Dinesh, S.; Menon, T.; Hanna, L.E.; Suresh, V.; Sathuvan, M.; Manikannan, M.M. In vitro anti-HIV-1 activity of fucoidan from *Sargassum swartzii*. *Int. J. Biol. Macromol.* **2016**, *82*, 83–88. [CrossRef] [PubMed]

58. Thanh, T.T.T.; Bui, M.L.; Tran, T.T.V.; Ngo, V.Q.; Ho, C.T.; Yue, Z.; Carole, S.D.; Bilan, M.U.A. Anti-HIV activity of fucoidans from three brown seaweed species. *Carbohydr. Polym.* **2015**, *115*, 122–128.

59. Shan, X.D.; Liu, X.; Hao, J.J.; Cai, C.; Fan, F.; Dun, Y.L.; Zhao, X.L.; Liu, X.X.; Li, C.X.; Yu, G.L. In vitro and in vivo hypoglycemic effects of brown algal fucoidans. *Int. J. Biol. Macromol.* **2016**, *82*, 249–255. [CrossRef] [PubMed]

60. Yang, W.Z.; Yu, X.F.; Zhang, Q.B.; Lu, Q.J.; Wang, J.; Cui, W.T.; Zheng, Y.Y.; Wang, X.M.; Luo, D.L. Attenuation of streptozotocin-induced diabetic retinopathy with low molecular weight fucoidan via inhibition of vascular endothelial growth factor. *Exp. Eye Res.* **2013**, *115*, 96–105. [CrossRef]
61. Cui, W.; Zheng, Y.; Zhang, Q.; Wang, J.; Wang, L.; Yang, W.; Guo, C.; Gao, W.; Wang, X.; Luo, D.L. Low-molecular-weight fucoidan protects endothelial function and ameliorates basal hypertension in diabetic Goto-Kakizaki rats. *Lab. Investig.* **2014**, *94*, 382–393. [CrossRef]
62. Jeong, Y.T.; Kim, Y.D.; Jung, Y.M.; Park, D.C.; Lee, D.S.; Ku, S.K.; Li, X.; Lu, Y.; Chao, G.H.; Kim, K.J. Low molecular weight fucoidan improves endoplasmic reticulum stress-reduced insulin sensitivity through AMP-Activated protein kinase activation in L6 myotubes and restores lipid homeostasis in a mouse model of type 2 diabetes. *Mol. Pharmacol.* **2013**, *84*, 147–157. [CrossRef]
63. Hu, S.W.; Xia, G.H.; Wang, J.F.; Wang, Y.M.; Li, Z.J.; Xue, C.H. Fucoidan from sea cucumber protects against high-fat high-sucrose diet-induced hyperglycaemia and insulin resistance in mice. *J. Funct. Foods* **2014**, *10*, 128–138. [CrossRef]
64. Chen, Q.; Liu, M.; Zhang, P.; Fan, S.; Huang, J.; Yu, S.; Zhang, C.; Li, H. Fucoidan and galacto-oligosaccharides ameliorate high-fat diet-induced dyslipidemia in rats by modulating the gut microbiota and bile acid metabolism. *Nutrition* **2019**, *65*, 50–59. [CrossRef] [PubMed]
65. Li, S.; Li, J.; Mao, G.; Wu, T.; Hu, Y.; Ye, X.; Tian, D.; Linhardt, R.J.; Chen, S. A fucoidan from sea cucumber *Pearsonothuria graeffei* with well-repeated structure alleviates gut microbiota dysbiosis and metabolic syndromes in HFD-fed mice. *Food Funct.* **2018**, *9*, 5371–5380. [CrossRef] [PubMed]
66. Parnell, J.A.; Reimer, R.A. Prebiotic fiber modulation of the gut microbiota improves risk factors for obesity and the metabolic syndrome. *Gut Microbes* **2012**, *3*, 29–34. [CrossRef]
67. Cheng, Y.; Luthuli, S.; Hou, L.F.; Jiang, H.J.; Chen, P.C.; Zhang, X.; Wu, M.; Tong, H.B. *Sargassum fusiforme* fucoidan modifies the gut microbiota during alleviation of streptozotocin-induced hyperglycemia in mice. *Int. J. Biol. Macromol.* **2019**, *131*, 1162–1170. [CrossRef]
68. Raskob, G.E.; Angchaisuksiri, P.; Blanco, A.N.; Buller, H.; Gallus, A.; Hunt, B.J.; Hylek, E.M.; Kakkar, A.; Konstantinides, S.V.; McCumber, M. Thrombosis: A major contributor to global disease burden. *Arterioscler. Thromb. Vasc. Biol.* **2014**, *34*, 2363–2371. [CrossRef] [PubMed]
69. Spyropoulos, A.C. Brave new world: The current and future use of novel anticoagulants. *Thromb. Res.* **2008**, *123*, 29–35. [CrossRef]
70. Moore, T.J.; Cohen, M.R.; Furberg, C.D. Serious adverse drug events reported to the Food and Drug Administration, 1998–2005. *Arch. Intern. Med.* **2007**, *167*, 1752–1759. [CrossRef] [PubMed]
71. Baroletti, S.A.; Goldhaber, S.Z. Heparin-induced thrombocytopenia. *Circulation* **2006**, *114*, 355–356. [CrossRef]
72. Clark, W.M.; Madden, K.P.; Lyden, P.D.; Zivin, J.A. Cerebral hemorrhagic risk of aspirin or heparin therapy with thrombolytic treatment in rabbits. *Stroke* **1991**, *22*, 872–876. [CrossRef] [PubMed]
73. Nishino, T.; Nagumo, T.; Kiyohara, H.; Yamada, H. Structural characterization of a new anticoagulant fucan sulfate from the brown seaweed *Ecklonia kurome*. *Carbohydr. Res.* **1991**, *211*, 77–90. [CrossRef]
74. Chandia, N.P.; Matsuhiro, B. Characterization of a fucoidan from *Lessonia vadosa* (Phaeophyta) and its anticoagulant and elicitor properties. *Int. J. Biol. Macromol.* **2008**, *42*, 235–240. [CrossRef] [PubMed]
75. Jin, W.H.; Zhang, Q.B.; Wang, J.; Zhang, W.J. A comparative study of the anticoagulant activities of eleven fucoidans. *Carbohydr. Polym.* **2013**, *91*, 1–6. [CrossRef] [PubMed]
76. Shanmugam, M.; Mody, K.H. Heparinoid-active sulphated polysaccharides from marine algae as potential blood anticoagulant agents. *Curr. Sci. India* **2000**, *79*, 1672–1683.
77. Wang, J.; Zhang, Q.B.; Zhang, Z.S.; Song, H.F.; Li, P.C. Potential antioxidant and anticoagulant capacity of low molecular weight fucoidan fractions extracted from *Laminaria japonica*. *Int. J. Biol. Macromol.* **2010**, *46*, 6–12. [CrossRef] [PubMed]
78. Obluchinksya, E.D.; Makarova, M.N.; Pozharitskaya, O.N.; Shikov, A.N. Effects of ultrasound treatment on the chemical composition and anticoagulant properties of dry *Fucus* extract. *Pharm. Chem. J.* **2015**, *49*, 183–186. [CrossRef]

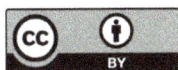

marine drugs

MDPI

Article

A Glycosaminoglycan Extract from *Portunus pelagicus* Inhibits BACE1, the β Secretase Implicated in Alzheimer's Disease

Courtney J. Mycroft-West [1], Lynsay C. Cooper [1], Anthony J. Devlin [1,2], Patricia Procter [1], Scott E. Guimond [1,3], Marco Guerrini [2], David G. Fernig [4], Marcelo A. Lima [1], Edwin A. Yates [1,4] and Mark A. Skidmore [1,3,4,*]

[1] Molecular & Structural Biosciences, School of Life Sciences, Keele University, Huxley Building, Keele, Staffordshire ST5 5BG, UK; c.j.mycroft-west@keele.ac.uk (C.J.M.-W.); l.c.cooper@keele.ac.uk (L.C.C.); a.devlin1@keele.ac.uk (A.J.D.); p.procter@keele.ac.uk (P.P.); s.e.guimond@keele.ac.uk (S.E.G.); mlimagb@gmail.com (M.A.L.); E.A.Yates@liverpool.ac.uk (E.A.Y.)
[2] Istituto di Ricerche Chimiche e Biochimiche G. Ronzoni, Via G. Colombo 81, 20133 Milan, Italy; guerrini@ronzoni.it
[3] Institute for Science and Technology in Medicine, Keele University, Keele, Staffordshire ST5 5BG, UK
[4] School of Biological Sciences, University of Liverpool, Crown Street, Liverpool L69 7ZB, UK; dgfernig@liverpool.ac.uk
* Correspondence: m.a.skidmore@keele.ac.uk; Tel.: +44-(0)1782-733945

check for updates

Received: 18 April 2019; Accepted: 9 May 2019; Published: 16 May 2019

Abstract: Therapeutic options for Alzheimer's disease, the most common form of dementia, are currently restricted to palliative treatments. The glycosaminoglycan heparin, widely used as a clinical anticoagulant, has previously been shown to inhibit the Alzheimer's disease-relevant β-secretase 1 (BACE1). Despite this, the deployment of pharmaceutical heparin for the treatment of Alzheimer's disease is largely precluded by its potent anticoagulant activity. Furthermore, ongoing concerns regarding the use of mammalian-sourced heparins, primarily due to prion diseases and religious beliefs hinder the deployment of alternative heparin-based therapeutics. A marine-derived, heparan sulphate-containing glycosaminoglycan extract, isolated from the crab *Portunus pelagicus*, was identified to inhibit human BACE1 with comparable bioactivity to that of mammalian heparin $(IC_{50} = 1.85\ \mu g\ mL^{-1}\ (R^2 = 0.94)$ and $2.43\ \mu g\ mL^{-1}\ (R^2 = 0.93)$, respectively), while possessing highly attenuated anticoagulant activities. The results from several structural techniques suggest that the interactions between BACE1 and the extract from *P. pelagicus* are complex and distinct from those of heparin.

Keywords: Alzheimer's disease; amyloid-β; BACE1; β-secretase; glycosaminoglycan; heparan sulphate; heparin; *Portunus pelagicus*

1. Introduction

Alzheimer's disease (AD), the most common form of dementia, is characterized by progressive neurodegeneration and cognitive decline [1]. The deposition and aggregation of toxic amyloid-β proteins (Aβ), the primary constituents of β-amyloid plaques, has been identified as one of the primary causative factors in the development of AD. Approximately 270 mutations within genes that are directly associated with Aβ production are currently linked to the early-onset development of AD [2]. Furthermore, additional genetic risk factors for late-onset AD have been identified, most notably the APOE polymorphism [1]. Other pathological hallmarks of AD include the presence of intraneuronal neurofibrillary tangles (NFTs), an enhanced inflammatory response, neurotransmitter depletion, metal cation accumulation and oxidative stress [3]. In light of the above, the multifaceted nature of AD has dictated strategies that are capable of modulating the multiple, distinct pathophysiological pathways associated with AD [4].

Amyloid-β peptides (Aβ) are produced through the sequential cleavage of the type 1 transmembrane protein, amyloid precursor protein (APP). APP is initially cleaved by the aspartyl protease, β-site amyloid precursor protein cleaving enzyme 1 (BACE1), the primary neuronal β-secretase [5], liberating a soluble N-terminal fragment (sAPPβ) and a membrane-bound C-terminal fragment (β-CTF or C99). The β-CTF/C99 fragment subsequently undergoes cleavage by γ-secretase within the transmembrane domain, releasing a 36–43 amino acid peptide (Aβ) into the extracellular space; the most predominant species of Aβ being Aβ40 [6,7]. An imbalance favouring the production of Aβ42 has been linked to the development of AD, owing to a higher propensity to oligomerize and form amyloid fibrils than the shorter Aβ40 [8].

As the rate-limiting step in Aβ production, BACE1 inhibition has emerged as a key drug target for the therapeutic intervention of the progression of AD in order to prevent the accumulation of toxic Aβ [9,10]. This is supported by the finding that BACE1-null transgenic mice models survive into adulthood with limited phenotypic abnormalities while exhibiting a reduction in brain Aβ levels [5,11–16]. Despite the therapeutic potential of BACE1 inhibition, the successful development of clinically approved pharmaceuticals has proven a challenge due to the large substrate-binding cleft of BACE1, and unfavourable in vivo pharmaceutical properties of potent peptide inhibitors, for example, oral bioavailability, half-life and blood–brain barrier (BBB) penetration [10,17].

Heparan sulphate (HS), and its highly-sulphated analogue heparin (Hp), are members of the glycosaminoglycan (GAG) family of linear, anionic polysaccharides. They share a repeating disaccharide backbone consisting of a uronic acid (D-glucuronic acid; GlcA or L-iduronic acid; IdoA) and D-glucosamine, which can be variably sulphated or N-acetylated. HS is synthesised attached to core protein-forming HS proteoglycans (HSPGs), which have been identified co-localized with BACE1 on cell surfaces in the Golgi complex and in endosomes [18]. HSPGs were reported to endogenously regulate BACE1 activity in vivo through either a direct interaction with BACE1 and/or by sequestration of the substrate APP [18]. The addition of exogenous HS or heparin was also shown to inhibit BACE1 activity in vitro and reduced the production of Aβ in cell culture [18–20]. Mouse models treated with low-molecular-weight heparin (LMWH) exhibit a reduction in Aβ burden [21] and display improved cognition [22], although the multifaceted modes of heparin interaction (including inflammation, apolipoprotein E, metal interactions, [23], Tau, Aβ and acetylcholinesterase) may present challenges when drawing definitive conclusions from in vivo mouse studies. That said, the ability of heparin to favourably modulate a multitude of potential AD-associated targets, beyond that of BACE-1 inhibition alone, would appear desirable. Furthermore, heparin oligosaccharides within the minimum size requirement for BACE1 inhibition [18,19] (<18-mers) possess the ability to cross the blood–brain barrier (BBB) [24] and can be made orally bioavailable depending on formulation and encapsulation methods [25]. Heparin analogues, therefore, hold therapeutic potential as a treatment against AD, which may also offer an advantage over small molecule and peptide inhibitors of BACE1.

Heparin has been utilized clinically as a pharmaceutical anticoagulant for over a century due to its ability to perturb the coagulation cascade, principally through interactions with antithrombin III via the pentasaccharide sequence [–4) α-D-GlcNS,6S (1–4) β-D-GlcA (1–4) α-D-GlcNS,3S,6S (1–4) α-L-IdoA2S (1–4) α-D-GlcNS,6S (1–]. The side effect of anticoagulation presents as an important consideration when determining the potential of a heparin-based pharmaceutical for the treatment of AD. It has been previously determined that the anticoagulation potential of heparin can be highly attenuated by chemical modifications, while retaining the favourable ability to inhibit BACE1 [18–20]. Polysaccharides in which the 6-O-sulphate had been chemically removed were reported to have attenuated BACE1 activity [18,19] although this correlates with an augmented rate of fibril formation [26].

Polysaccharides analogous to GAGs have been isolated from a number of marine invertebrate species that offer rich structural diversity and display highly attenuated anticoagulant activities compared to mammalian counterparts (for further detail, the reader is referred to the following reviews; [27,28]). The largely unexplored chemical diversity of marine-derived GAGs provides a vast reservoir for the discovery of novel bioactive compounds, some of which have been identified to exhibit antiviral [29,30], anti-parasitic [31,32], anti-inflammatory [33,34], anti-metastasis [35–37], anti-diabetic [38], anti-thrombotic [39] and neurite outgrowth-promoting activities [40]. Also, these compounds may be obtained from waste material, which makes their exploitation both economically and environmentally appealing. Here, a GAG extract isolated from the crab *Portunus pelagicus* has been found to possess attenuated anticoagulant activity while potently inhibiting the AD relevant β-secretase, BACE1, in vitro.

2. Results

2.1. Isolation and Characterisation of a Glycosaminoglycan Extract from the Crab Portunus Pelagicus

A glycosaminoglycan extract isolated from the crab *Portunus pelagicus* via proteolysis was fractionated by DEAE-Sephacel anion-exchange chromatography utilizing a stepwise sodium chloride gradient. The eluent at 1 M NaCl (fraction 5; designated *P. pelagicus* F5) was observed to have similar electrophoretic mobility in 1,3-diaminopropane buffer (pH 9.0) to mammalian HS/Hp, with no bands observed corresponding to monosulphated chondroitin sulphate (CSA/CSC), disulphated chondroitin sulphate (CSD) or dermatan sulphate (DS) (Figure 1).

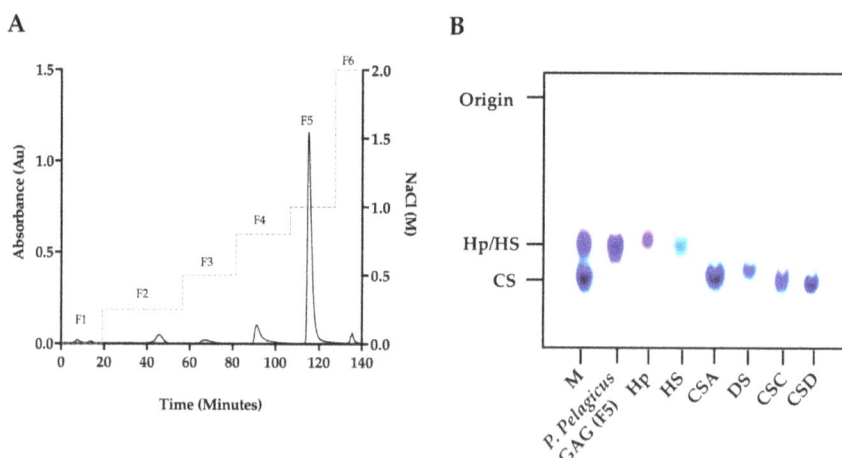

Figure 1. (**A**) DEAE purification of *P. pelagicus* crude glycosaminoglycan. Fractions 1–6 (F1–6; λ_{Abs} = 232 nm, solid line) were eluted using a stepwise NaCl gradient with HPAEC (dashed line). (**B**) Agarose gel electrophoresis of *P. pelagicus* F5. The electrophoretic mobility of *P. pelagicus* F5 was compared to that of bone fide glycosaminoglycan standards, heparin (Hp), heparan sulphate (HS), dermatan sulphate (DS) and chondroitin sulphate A, C and D (CSA, CSC and CSD, respectively). M: CSA, Hp and HS mixture.

In order to corroborate the Hp/HS like structural characteristics of *P. pelagicus* F5, the ATR-FTIR spectra has been compared with that of Hp. Both *P. pelagicus* F5 and Hp were shown to share similar spectral features, for instance bands at 1230, 1430 and 1635 cm^{-1}, which are associated with S=O stretches, symmetric carbonyl stretching and asymmetric stretches, respectively, indicative of common structural motifs. An additional peak and a peak shoulder located at ~1750 and ~1370 cm^{-1} were observed in *P. pelagicus* F5, but absent in Hp. The peak shoulder at ~1370 cm^{-1} is indicative of a Hp and CS mixture. The differences observed between the spectra of *P. pelagicus* F5 and Hp in the variable

OH region (>3000 cm^{-1}) are likely to be associated with changeable moisture levels present during sample acquisition (Figure 2A) as opposed to underlying differences within the glycan structure [41].

Post-acquisition, the ATR-FTIR spectrum of *P. pelagicus* F5 was interrogated against a library of known GAGs comprising: 185 Hps, 31 HSs, 44 CSs and DSs, 11 hyaluronic acids (HAs) and 6 oversulphated chondroitin sulphates (OSCSs) using principal component analysis (PCA; Figure 2B) [41]. Principal component 1 (PC1), which covers 57% of the total variance, indicates that *P. pelagicus* F5 locates within the region containing mammalian Hp/HS. Through comparison of PC1 and PC2, comprising >70% of the total variance, *P. pelagicus* F5 lies towards the CS region, a location previously identified with Hps containing small amounts of CS/DS [41] analogous to crude, pharmaceutical Hp.

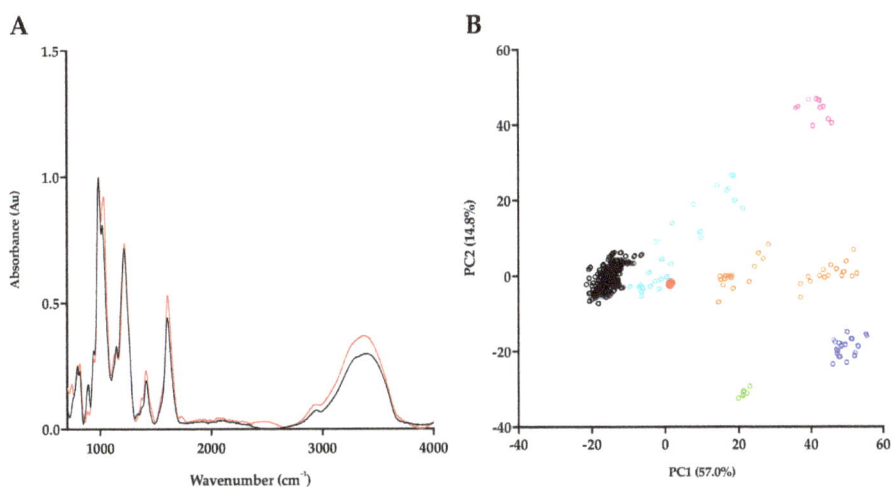

Figure 2. (**A**) ATR-FTIR spectra of porcine mucosal Hp (black) and *P. pelagicus* F5; (red), n = 5. (**B**) Principal component analysis (PCA) Score Plot for PC1 vs. PC2 of *P. pelagicus* F5 against a bone fide GAG library. Hp, black; HS, cyan; CS, orange; DS, blue; hyaluronic acid (HA), magenta; oversulphated-CS, light green and *P. pelagicus* F5, red (filled circle).

P. pelagicus F5 was subsequently subjected to exhaustive enzymatic cleavage with *Flavobacterium heparinum* lyases I, II and III. The digest products from Hp control (Figure 3, Table 1) and *P. pelagicus* F5 (Figure 4, Table 1), were analysed using strong anion-exchange chromatography and the retention times compared to those of the eight common Δ-disaccharide standards present within both Hp and HS [42].

The digest products detected for Hp were in agreement with a typical mammalian Hp disaccharide profile [42], with 51.5% of the total products attributable to the trisulphated Δ-UA(2S)-GlcNS(6S) and 22.9% to Δ-UA-GlcNS(6S). A minimal proportion of mono- or unsulphated disaccharides, accounting for 12.3 and 4.3%, respectively, were also observed for Hp. In comparison, a more disperse sulphation profile was observed for *P. pelagicus* F5 than Hp (Table 1), with a comparatively lower proportion of trisulphated disaccharides, 23.1%. The *P. pelagicus* F5 contained 24.4% monosulphated disaccharides, of which 16.5% was accounted for by Δ-UA(2S)-GlcNAc. A higher proportion of Δ-UA(2S)-GlcNS (23.5%) was also detected in *P. pelagicus* F5 than Hp (5.9%), indicating that the compound displays distinct structural characteristics. Such features also contrast with that of HS, where ~50–70% of disaccharides are comprised of Δ-UA-GlcNAc/Δ-UA-GlcNS [42–45]. Also, *P. pelagicus* F5 presents a significant higher proportion of trisulphated disaccharides than commonly present in mammalian HS, a typical marker of more heparin-like structures.

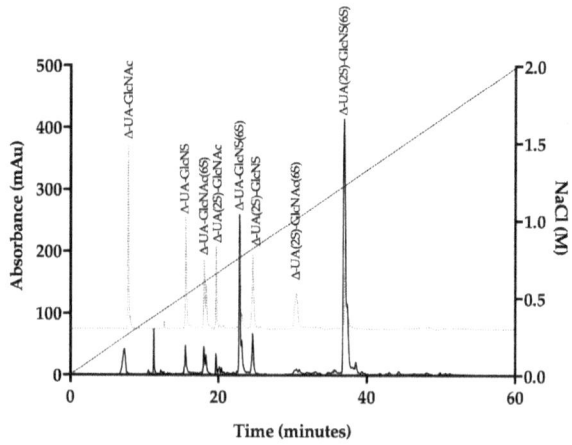

Figure 3. UV-SAX HPLC disaccharide composition analysis was performed on the bacterial lyase digest of Hp (λ_{Abs} = 232 nm) eluting with a linear gradient of 0–2 M NaCl (dashed line). Eluted Δ-disaccharides were referenced against the eight common standards present within Hp and HS (light grey, dotted line).

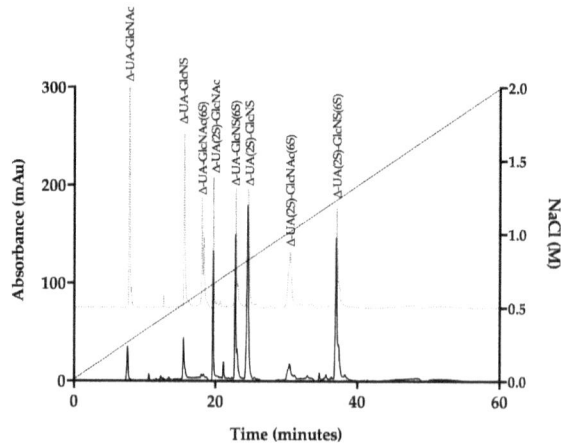

Figure 4. UV-SAX HPLC disaccharide composition analysis was performed on the bacterial lyase digest of the *P.pelagicus* F5 (λ_{Abs} = 232 nm), eluting with a linear gradient of 0–2 M NaCl (dashed line). Eluted Δ-disaccharides were referenced against the eight common standards present within Hp and HS (light grey, dotted line).

Table 1. Corrected disaccharide composition analysis of *P. pelagicus* F5 and Hp.

Δ-Disaccharide	*P. pelagicus* F5 (%)	Hp (%)
Δ-UA-GlcNAc	2.8	4.3
Δ-UA-GlcNS	5.6	4.2
Δ-UA-GlcNAc(6S)	2.3	5.0
Δ-UA(2S)-GlcNAc	16.5	3.1
Δ-UA-GlcNS(6S)	20.2	22.9
Δ-UA(2S)-GlcNS	23.5	5.9
Δ-UA(2S)-GlcNAc(6S)	6.0	3.1
Δ-UAs(2S)-GlcNS(6S)	23.1	51.5

Proton and Heteronuclear Single-Quantum Correlation (HSQC) NMR was employed to confirm the GAGs composition of *P. pelagicus* F5. ^{1}H NMR can indicate the major signals associated with HS as well as signals that arise from galactosaminoglycans such as CS. The presence of both (Figure 5A insert) is easily identified by the two N-acetyl signals at 2.02 ppm (CS) and 2.04 ppm (HS). ^{1}H–^{13}C HSQC NMR (Figure 5B) has been used to resolve overlapping signals and saccharide composition estimates using peak volume integration. The integration of N-acetyl signals revealed that the extract is composed of approximately 60% HS and 40% CS. The combined integration of the N-acetyl and A2 signals from the HS showed that *P. pelagicus* F5 possesses a high NS content of approximately 76%, which supports the HPLC-based empirical disaccharide analysis (Figure 4 and Table 1). Together, this data establishes that the HS of *P. pelagicus* F5 is considerably more sulphated (Table 1) than that commonly extracted from mammalian sources [45]. With regard to the CS element of *P. pelagicus* F5, signals typical of the CS backbone are present although sulhation is generally low, with galactosamine 6-O-sulphation occurring in approximately 35% of all CS residues. The lack of non-overlapping signals for galactosamine 4-O-sulphation indicates that all but negligible levels of such a modification are present within the CS component.

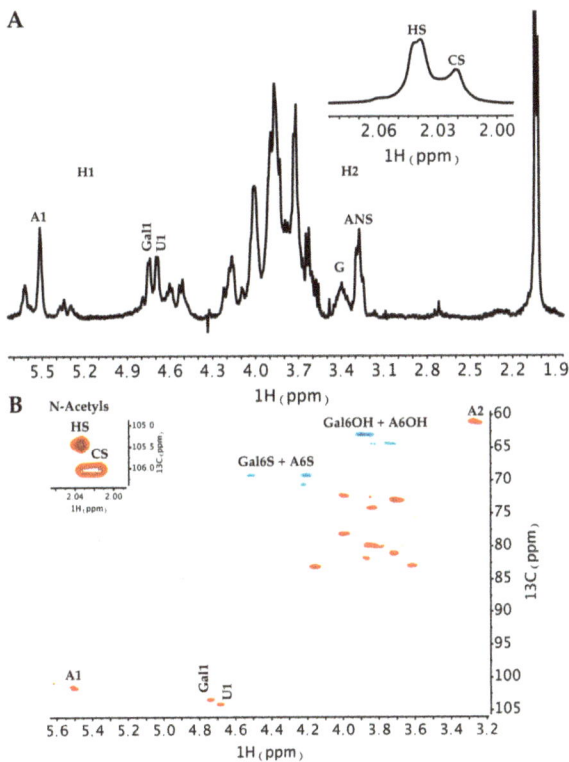

Figure 5. (**A**) ^{1}H and (**B**) ^{1}H-^{13}C HSQC NMR spectra of *P. pelagicus* F5. Major signals associated with HS and CS are indicated. Spectral integration was performed on the HSQC using labelled signals. Key: glucosamine, A; uronic acid, U; N-Acetyl, Nac and galactosamine, Gal.

2.2. *P. pelagicus F5 Inhibits the Alzheimer's Disease-Relevant β-Secretase 1*

P. pelagicus F5 was assayed for inhibitory potential against BACE1, utilizing a fluorogenic peptide cleavage FRET assay, based on the APP Swedish mutation. Reactions were performed at pH 4.0, within the optimal pH range for BACE1 activity (Figure 6). A maximal level of BACE1 inhibition of

90.7 ± 2.9% (n = 3) was observed in the presence of 5 µg mL^{-1} *P. pelagicus* F5, with an IC$_{50}$ value of 1.9 µg mL^{-1} (R^2 = 0.94). This was comparable to the activity of Hp, which exhibited a maximal level of BACE1 inhibition of 92.5 ± 1.5% (n = 3) at 5 µg mL^{-1}, with an IC$_{50}$ of 2.4 µg mL^{-1} (R^2 = 0.93).

In the presence of low concentrations of Hp, an increase in BACE1 activity was observed (Figure 6A,B), with maximal activation occurring at 625 ng mL^{-1} (57.5 ± 3.7%, n = 3). The BACE1 utilised in this study consisted of the zymogen form (Thr^{22}–Thr^{457}), containing the prodomain sequence. This is in accordance with previous reports that demonstrate low concentrations (~1 µg mL^{-1}) of heparin can stimulate proBACE1 activity [46,47]. A maximum increase in BACE1 activity was also detected in the presence of 625 ng mL^{-1} of *P. pelagicus* F5 (38.5 ± 1.4%, n = 3), although significantly diminished promotion was displayed compared to the same concentration of Hp (57.5 ± 3.7%, n = 3); t(4) = 4.859, *p* = 0.0083. This indicates that although *P. pelagicus* F5 exhibits stimulatory activity, it is significantly less than that of Hp. The percent activity level returned to that of the negative control value at concentrations lower than 312.5 ng mL^{-1}, indicating that both inhibitory and stimulatory effects are dose dependent. For both Hp and *P. pelagicus* F5, BACE1 promotion was followed by enzyme inhibition, as previously reported (Figure 6B,C; [47]). The rate of BACE1 activity between 60 and 90 min was significantly different from controls lacking either Hp (n = 3–6; t(4) = 7, *p* < 0.003) or *P. pelagicus* F5 (n = 3–6; t(6) = 7, *p* < 0.004) at 625 ng mL^{-1}, indicating that inhibition was not due to substrate limitations.

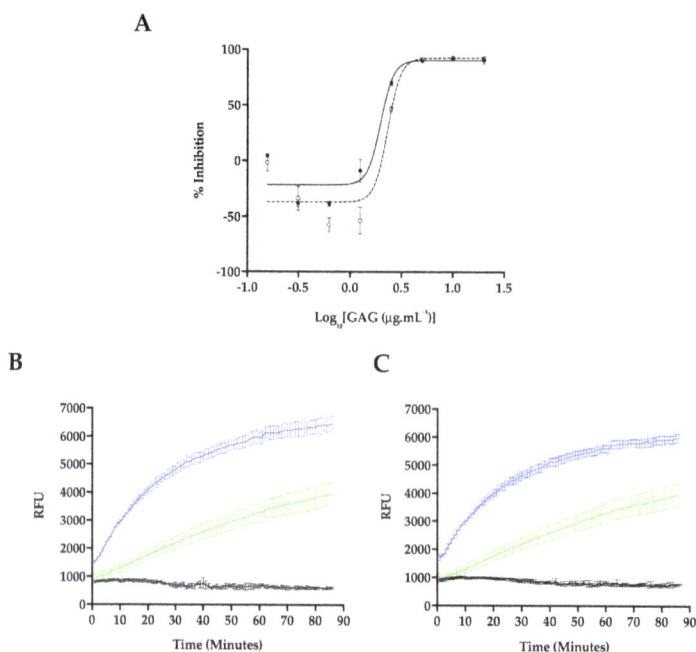

Figure 6. Inhibition of human BACE1 by Hp or *P. pelagicus* F5. (**A**) Dose response of Hp (dashed line, open circles) or *P. pelagicus* F5 (solid line, filled circles) as determined using FRET. *P. pelagicus* F5, IC$_{50}$ = 1.9 µg mL^{-1} (R^2 = 0.94); Hp, IC$_{50}$ = 2.4 µg mL^{-1} (R^2 = 0.93). (**B**) Time-course activation or inhibition of BACE1 by 5 µg mL^{-1} (black) or 625 ng mL^{-1} (blue) Hp, compared to water control (green). (**C**) The same as (**B**) for *P. pelagicus* F5.

2.3. Heparin Binding Induces a Conformational Change in the Alzheimer's Disease β-Secretase, BACE1

Hp binding has been proposed to occur at a location close to the active site of BACE1 [18], possibly within or adjacent to the prodomain sequence [46]. In light of the contrasting and concentration-dependant BACE1:GAG bioactivities, the ability of Hp and *P. pelagicus* F5 to induce structural changes in BACE1 has been investigated utilising circular dichroism (CD) spectroscopy at a range of *w/w* ratios; this also negates the intrinsic effect of the significant polydispersity for this class of biomolecules.

The CD spectra of BACE1 at pH 4.0 has previously been shown to contain a greater proportion of β-sheet and reduced α-helical content, compared to spectra obtained at pH 7.4, indicating that at an acidic pH, where BACE1 is most active, a conformational change can be observed by CD [50]. Consistent with this, the CD spectra of BACE1 in 50 mM sodium acetate buffer at pH 4.0 (Figures 7 and 8) featured a positive peak at wavelengths below 200 nm, which can be attributed to a sum of α-helical and β- sheet structures [51]. The broad, negative band observed between wavelengths 250 and 200 nm, contains a peak at λ = 218 nm ~ 208 nm, commonly associated with antiparallel β-sheets and α-helical structures, respectively [51] (Figures 7 and 8). The CD spectra of BACE1 at pH 4.0 can be estimated to have a secondary structural composition of 9% α-helix, 31% antiparallel β-sheet, 16% turn and 44% other (NRMSD < 0.1) when fitted against a library of representative proteins using BeStSel [48]. This was in close agreement with the BestSel secondary structure prediction based on x-ray crystallography of BACE1 at pH 4.0 (PDB accession no 2ZHS, [52] of 7% α-helix, 30% antiparallel, 4% parallel, 12% turn and 47% other). Deviations between secondary structure predictions may be accounted for by subtle differences present within the BACE1 primary sequences.

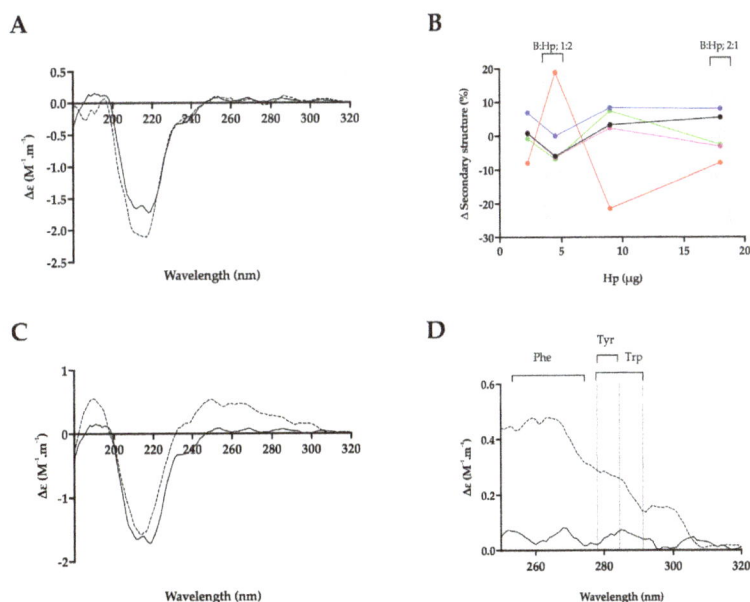

Figure 7. The structural change of BACE1 observed in the presence of Hp by circular dichroism (CD) spectroscopy. (**A**) CD spectra of BACE1 alone (solid line) or with Hp at a ratio of 1:2 (*w/w*; dashed line; B:Hp 1:2); (**B**) Δ secondary structure (%) of BACE1 upon the addition of increasing amounts of Hp; α-helix (black), antiparallel (red), parallel (blue), turn (magenta) and others (green) [48]. % structural change of B:Hp; 1:2 or 2:1 (*w/w*) ratio are highlighted in grey. (**C**) CD spectra of BACE1 alone (solid line) with Hp (dashed line) at a ratio of 2:1 *w/w* (**D**) Near-UV CD spectra of (**C**); respective absorption regions of aromatic amino acids are indicated [49]. Spectra were recorded in 50 mM sodium acetate buffer at pH 4.0 in all panels.

In the presence of a BACE1:Hp (B:Hp), ratio of 1:2 (*w/w*) where maximal inhibition was observed in FRET assays, the CD spectra of BACE1 exhibited increased negative ellipticity below λ = 222 nm, resulting in an estimated increase in α-helix (+6%) and a reduction in antiparallel β-sheet (−8%) (NRMSD < 0.1) [48] (Figure 7A,B). In comparison to Hp, BACE1 in the presence of *P. pelagicus* F5 (B:F5), at the same ratio (1:2; *w/w*), exhibited a slight increase in positive ellipticity between λ = 222–200 nm and decreases at λ < 200 nm, resulting in an estimated change in α-helical content of +1% accompanied by a decrease in antiparallel β-sheet content of 8% (Figure 8A,B). This is in contrast to CD studies in the presence of peptide inhibitors, which did not reveal a secondary structural change in BACE1 [50].

The conformational change of BACE1 upon binding to Hp and *P. pelagicus* F5 was assessed over a range of ratios (Figures 7B and 8B). At a B:Hp ratio of 2:1 (*w/w*), a change in the characteristics of the CD spectrum of BACE1 was observed in the far-UV region (λ < 250 nm; Figure 7C) that was identified as a reduction in α-helix by 6% and an increase in antiparallel β-sheet structures 19% (NRMSD < 0.1) [48]. In addition, an increase in positive ellipticity was observed in the near-UV region (250–300 nm; Figure 7C,D) following the addition of Hp, which may be attributed to a change in the tertiary structure of BACE1 involving aromatic amino acids [49,53]. In contrast, B:F5 at the same ratio of 2:1 (*w/w*), exhibited a decrease in ellipticity in the near- and far- UV region (λ < 300 nm; Figure S1).

The increase in positive ellipticity observed in the CD spectra of BACE1 in the near-UV region at a B:Hp ratio of 2:1 (*w/w*) was also observed at a 1:1 (*w/w*) ratio of B:F5 (Figure 8C,D). The secondary structural change in the far-UV CD spectrum of BACE1 at a B:F5 ratio of 1:1 (*w/w*) for λ= 250–190 nm corresponded to a decrease in α-helix by 8% and an increase in antiparallel β-sheet structures by 15%.

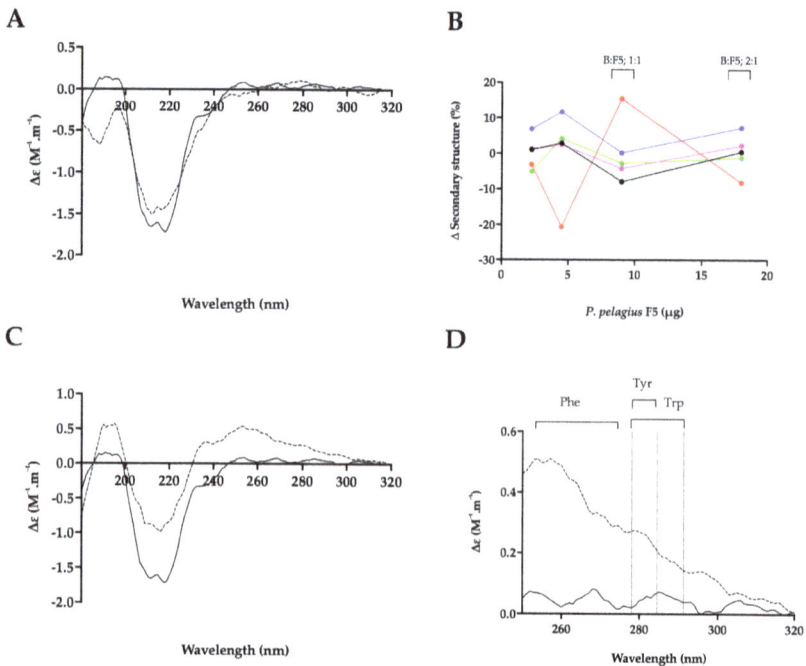

Figure 8. The structural change of BACE1 observed in the presence of *P. pelagicus* F5 by CD spectroscopy. (**A**) CD spectra of BACE1 alone (solid line) with *P. pelagicus* F5 (dashed line; ratio of 1:2 *w/w*; B:F5); (**B**) Δ secondary structure (%) of BACE1 upon the addition of increasing amounts of *P. pelagicus* F5; α-helix (black), antiparallel (red), parallel (blue), turn (magenta) and others (green) [48] % structural change of B:F5; 1:2 or 1:1 ratio are highlighted in grey. (**C**) CD spectra of BACE1 alone (solid line) or with *P. pelagicus* F5 (dashed line; ratio of 1:1 *w/w*); (**D**) Near-UV CD spectra of (**C**); respective absorption regions of aromatic amino acids are indicated [49]. Spectra were recorded in 50 mM sodium acetate buffer at pH 4.0 in all panels.

2.4. Heparin and P. pelagicus F5 Destabilise the Alzheimer's Disease β-Secretase, BACE1

Both Hp and *P. pelagicus* F5 were shown to induce a conformational change in BACE1, in contrast to previous CD studies in the presence of peptide inhibitors [50]. Therefore, to explore whether the binding of Hp or *P. pelagicus* F5 alters the stability of BACE1 in a mechanism similar to known inhibitors, differential scanning fluorimetry (DSF) was employed to monitor the change in thermal stability. Previously identified BACE1 inhibitors have been shown to stabilize BACE1, exemplified by an increase in T_M values obtained through DSF measurements [54]. In the presence of a BACE1:Hp or *P. pelagicus* F5 ratio of 1:2, a decrease in the T_M of BACE1 by 11 °C and 10 °C, respectively was observed (Figure 9A). The change in T_M of BACE1 induced by binding of either Hp or *P. pelagicus* F5 was not significantly different, (p = 0.1161 t= 2 df = 4). The destabilisation of BACE1 in the presence of both Hp and *P. pelagicus* F5 was found to be concentration dependent (Figure 9B).

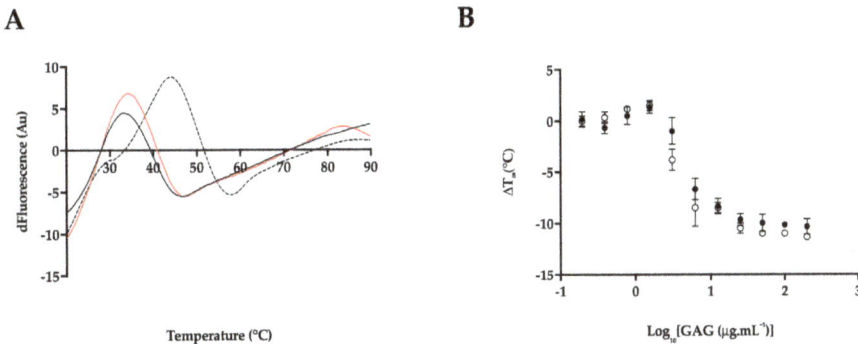

Figure 9. (**A**) First differential of the DSF thermal stability profile of BACE1 alone (1 µg; dashed line), and with Hp (2 µg; black line) or *P. pelagicus* F5 (2 µg; red line) in 50 mM sodium acetate, pH 4.0; (**B**) Δ T_m of BACE1 with increasing [Hp] or [*P. pelagicus* F5] (open or closed circles, respectively).

2.5. Attenuated Anticoagulant Activities of the P. pelagicus Glycosaminoglycan Extract

An important consideration when determining the therapeutic potential of a heparin-like polysaccharide against AD is the likely side effect of anticoagulation. The prothrombin time (PT) and activated partial thromboplastin time (aPTT) of *P. pelagicus* F5 were measured compared to Hp (193 IU mg^{-1}), to determine the overall effect on the extrinsic and intrinsic coagulation pathways, respectively (both assays also include the common coagulation pathway). In comparison to Hp, *P. pelagicus* F5 exhibited reduced anticoagulant activity in both the PT (Figure 10A; EC$_{50}$ of 420.2 µg mL^{-1} compared to 19.53 µg mL^{-1}, respectively) and aPTT (Figure 10B; EC$_{50}$ 43.21 µg mL^{-1} compared to 1.66 µg mL^{-1}, respectively) coagulation assays. Both results show that the extract presents a negligible anticoagulant activity.

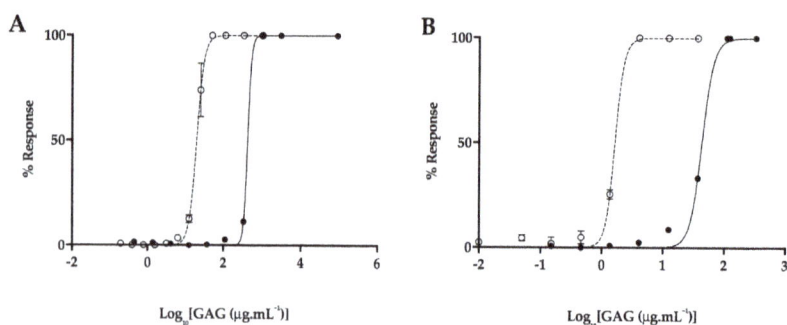

Figure 10. (**A**) Prothrombin time (PT) and (**B**) activated partial thromboplastin time (aPTT) inhibitory response ($\bar{x}$%, ± SD, n = 3) for Hp (open circle, dashed line) and *P. pelagicus* F5 (closed circle, solid line); PT: Hp EC_{50} = 19.53 µg mL^{-1}; *P. pelagicus* F5, EC_{50} = 420.2 µg mL^{-1}. aPTT: Hp EC_{50} = 1.66 µg mL^{-1}; *P. pelagicus* F5, EC_{50} = 43.21 µg mL^{-1}.

3. Discussion

The glycosaminoglycan extract isolated from *P. pelagicus* was observed to possess similar electrophoretic behaviour to mammalian HS and Hp, with no bands identified corresponding to CS or DS standards. In contrast, the FTIR and HSQC analyses of *P. pelagicus* F5 identified regions corresponding to both HS and CS saccharides within the extract. PCA analysis of the FTIR spectra revealed *P. pelagicus* F5 contained features associated with both HS/Hp and CS/DS, which are typical of crude heparin preparations [41]. This was confirmed by HSQC NMR, which identified N-acetyl peaks associated with both galactosamine (CS) and glucosamine (HS). The absence of an IdoA signal from the NMR spectra suggests that *P. pelagicus* F5 resembles HS and CS more closely than DS/Hep [55,56]. Peaks corresponding to Gal-6S and 6-OH were identified by NMR analysis, with no detectable 4-O-sulphation, indicating that the CS component of *P. pelagicus* F5 resembles CSC saccharides. The HS component possesses >70% N-sulphated moieties, which is greater than mammalian HSs published previously, but is not as heavily N-sulphated as mammalian heparins. An intermediate proportion of trisulphated Δ-disaccharides were also identified post-bacterial lyase digestion in *P. pelagicus* F5 when compared to mammalian HS and Hp samples. Furthermore, the *P. pelagicus* F5 extract contained a low proportion of Δ-UA-GlcNAc/Δ-UA-GlcNS, which is typical of more heparin-like structures. This suggests that the HS/Hp component of *P. pelagicus* F5 consists of a hybrid structure lacking the domain structure of HS and the highly-sulphated regions of Hp.

The absence of a band migrating in a similar manner to that of CS when *P. pelagicus* F5 was subjected to agarose gel electrophoresis suggests that the polysaccharide is not a mixture of HS and CS chains. The simplicity of the signals in the HSQC spectrum suggests either two separate populations or two distinct domains, while the former is not consistent with the agarose gel electropherogram mentioned previously. The PCA of the FTIR spectra is also in agreement with the presence of discrete, rather than mixed, HS/CS sequences. The precise nature of the arrangement of these stretches remains unknown, although it is well documented that marine-derived GAGs harbour significant and unusual structural features, when compared to those present within their mammalian counterparts [33,43,57–66]. Studies to resolve this technically demanding question are currently in progress.

The *P. pelagicus* F5 extract was found to possess significant inhibitory potential against human BACE1, in a manner akin to that of mammalian Hp, as demonstrated by comparable IC_{50} concentrations determined via FRET. The ability of *P. pelagicus* F5 to promote BACE1 bioactivity at lower concentrations, owing to the presence of the BACE1 pro-domain [46,47], appears to be at a diminished level compared to mammalian Hp, suggesting differences between these GAGs and the nature of their interactions with human BACE1. This was exemplified when the secondary structural changes in BACE1 (evident from CD) in the presence of Hp or *P. pelagicus* F5 were examined.

BACE1 has previously been observed to adopt a unique secondary structure at pH 4.0, where catalytic activity is increased, resulting in a predicted increase in beta-sheet and a reduction in alpha-helical structures [50]. When the changes in the secondary structure (evident from CD) of BACE1 in the presence of high concentrations of Hp (BACE1:Hp ratio of 1:2) was examined, a shift towards the structural features observed for BACE1 alone at pH 7.4 was observed (increase in alpha-helical and reduction in beta sheet structures). At high concentrations (B:F5 ratio of 1:2), the *P. pelagicus* F5 extract induced similar, but not identical, changes to the secondary structure of human BACE1, when compared to those of Hp at the same ratio.

In contrast, the CD spectra observed for B:Hp complexes under conditions that facilitate BACE1 promotion (i.e., low Hp concentrations) demonstrated evidence of an interaction that involves the aromatic amino acids (near UV CD). Tyr-71 is located within the BACE1 flap that has previously been identified to change conformation between the flap-open and flap-closed states [67]. Unfortunately, due to the location of the aromatic residues on the surface of the protein, it is not possible to conclude definitely whether interaction(s) of Hp-based inhibitors with human BACE1 occur at, or near to, the active site. This interpretation is consistent with the previous reports that a conformational change in BACE1 may occur upon heparin binding, which would be required to allow access into the active site [46]. In addition, the increase in BACE1 activity by heparin has been shown to be followed by BACE1 inhibition [47], which may suggest this arrangement is required to allow access to the active site. The results also support the work by Scholefield et al. [18] who showed that the mode of Hp inhibition is non-competitive, and can prevent access of the substrate.

At lower GAG concentrations, differences in BACE1 secondary structure were observed between the B:Hp and B:F5 complexes in the CD spectra, although a similar change in the near UV CD spectra of BACE1 was observed with increased amounts of *P. pelagicus* F5. This may be accounted for by the reduced potency of *P. pelagicus* F5 with regard to activating BACE1, or indicative of an alternative interaction. The conformational change induced in the near-UV CD spectra of BACE1 is solely the result of the HS/Hp-like component of the *P. pelagicus* F5 extract. CS has previously been shown to possess diminished BACE1 promotion activity compared to Hp/HS [46].

From a mechanistic standpoint, the decrease in the T_ms observed using DSF for both the human BACE1 protein in the presence of either Hp or the *P. pelagicus* F5 extract, when compared to human BACE1 alone, suggests that the mode of BACE1 inhibition by this class of carbohydrates could both involve structural destabilisation. The Hp-induced thermal instability of human BACE1 occurs in a concentration dependent manner, akin to that of the inhibitory potential of Hp in the FRET-based bioactivity assay. As for the FRET-based, BACE1 inhibition assays, *P. pelagicus* [F5] also induces comparable destabilisation of BACE1 with similar T_m values. A graph of BACE1:GAG T_m vs. concentration demonstrates similar profiles for the *P. pelagicus* GAG extract and that of mammalian Hp. The relationship between Hp and *P. pelagicus* F5 concentration and biological properties that coexists for both FRET-based, BACE1 inhibition and DSF is not mirrored at defined concentrations of Hp and *P. pelagicus* F5 with regard to their distinct CD spectra and predicted secondary structure. This would suggest that complex and distinct modes of interactions are present.

One of the major obstacles that precludes the use of mammalian Hp compounds as potential BACE1 inhibitors and pharmaceutical candidates in general is that of the significant anticoagulant potential residual within the biomolecule. This anticoagulant potential is afforded by the propensity of Hp to interact with antithrombin and thereby inhibit the human coagulation pathway, which unperturbed, ultimately results in fibrin clot formation. The anticoagulant potential of *P. pelagicus* F5 has been shown to be highly attenuated in contrast to mammalian Hp, as measured by both the aPTT and PT clotting assays. These coagulation assays are routinely employed, in clinical settings, to screen for the common pathway in combination with either the intrinsic (aPTT) or extrinsic pathways (PT).

4. Materials and Methods

4.1. Extraction of Glycosaminoglycans from Portunus pelagicus

A total of 2.4 kg *Portunus pelagicus* tissue (Yeuh Chyang Canned Food Co., Ltd., Nhut Chanh, Vietnam) was homogenised with excess acetone (VWR, UK) and agitated for 24 h at r.t. Defatted *P. pelagicus* tissue was recovered via centrifugation, 5670 rcf at r.t. for 10 min, and allowed to air dry. The tissue was then subjected to extensive proteolytic digestion (Alcalase®; Novozymes, Bagsværd, Denmark) using 16.8 U kg^{-1} dried tissue mass, in PBS (*w/v*; Gibco, Loughborough, UK) made up to a final concentration of 1 M NaCl (Fisher Scientific, UK), pH 8.0, and incubated at 60 °C for 24 h. Post-digestion, the supernatant was collected via centrifugation (5670× *g* for 10 min, r.t.), and subjected to ion exchange chromatography employing Amberlite IRA-900 resin (Sigma-Aldrich, Dorset, UK; hydroxide counterion form) for 24 h under constant agitation at r.t. Ion exchange resin was recovered by filtration and washed successively with distilled H$_2$O (Fisher Scientific, Loughborough, UK) at 60 °C with two volumes of water and 10 volumes of 1 M NaCl at r.t. The ion exchange resin was then re-suspended in 1 L 3 M NaCl and agitated for 24 h at r.t. The ion exchange resin was removed and the filtrate was added to ice cold methanol (VWR, Lutterworth, UK), 1:1 (*v/v*), prior to incubation for 48 h at 4 °C. The precipitate formed was recovered by centrifugation at 4 °C, 15,400× *g* for 1 h and re-suspended in distilled H$_2$O. The crude *P. pelagicus* extract was dialysed against distilled H$_2$O (3.5 kDa MWCO membrane; Biodesign, Carmel, NY, USA) for 48 h prior to syringe filtration (0.2 μm) and lyophilisation. The crude GAG extract was re-suspended in 1 mL HPLC-grade H$_2$O and loaded onto a pre-packed DEAE-Sephacel column (10 mm I.D. × 10 cm; GE Healthcare, Buckinghamshire, UK) at a flow rate of 1 mL min^{-1}. The column was eluted using a stepwise NaCl gradient of 0, 0.25, 0.5, 0.8, 1 and 2 M NaCl at a flow rate of 1 mL min^{-1}, with elution monitored in-line at λ_{abs} = 232 nm (using a UV/Vis, binary gradient HPLC system; Cecil Instruments, Cambridge, UK), resulting in six fractions (F1–F6, respectively). Each of the eluted fractions was dialysed against distilled H$_2$O, employing a 3.5-kDa MWCO (Biodesign, Carmel, NY, USA) for 48 h under constant agitation. The retentate obtained for F5 was lyophilised and stored at 4 °C prior to use.

4.2. Agarose Gel Electrophoresis

Agarose gel electrophoresis was performed in 0.55% (*w/v*) agarose gels (8 × 8 cm, 1.5 mm thick) prepared in 1,3-diaminopropane-acetate buffer at pH 9.0 (VWR, Lutterworth, UK), 2–7.5 μg *P. pelagicus* F5 or GAG standards were subjected to electrophoresis utilizing a X-Cell SureLock™ Mini-Cell Electrophoresis System (ThermoFisher, Altrincham, UK). Electrophoresis was performed in 0.5 M 1,3-diaminopropane-acetate buffer (pH 9.0), at a constant voltage of 150 V (~100 mA) for ~30 min or until the dye front had migrated ~8 cm from the origin. The gels were then precipitated with 0.1% *w/v* cetyltrimethylammonium bromide solution (VWR, Lutterworth, UK) for a minimum of 4 h and then stained for 1 h in 0.1% toluidine blue dissolved in acetic acid:ethanol:water (0.1:5:5). Gels were de-stained in acetic acid:ethanol:water (0.1:5:5 *v/v*) for ~30 min prior to image acquisition with GIMP software (v2.8, Berkeley, CA, USA) and processing with ImageJ (v1.51(100), Madison, WI, USA).

4.3. Attenuated FTIR Spectral Analysis of Marine-Derived Glycosaminoglycans

Samples (10 mg, lyophilised) were recorded using a Bruker Alpha I spectrometer in the region of 4000 to 400 cm^{-1} for 32 scans at a resolution of 2 cm^{-1} (approx 70 seconds acquisition time), 5 times. Spectral acquisition was carried out using OPUS software (v8.1, Bruker, Coventry, UK) with correction to remove the residual spectrum of the sampling environment.

Spectral processing and subsequent data analyses were performed using an Asus Vivobook Pro (M580VD-EB76, Taipei, Taiwan) equipped with an intel core i7-7700HQ. Spectra were smoothed, employing a Savitzky–Golay smoothing algorithm (R studio v1.1.463; *signal* package, *sgolayfilter*), to a 2nd-degree polynomial with 21 neighbours prior to baseline correction employing a 7th-order polynomial and subsequent normalisation (0–1). CO$_2$ and H$_2$O regions were removed prior to further analysis in order to negate environmental variability (<700 cm^{-1}, between 2000 and 2500 cm^{-1} and >3600 cm^{-1}). Second derivatives plots were calculated using the Savitzky–Golay algorithm, with 41 neighbours and a 2nd-order polynomial.

The normalised and corrected matrix of intensities was subject to PCA using singular value decomposition in R studio (v1.1.463, Boston, MA, USA) with the mean-centred, *base prcomp* function deployed.

4.4. Nuclear Magnetic Resonance (NMR)

NMR experiments were performed upon *P. pelagicus* F5 (5 mg) dissolved in D$_2$O (600 µL; VWR, São Paulo, Brazil) containing TMSP (0.003% *v/v*; VWR, Brazil) at 343 K using a 500-MHz Avance Neo spectrometer fitted with a 5-mm TXI Probe (Bruker, São Paulo, Brazil)). In addition to 1-dimensional (^{1}H) spectra, ^{1}H–^{13}C Heteronuclear Single-Quantum Correlation (HSQC) 2-dimensional spectra were collected using standard pulse sequences available. Spectra were processed and integrated using TopSpin (Bruker, São Paulo, Brazil)

4.5. Constituent Δ-Disaccharide Analysis of Hp/HS-Like, Marine-Derived Carbohydrates

Pharmaceutical (API) grade, porcine intestinal mucosal heparin (193 IU mg^{-1}; Celsus, Cincinnati, OH, USA) and *P. pelagicus* F5 carbohydrate samples were re-suspended in lyase digestion buffer (50 µL; 25 mM sodium acetate, 5 mM calcium acetate (VWR, Lutterworth, UK), pH 7) prior to exhaustive digestion by the sequential addition of a cocktail of the three recombinantly expressed heparinase enzymes (I, III and II) from the soil bacterium *Flavobacterium heparinum* (2.5 mIU mg^{-1}; Iduron, Alderley Edge, UK). Samples were incubated for 4 h at 37 °C prior to a further addition of the same quantity of enzymes and an additional overnight incubation. Samples were then heated briefly at 95 °C post-enzyme digestion (5 min) and allowed to cool.

Denatured heparinase enzymes were removed from the sample solution by immobilisation upon a pre-washed (50% methanol (aq.) followed by HPLC-grade H$_2$O) C^{18} spin column (Pierce, Altrincham, UK), whereby the newly liberated Δ-disaccharides were present in the column eluate upon washing with HPLC-grade H$_2$O.

Lyophilised Δ-disaccharide samples from Hp and *P. pelagicus* F5 were desalinated by immobilisation up on graphite spin columns (Pierce, Altrincham, UK) that had been extensively prewashed with 80% acetonitrile, 0.5% (aq.) trifluoroacetic acid and HPLC-grade H$_2$O prior to use. Δ-disaccharides liberated from the exhaustive, heparinase digestion were separated from buffer salts by extensive washing with HPLC-grade H$_2$O prior to elution with a solution of 40% acetonitrile, 0.5% trifluoroacetic acid (aq.). Contaminant, non Δ-disaccharide components of the spin column eluate were removed by serial lyophilization prior to chromatographic separation, using high performance anion exchange chromatography (HPAEC).

Heparinase digested samples (50 µg) were made up in HPLC-grade H$_2$O (1 mL) immediately before injection onto a ProPac PA-1 analytical column (4 × 250 mm, ThermoFisher Scientific, Altrincham, UK), and pre-equilibrated in HPLC-grade H$_2$O at a flow rate of 1 mL min^{-1}. The column was held under isocratic flow for 10 min prior to developing a linear gradient from 0 to 2 M NaCl (HPLC grade; VWR, UK) over 60 min. Eluted Δ-disaccharides were detected absorbing within the UV range λ_{abs} = 232 nm via the unsaturated C=C bond, present between C$_4$ and C$_5$ of the uronic acid residues, introduced as a consequence of lyase digestion.

Authentic Δ-disaccharide reference standards, comprising the 8 common standards found in Hp and HS (Iduron, Alderley Edge, UK), were employed as a mixture (each at 5 µg mL^{-1}) and served as chromatographic references with elution times cross-correlated with Hp and *P. pelagicus* F5 samples. The column was washed extensively with 2 M NaCl and HPLC-grade H$_2$O prior to use and between runs.

4.6. Determination of Human BACE1 Inhibitory Activity Using Förster Resonance Energy Transfer

P. pelagicus F5 and Hp were assayed for inhibitory potential against human β-secretase, tag free (BACE1; ACRO Biosystems, Cambridge, MA, USA), using the fluorescence resonance energy transfer (FRET) inhibition assay, essentially as described by Patey et al. (2006) [19]. Human BACE1 (312.5 ng), and *P. pelagicus* F5 or Hp were incubated in 50 mM sodium acetate at pH 4.0 at 37 °C for 10 min, followed by the addition a quenched fluorogenic peptide substrate (6.25 µM; Biomatik, Cambridge, Ontario, Canada; MCA-SEVNLDAEFRK(DNP)RR-NH$_2$; pre-incubated at 37 °C for 10 min) to a final well volume of 50 µL. Fluorescent emission was recorded using a Tecan Infinite® M200 Pro multi-well plate reader (Tecan Group Ltd., Männedorf, Switzerland) with i-control™ software (λ_{ex} = 320 nm, λ_{em} = 405 nm) over 90 min. The relative change in fluorescence per minute was calculated in the linear range of the no inhibitor control, with normalized percentage inhibition calculated (% ± SD, n = 3) compared to the $\bar{x}$ of substrate only and no inhibitor control, followed by fitting to a four-parameter logistics model using Prism 7 (GraphPad Software, San Diego, CA, USA).

4.7. Secondary Structure Determination of Human BACE1 by Circular Dichroism Spectroscopy

The circular dichroism (CD) spectra of native, human BACE1 (6.12 µM, 30 µL; Acro Biosystems, USA) in 50 mM sodium acetate (pH 4.0; VWR, Lutterworth, UK) was obtained using a J-1500 Jasco CD spectrometer and Spectral Manager II software, equipped with a 0.2-mm path length quartz cuvette (Hellma, Plainview, NY, USA) operating at a scan speed of 100 nm min^{-1} with 1-nm resolution over the range λ = 190–320 nm. Spectra obtained were the mean of five independent scans. Human BACE1 was buffer exchanged (in order to remove commercially supplied buffer) prior to spectral analysis using a 10-kDa Vivaspin centrifugal filter (Sartorius, Goettingen, Germany) at 12,000× *g* washed thrice. Collected data was processed using Spectral Manager II software and data analysis was carried out with GraphPad Prism 7, employing a 2nd-order polynomial smoothed to 9 neighbours. Secondary structure prediction was performed utilizing the BeStSel analysis server on the unsmoothed data [48]. To ensure the CD spectral change of BACE1 in the presence of each GAG was not altered owing to the addition of the GAG alone, which are known to possess CD spectra at high concentrations [68,69] GAG control spectra were subtracted before analysis. In addition, the theoretical, summative CD spectra was confirmed to differ from the observed experimental CD spectra, thereby indicating that the change in the CD spectra compared to that of BACE1 alone is a result of a conformational change upon binding to the GAG. The conformational change observed is believed to occur as a result of changes solely in BACE1 secondary structure, as GAG controls exhibited negligible spectra at the concentration used. All CD data has been presented with GAG controls subtracted.

4.8. Investigating the Thermal Stability of Human BACE1 with Differential Scanning Fluorimetry

Differential scanning fluorimetry (DSF) was carried out using the method of Uniewicz et al. (2010) [70] based on a modification to the original method of Niesen et al. (2007) [71]. DSF was performed on human BACE1 (1 µg) using 96-well qPCR plates (AB Biosystems, Warrington, UK) with 20X Sypro Orange (Invitrogen, Warrington, UK) in 50 mM sodium acetate, pH 4.0, in a final well volume of 40 µl. Hp or mGAG were included, as necessary, to a maximal concentration of 200 µg mL^{-1}. An AB Biosystems StepOne plus qPCR machine, with the TAMRA filter set deployed, was used to carry out melt curve experiments, with an initial incubation phase of 2 min at 20 °C increasing by 0.5 °C increments every 30 s up to a final temperature of 90 °C. Data analysis was completed using Prism 7 (GraphPad Software, San Diego, CA, USA) with the first derivative plots smoothed to 19 neighbours, using a 2nd-order polynomial (Savitzky-Golay). The peak of the first derivatives (yielding T_ms) was determined using MatLab software (R20018a, MathWorks, Cambridge, UK).

4.9. Activated Partial Thromboplastin Time (aPTT)

Serially diluted GAG samples (25 µL) were incubated with pooled, normal human citrated plasma (50 µL; Technoclone, Surrey, UK) and Pathromtin SL reagent (50 µL; Siemens, Erlangen, Germany) for 2 mins at 37 °C prior to the addition of calcium chloride (25 µL, 50 mM; Alfa Aesar, Heysham, UK). The time taken for clot formations to occur (an upper maximal of 2 mins was imposed, represented as 100% inhibition of clotting) was recorded using a Thrombotrak Solo coagulometer (Axis-Shield). HPLC-grade H_2O (0% inhibition of clotting, representing a normal aPTT clotting time, of $\approx$ 37–40 seconds) and porcine mucosal heparin (193 IU mg^{-1}; Celsus, Cincinnati, OH, USA) were screened as controls. The EC_{50} values of all test and control samples were determined using a sigmoidal dose response curve fitted with Prism 7 (GraphPad Software, San Diego, CA, USA).

4.10. Prothrombin Time (PT)

Serially diluted GAGs (50 µL) or control (H_2O, HPLC grade) were incubated with pooled, normal human citrated plasma (50 µL) for 1 minute at 37 °C prior to the addition of Thromborel S reagent (50 µL; Siemens, Erlangen, Germany). The time taken for clot formations to occur (an upper maximal of 2 min was imposed, representing 100% inhibition of clotting) was recorded using a Thrombotrak Solo coagulometer. HPLC-grade H_2O (0% inhibition of clotting, representing a normal PT clotting time of $\approx$ 13–14 s) and porcine mucosal heparin (193 IU mg^{-1}; Celsus, Cincinnati, OH, USA) were screened as controls. The EC_{50} values of all test and control samples were determined using a sigmoidal dose response curve fitted with Prism 7 (GraphPad Software, San Diego, CA, USA).

5. Conclusions

While the search for effective AD treatments is still on-going, GAGs offer a route to BACE1 inhibition that surmounts the challenge presented by the large substrate-binding cleft of the enzyme and the unfavourable pharmokinetics of peptide-based inhibitors. Heparin, a GAG from mammalian sources (usually porcine or bovine intestinal tissue), has long been known to possess potent BACE1 inhibitory activity [18–20] but also exhibits undesirable anticoagulant properties. The *P. pelagicus* GAG of the present study largely circumvents the anticoagulant limitations of mammalian heparins while maintaining comparable, low IC_{50} BACE1 inhibition values. Additional advantages with marine-derived GAGs is that they offer sources, derived from waste material of otherwise very low economic value, that are free from contamination with mammalian pathogens (e.g., BSE) and avoid many of the religious and social issues associated with mammalian products [72]. Interestingly, the mechanism by which the present product from *P. pelagicus* inhibits BACE1 is complex, concentration dependent and appears to be distinct from that of mammalian heparin, suggesting marine GAGs as a potential starting point for future drug development. Furthermore, as heparin has been shown to positively modulate distinct pathophysiological processes associated with AD [23], this class of molecules may hold the potential for the delivery of a multi-target AD therapeutic. The present contribution highlights the potential offered by the largely unexplored chemical space defined by marine-derived GAGs.

Supplementary Materials: The following are available online at http://www.mdpi.com/1660-3397/17/5/293/s1, Figure S1: The CD structural change of BACE1 observed in the presence of *P. pelagicus* F5 with a ratio of 2:1 *w/w*.

Author Contributions: M.S., C.M.-W., L.C., S.G. and E.Y. designed and conceived the project. C.M.-W. performed all experimentation with the technical assistance of L.C., P.P., S.G. and D.F. A.D. performed FTIR and carried out principal component analysis on data sets and M.L. and M.G. performed and analysed the NMR data. M.S., C.M.-W., L.C., S.G. and E.Y. wrote the manuscript and all authors contributed to the final version of the manuscript.

Funding: The authors would like to thank the Engineering and Physical Sciences Research Council, UK (M.S.), the Biotechnology and Biological Sciences Research Council, UK (M.S. and E.Y.), the Medical Research Council, UK (M.S., L.C. and E.Y.), Intellihep Ltd., UK (C.M.-W. and M.S.), MI Engineering Ltd., UK (A.D. and M.S.) and Financiadora de Estudos e Projetos (FINEP) (M.L.) for financial support.

Acknowledgments: The authors would like to thank Sarah Taylor for technical assistance with the use of CD instrumentation.

Conflicts of Interest: The funders had no role in the study design, data collection and interpretation, or the decision to submit the work for publication.

References

1. Lane, C.; Hardy, J.; Schott, J.M. Alzheimer's disease. *Eur. J. Neurol.* **2017**, *25*, 59–70. [CrossRef]
2. Cruts, M.; Theuns, J.; Van Broeckhoven, C. Locus-specific mutation databases for neurodegenerative brain diseases. *Hum. Mutat.* **2012**, *33*, 1340–1344. [CrossRef] [PubMed]
3. Carreiras, M.; Mendes, E.; Perry, M.; Francisco, A.; Marco-Contelles, J. The Multifactorial Nature of Alzheimer's Disease for Developing Potential Therapeutics. *Curr. Top. Med. Chem.* **2014**, *13*, 1745–1770. [CrossRef]
4. Ibrahim, M.M.; Gabr, M.T. Multitarget therapeutic strategies for Alzheimer's disease. *Neural Regen. Res.* **2019**, *14*, 437–440.
5. Cai, H.; Wang, Y.; McCarthy, D.; Wen, H.; Borchelt, D.R.; Price, D.L.; Wong, P.C. BACE1 is the major β-secretase for generation of Aβ peptides by neurons. *Nat. Neurosci.* **2001**, *4*, 233–234. [CrossRef] [PubMed]
6. Querfurth, H.W.; LaFerla, F.M. Alzheimer's Disease. *N. Engl. J. Med.* **2010**, *362*, 329–344. [CrossRef]
7. Lichtenthaler, S.F.; Haass, C.; Steiner, H. Regulated intramembrane proteolysis—Lessons from amyloid precursor protein processing. *J. Neurochem.* **2011**, *117*, 779–796. [CrossRef] [PubMed]
8. Walsh, D.M.; Selkoe, D.J. Aβ Oligomers—A decade of discovery. *J. Neurochem.* **2007**, *101*, 1172–1184. [CrossRef]
9. Thinakaran, G.; Koo, E.H. Amyloid precursor protein trafficking, processing, and function. *J. Biol. Chem.* **2008**, *283*, 29615–29619. [CrossRef] [PubMed]
10. Vassar, R. BACE1 inhibition as a therapeutic strategy for Alzheimer's disease. *J. Sport Health Sci.* **2016**, *5*, 388–390. [CrossRef] [PubMed]
11. Roberds, S.L.; Anderson, J.; Basi, G.; Bienkowski, M.J.; Branstetter, D.G.; Chen, K.S.; Freedman, S.B.; Frigon, N.L.; Games, D.; Hu, K.; et al. BACE knockout mice are healthy despite lacking the primary beta-secretase activity in brain: Implications for Alzheimer's disease therapeutics. *Hum. Mol. Genet.* **2001**, *10*, 1317–1324. [CrossRef]
12. Luo, Y.; Bolon, B.; Kahn, S.; Bennett, B.D.; Babu-Khan, S.; Denis, P.; Fan, W.; Kha, H.; Zhang, J.; Gong, Y.; et al. Mice deficient in BACE1, the Alzheimer's β-secretase, have normal phenotype and abolished β-amyloid generation. *Nat. Neurosci.* **2001**, *4*, 231–232. [CrossRef] [PubMed]
13. Dominguez, D.; Tournoy, J.; Hartmann, D.; Huth, T.; Cryns, K.; Deforce, S.; Serneels, L.; Camacho, I.E.; Marjaux, E.; Craessaerts, K.; et al. Phenotypic and Biochemical Analyses of BACE1- and BACE2-deficient Mice. *J. Biol. Chem.* **2005**, *280*, 30797–30806. [CrossRef]
14. Ohno, M.; Sametsky, E.A.; Younkin, L.H.; Oakley, H.; Younkin, S.G.; Citron, M.; Vassar, R.; Disterhoft, J.F. BACE1 deficiency rescues memory deficits and cholinergic dysfunction in a mouse model of Alzheimer's disease. *Neuron* **2004**, *41*, 27–33. [CrossRef]
15. Ohno, M.; Cole, S.L.; Yasvoina, M.; Zhao, J.; Citron, M.; Berry, R.; Disterhoft, J.F.; Vassar, R. BACE1 gene deletion prevents neuron loss and memory deficits in 5XFAD APP/PS1 transgenic mice. *Neurobiol. Dis.* **2007**, *26*, 134–145. [CrossRef] [PubMed]
16. McConlogue, L.; Buttini, M.; Anderson, J.P.; Brigham, E.F.; Chen, K.S.; Freedman, S.B.; Games, D.; Johnson-Wood, K.; Lee, M.; Zeller, M.; et al. Partial Reduction of BACE1 Has Dramatic Effects on Alzheimer Plaque and Synaptic Pathology in APP Transgenic Mice. *J. Biol. Chem.* **2007**, *282*, 26326–26334. [CrossRef] [PubMed]
17. Vassar, R. BACE1 inhibitor drugs in clinical trials for Alzheimer's disease. *Alzheimer's Res. Ther.* **2014**, *6*, 89. [CrossRef] [PubMed]
18. Scholefield, Z.; Yates, E.A.; Wayne, G.; Amour, A.; McDowell, W.; Turnbull, J.E. Heparan sulfate regulates amyloid precursor protein processing by BACE1, the Alzheimer's beta-secretase. *J. Cell Biol.* **2003**, *163*, 97–107. [CrossRef] [PubMed]

19. Patey, S.J.; Edwards, E.A.; Yates, E.A.; Turnbull, J.E. Heparin derivatives as inhibitors of BACE-1, the Alzheimer's β-secretase, with reduced activity against factor Xa and other proteases. *J. Med. Chem.* **2006**, *49*, 6129–6132. [CrossRef]
20. Patey, S.J.; Edwards, E.A.; Yates, E.A.; Turnbull, J.E. Engineered heparins: Novel beta-secretase inhibitors as potential Alzheimer's disease therapeutics. *Neurodegener. Dis.* **2008**, *5*, 197–199. [CrossRef]
21. Bergamaschini, L.; Rossi, E.; Storini, C.; Pizzimenti, S.; Distaso, M.; Perego, C.; De Luigi, A.; Vergani, C.; De Simoni, M.G. Peripheral Treatment with Enoxaparin, a Low Molecular Weight Heparin, Reduces Plaques and β-Amyloid Accumulation in a Mouse Model of Alzheimer's Disease. *J. Neurosci.* **2004**, *24*, 4181–4186. [CrossRef]
22. Timmer, N.M.; van Dijk, L.; van der Zee, C.E.; Kiliaan, A.; de Waal, R.M.; Verbeek, M.M. Enoxaparin treatment administered at both early and late stages of amyloid β deposition improves cognition of APPswe/PS1dE9 mice with differential effects on brain Aβ levels. *Neurobiol. Dis.* **2010**, *40*, 340–347. [CrossRef] [PubMed]
23. Bergamaschini, L.; Rossi, E.; Vergani, C.; De Simoni, M.G. Alzheimer's disease: Another target for heparin therapy. *Sci. World J.* **2009**, *9*, 891–908. [CrossRef]
24. Leveugle, B.; Ding, W.; Laurence, F.; Dehouck, M.P.; Scanameo, A.; Cecchelli, R.; Fillit, H. Heparin oligosaccharides that pass the blood-brain barrier inhibit beta-amyloid precursor protein secretion and heparin binding to beta-amyloid peptide. *J. Neurochem.* **1998**, *70*, 736–744. [CrossRef] [PubMed]
25. Hoffart, V.; Lamprecht, A.; Maincent, P.; Lecompte, T.; Vigneron, C.; Ubrich, N. Oral bioavailability of a low molecular weight heparin using a polymeric delivery system. *J. Control. Release* **2006**, *113*, 38–42. [CrossRef]
26. Stewart, K.L.; Hughes, E.; Yates, E.A.; Middleton, D.A.; Radford, S.E. Molecular Origins of the Compatibility between Glycosaminoglycans and Aβ40 Amyloid Fibrils. *J. Mol. Biol.* **2017**, *429*, 2449–2462. [CrossRef] [PubMed]
27. Mycroft-West, C.J.; Yates, E.A.; Skidmore, M.A. Marine glycosaminoglycan-like carbohydrates as potential drug candidates for infectious disease. *Biochem. Soc. Trans.* **2018**, *46*, 919–929. [CrossRef] [PubMed]
28. Valcarcel, J.; Nova-Carballal, R.; Perez-Martin, I.R.; Reis, L.R.; Vazeuez, A.J. Glycosaminoglycans from Marine Sources as therapeutic Agents. *Biotechnol. Adv.* **2017**, *35*, 711–725. [CrossRef]
29. Bergefall, K.; Trybala, E.; Johansson, M.; Uyama, T.; Yamada, S.; Kitagawa, H.; Sugahara, K.; Bergstrom, T. Chondroitin sulfate characterized by the E-disaccharide unit is a poten inhibtor of herpes simplex virus infectivity and provides the virus binding sites on gro2C cells. *J. Biol. Chem.* **2005**, *280*, 32193–32199. [CrossRef]
30. Huang, N.; Wu, M.Y.; Zheng, C.B.; Zhu, L.; Zhao, J.H.; Zheng, Y.T. The depolymerized fucosylated chondroitin sulfate from sea cucumber potently inhibits HIV replication via interfering with virus entry. *Carbohydr. Res.* **2013**, *380*, 64–69. [CrossRef]
31. Bastos, F.M.; Albrecht, L.; Kozlowski, O.E.; Lopes, P.C.S.; Blanco, C.Y.; Carlos, C.B.; Castineiras, C.; Vicente, P.C.; Werneck, C.C.; Gerhard, W.; et al. Fucosylated Chondroitin Sulphate Inhibits *Plasmodium falciparum* Cytoadhesion and Merozoite Invasion. *Antimicrob. Agents Chemother.* **2014**, *58*, 1862–1871. [CrossRef] [PubMed]
32. Marques, J.; Vilanova, E.; Mourao, S.A.P.; Fernandez-Busquets, X. Marine organism sulfated polysaccharides exhibiting significant antimalarial activity and inhibition of red blood cell invasion by plasmodium. *Sci. Rep.* **2016**, *6*, 24368. [CrossRef]
33. Brito, A.S.; Arimatéia, D.S.; Souza, L.R.; Lima, M.A.; Santos, V.O.; Medeiros, V.P.; Ferreira, P.A.; Silva, R.A.; Ferreira, C.V.; Justo, G.Z.; et al. Anti-inflammatory properties of a heparin-like glycosaminoglycan with reduced anti-coagulant activity isolated from a marine shrimp. *Bioorg. Med. Chem.* **2008**, *16*, 9588–9595. [CrossRef]
34. Suleria, H.A.R.; Masci, P.P.; Addepalli, R.; Chen, W.; Gobe, G.C.; Osborne, S.A. In vitro anti-thrombotic and anti-coagulant properties of blacklip abalone (*Haliotis rubra*) viscera hydrolysate. *Anal. Bioanal. Chem.* **2017**, *409*, 4195–4205. [CrossRef]
35. Gomes, A.M.; Kozlowski, E.O.; Borsig, L.; Teixeira, F.C.; Vlodavsky, I.; Pavão, M.S.G. Antitumor properties of a new non-anticoagulant heparin analog from the mollusk *Nodipecten nodosus*: Effect on P-selectin, heparanase, metastasis and cellular recruitment. *Glycobiology* **2015**, *25*, 386–393. [CrossRef] [PubMed]
36. Khurshid, C.; Pye, D.; Khurshid, C.; Pye, D.A. Isolation and Composition Analysis of Bioactive Glycosaminoglycans from Whelk. *Mar. Drugs* **2018**, *16*, 171. [CrossRef] [PubMed]

37. Aldairi, A.F.; Ogundipe, O.D.; Pye, D.A.; Aldairi, A.F.; Ogundipe, O.D.; Pye, D.A. Antiproliferative Activity of Glycosaminoglycan-Like Polysaccharides Derived from Marine Molluscs. *Mar. Drugs* **2018**, *16*, 63. [CrossRef]

38. Hu, S.; Jiang, W.; Li, S.; Song, W.; Ji, L.; Cai, L.; Liu, X. Fucosylated chondroitin sulphate from sea cucumber reduces hepatic endoplasmic reticulum stress-associated inflammation in obesity mice. *J. Funct. Foods* **2015**, *16*, 352–363. [CrossRef]

39. Gomes, A.M.; Kozlowski, E.O.; Pomin, V.H.; de Barros, C.M.; Zaganeli, J.L.; Pavão, M.S. Unique Extracellular Matrix Heparan Sulfate from the Bivalve *Nodipecten nodosus* (Linnaeus, 1758) Safely Inhibits Arterial Thrombosis after Photochemically Induced Endothelial Lesion. *J. Biol. Chem.* **2010**, *285*, 7312–7323. [CrossRef]

40. Hikino, M.; Mikami, T.; Faissner, A.; Vilela-Silva, A.-C.E.; Pavão, M.S.G.; Sugahara, K. Oversulfated Dermatan Sulfate Exhibits Neurite Outgrowth-promoting Activity toward Embryonic Mouse Hippocampal Neurons. *J. Biol. Chem.* **2003**, *278*, 43744–43754. [CrossRef] [PubMed]

41. Devlin, A.; Mycroft-west, c.J.; Guerrini, M.; Yates, E.A. Analysis of solid-state heparin samples by ATR-FTIR spectroscopy. *bioRxiv* **2019**. [CrossRef]

42. Skidmore, M.A.; Guimond, S.E.; Turnbull, J.E.; Dumax-Vorzet, A.F.; Yates, E.A.; Atrih, A. High sensitivity separation and detection of heparan sulfate disaccharides. *J. Chromatogr. A* **2006**, *1135*, 52–56. [CrossRef]

43. Andrade, P.V.G.; Lima, A.M.; de Souza Junior, A.A.; Fareed, J.; Hoppensteadt, A.D.; Santos, E.; Chavante, F.S.; Oliveira, W.F.; Rocha, A.O.H.; Nader, B.H. A heparin-like compound isolated from a marine crab rich in glucuronic acid 2-O-sulfate presents low anticoagulant activity. *Carbohydr. Polym.* **2013**, *94*, 647–654. [CrossRef] [PubMed]

44. Dietrich, C.P.; Tersariol, I.L.; Toma, L.; Moraes, C.T.; Porcionatto, M.A.; Oliveira, F.W.; Nader, H.B. Structure of heparan sulfate: Identification of variable and constant oligosaccharide domains in eight heparan sulfates of different origins. *Cell. Mol. Biol.* **1998**, *44*, 417–429.

45. Zhang, Z.; Xie, J.; Liu, H.; Liu, J.; Linhardt, R.J. Quantification of heparan sulfate disaccharides using ion-pairing reversed-phase microflow high-performance liquid chromatography with electrospray ionization trap mass spectrometry. *Anal. Chem.* **2009**, *81*, 4349–4355. [CrossRef]

46. Klaver, D.W.; Wilce, M.C.J.; Gasperini, R.; Freeman, C.; Juliano, J.P.; Parish, C.; Foa, L.; Aguilar, M.-I.; Small, D.H. Glycosaminoglycan-induced activation of the β-secretase (BACE1) of Alzheimer's disease. *J. Neurochem.* **2010**, *112*, 1552–1561. [CrossRef]

47. Beckman, M.; Holsinger, R.M.D.; Small, D.H. Heparin activates β-secretase (BACE1) of Alzheimer's disease and increases autocatalysis of the enzyme. *Biochemistry* **2006**, *45*, 6703–6714. [CrossRef] [PubMed]

48. Micsonai, A.; Wien, F.; Kernya, L.; Lee, Y.-H.; Goto, Y.; Réfrégiers, M.; Kardos, J. Accurate secondary structure prediction and fold recognition for circular dichroism spectroscopy. *Proc. Natl. Acad. Sci. USA* **2015**, *112*, E3095–E3103. [CrossRef] [PubMed]

49. Gasymov, O.K.; Abduragimov, A.R.; Glasgow, B.J. Probing tertiary structure of proteins using single Trp mutations with circular dichroism at low temperature. *J. Phys. Chem. B* **2014**, *118*, 986–995. [CrossRef] [PubMed]

50. De Simone, A.; Mancini, F.; Real Fernàndez, F.; Rovero, P.; Bertucci, C.; Andrisano, V. Surface plasmon resonance, fluorescence, and circular dichroism studies for the characterization of the binding of BACE-1 inhibitors. *Anal. Bioanal. Chem.* **2013**, *405*, 827–835. [CrossRef] [PubMed]

51. Greenfield, N.J. Using circular dichroism spectra to estimate protein secondary structure. *Nat. Protoc.* **2006**, *1*, 2876. [CrossRef] [PubMed]

52. Shimizu, H.; Tosaki, A.; Kaneko, K.; Hisano, T.; Sakurai, T.; Nukina, N. Crystal Structure of an Active Form of BACE1, an Enzyme Responsible for Amyloid β Protein Production. *Mol. Cell. Biol.* **2008**, *28*, 3663–3671. [CrossRef]

53. Sreerama, N.; Woody, R.W. On the analysis of membrane protein circular dichroism spectra. *Protein Sci.* **2004**, *13*, 100–112. [CrossRef] [PubMed]

54. Lo, M.-C.; Aulabaugh, A.; Jin, G.; Cowling, R.; Bard, J.; Malamas, M.; Ellestad, G. Evaluation of fluorescence-based thermal shift assays for hit identification in drug discovery. *Anal. Biochem.* **2004**, *332*, 153–159. [CrossRef]

55. Casu, B.; Grazioli, G.; Razi, N.; Guerrini, M.; Naggi, A.; Torri, G.; Oreste, P.; Tursi, F.; Zoppetti, G.; Lindahl, U. Heparin-like compounds prepared by chemical modification of capsular polysaccharide from *E. coli* K5. *Carbohydr. Res.* **1994**, *263*, 271–284. [CrossRef]

56. Yates, E.A.; Santini, F.; Guerrini, M.; Naggi, A.; Torri, G.; Casu, B. 1H and 13C NMR spectral assignments of the major sequences of twelve systematically modified heparin derivatives. *Carbohydr. Res.* **1996**, *294*, 15–27. [CrossRef]

57. Cavalcante, R.S.; Brito, A.S.; Palhares, L.C.; Lima, M.A. 2,3-Di-O-sulfo glucuronic acid: An unmodified and unusual residue in a highly sulfated chondroitin sulfate from *Litopenaeus vannamei*. *Carbohydr. Polym.* **2018**, *183*, 192–200. [CrossRef]

58. Vasconcelos, A.; Pomin, V.H. The Sea as a Rich Source of Structurally Unique Glycosaminoglycans and Mimetics. *Microorganisms* **2017**, *5*, 51. [CrossRef] [PubMed]

59. Pavão, M.S. Glycosaminoglycans analogs from marine invertebrates: Structure, biological effects, and potential as new therapeutics. *Front. Cell. Infect. Microbiol.* **2014**, *4*, 123. [CrossRef]

60. Dietrich, C.P.; Paiva, J.F.; Castro, R.A.B.; Chavante, S.F.; Jeske, W.; Fareed, J.; Gorin, P.A.J.; Mendes, A.; Nader, H.B. Structural features and anticoagulant activities of a novel natural low molecular weight heparin from the shrimp *Penaeus brasiliensis*. *Biochim. Biophys. Acta Gen. Subj.* **1999**, *1428*, 273–283. [CrossRef]

61. Medeiros, G.F.; Mendes, A.; Castro, R.A.B.; Baú, E.C.; Nader, H.B.; Dietrich, C.P. Distribution of sulfated glycosaminoglycans in the animal kingdom: Widespread occurrence of heparin-like compounds in invertebrates. *Biochim. Biophys. Acta Gen. Subj.* **2000**, *1475*, 287–294. [CrossRef]

62. Brito, A.S.; Cavalcante, R.S.; Palhares, L.C.; Hughes, A.J.; Andrade, G.P.V.; Yates, E.A.; Nader, H.B.; Lima, M.A.; Chavante, S.F. A non-hemorrhagic hybrid heparin/heparan sulfate with anticoagulant potential. *Carbohydr. Polym.* **2014**, *99*, 372–378. [CrossRef]

63. Chavante, S.F.; Brito, A.S.; Lima, M.; Yates, E.; Nader, H.; Guerrini, M.; Torri, G.; Bisio, A. A heparin-like glycosaminoglycan from shrimp containing high levels of 3-O-sulfated D-glucosamine groups in an unusual trisaccharide sequence. *Carbohydr. Res.* **2014**, *390*, 59–66. [CrossRef] [PubMed]

64. Chavante, S.F.; Santos, E.A.; Oliveira, F.W.; Guerrini, M.; Torri, G.; Casu, B.; Dietrich, C.P.; Nader, H.B. A novel heparan sulphate with high degree of N-sulphation and high heparin cofactor-II activity from brine shrimp *Artemia franciscana*. *Int. J. Biol. Macromol.* **2000**, *27*, 49–57. [CrossRef]

65. Lima, M.; Rudd, T.; Yates, E. New Applications of Heparin and Other Glycosaminoglycans. *Molecules* **2017**, *22*, 749. [CrossRef] [PubMed]

66. Pomin, V.H. Holothurian fucosylated chondroitin sulfate. *Mar. Drugs* **2014**, *12*, 232–254. [CrossRef] [PubMed]

67. Spronk, S.A.; Carlson, H.A. The role of tyrosine 71 in modulating the flap conformations of BACE1. *Proteins Struct. Funct. Bioinform.* **2011**, *79*, 2247–2259. [CrossRef] [PubMed]

68. Rudd, T.R.; Guimond, S.E.; Skidmore, M.A.; Duchesne, L.; Guerrini, M.; Torri, G.; Cosentino, C.; Brown, A.; Clarke, D.T.; Turnbull, J.E.; et al. Influence of substitution pattern and cation binding on conformation and activity in heparin derivatives. *Glycobiology* **2007**, *17*, 983–993. [CrossRef] [PubMed]

69. Rudd, T.; Skidmore, M.; Guimond, S.; Holman, J.; Turnbull, J. The potential for circular dichroism as an additional facile and sensitive method of monitoring low-molecular-weight heparins and heparinoids. *Thromb. Haemost.* **2009**, *102*, 874–878. [PubMed]

70. Uniewicz, K.A.; Ori, A.; Xu, R.; Ahmed, Y.; Fernig, D.G.; Yates, E.A. Differential Scanning Fluorimetry measurement of protein stability changes upon binding to glycosaminoglycans: A rapid screening test for binding specificity. *Anal. Chem.* **2010**, *82*, 3796–3802. [CrossRef]

71. Niesen, F.H.; Berglund, H.; Vedadi, M. The use of differential scanning fluorimetry to detect ligand interactions that promote protein stability. *Nat. Protoc.* **2007**, *2*, 2212–2221. [CrossRef] [PubMed]

72. Van der Meer, J.Y.; Kellenbach, E.; van den Bos, L. From Farm to Pharma: An Overview of Industrial Heparin Manufacturing Methods. *Molecules* **2017**, *22*, 1025. [CrossRef] [PubMed]

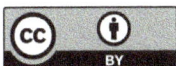

marine drugs

MDPI

Article

Physicochemical Characteristics and Anticoagulant Activities of the Polysaccharides from Sea Cucumber *Pattalus mollis*

Wenqi Zheng [1], Lutan Zhou [2,3], Lisha Lin [2,3], Ying Cai [2,3], Huifang Sun [2,3], Longyan Zhao [1],
Na Gao [1], Ronghua Yin [2,*] and Jinhua Zhao [1,2,*]

[1]   School of Pharmaceutical Sciences, South-Central University for Nationalities, Wuhan 430074, China;
      zwq_scuec@126.com (W.Z.); zhaolongyan@mail.scuec.edu.cn (L.Z.); gn2008.happy@163.com (N.G.)
[2]   State Key Laboratory of Phytochemistry and Plant Resources in West China, Kunming Institute of Botany,
      Chinese Academy of Sciences, Kunming 650201, China; zhoulutan@mail.kib.ac.cn (L.Z.);
      linlisha@mail.kib.ac.cn (L.L.); caiying@mail.kib.ac.cn (Y.C.); sunhuifang@mail.kib.ac.cn (H.S.)
[3]   University of Chinese Academy of Sciences, Beijing 100049, China
*   Correspondence: yinronghua@mail.kib.ac.cn (R.Y.); zhao.jinhua@yahoo.com (J.Z.);
      Tel.: +86-871-65226278 (J.Z.)

Received: 5 March 2019; Accepted: 25 March 2019; Published: 29 March 2019

check for
updates

Abstract: Sulfated polysaccharides from sea cucumbers possess distinct chemical structure and various biological activities. Herein, three types of polysaccharides were isolated and purified from *Pattalus mollis*, and their structures and bioactivities were analyzed. The fucosylated glycosaminoglycan (PmFG) had a CS-like backbone composed of the repeating units of {-4-D-GlcA-β-1,3-D-GalNAc$_{4S6S}$-β-1-}, and branches of a sulfated α-L-Fuc (including Fuc$_{2S4S}$, Fuc$_{3S4S}$ and Fuc$_{4S}$ with a molar ratio of 2:2.5:1) linked to O-3 of each D-GlcA. The fucan sulfate (PmFS) had a backbone consisting of a repetitively linked unit {-4-L-Fuc$_{2S}$-α-1-}, and interestingly, every trisaccharide unit in its backbone was branched with a sulfated α-L-Fuc (Fuc$_{4S}$ or Fuc$_{3S}$ with a molar ratio of 4:1). Apart from the sulfated polysaccharides, two neutral glycans (PmNG-1 & -2) differing in molecular weight were also obtained and their structures were similar to animal glycogen. Anticoagulant assays indicated that PmFG and PmFS possessed strong APTT prolonging and intrinsic factor Xase inhibition activities, and the sulfated α-L-Fuc branches might contribute to the anticoagulant and anti-FXase activities of both PmFG and PmFS.

Keywords: *Pattalus mollis*; fucosylated glycosaminoglycan; fucan sulfate; physicochemical characteristics; anticoagulant activities

1. Introduction

Some sea cucumbers (*Echinodermata, Holothuroidea*) are popular tonic foods and traditional Chinese medicines in China for centuries [1]. Sulfated polysaccharides such as fucosylated glycosaminoglycan (FG) and fucan sulfate (FS) are the main components of polysaccharides extracted from sea cucumbers, and have attracted considerable attention due to their unique structures and extensive bioactivities [2–6].

FG is a distinct glycosaminoglycan (GAG) found exclusively so far in sea cucumbers [2]. Due to its multiple pharmacological activities such as antitumor, anti-thrombosis and anti-inflammation [7–9], and especially potent anticoagulation by inhibiting the intrinsic factor Xase complex (FXase) [8,10,11], FG has attracted increasing attention. It is generally agreed that FG possesses a chondroitin sulfate (CS)-like backbone which consists of the disaccharide repeating units {-4-D-GalNAcS-β-1,3-D-GlcA-β-1-}, and the backbone is branched with fucose sulfate (FucS) [2,10]. Factually, the structures of some FG, especially with various types of FucS branches, are still ill-defined [12–17]. For instance, early research showed that FG from *Stichopus japonicas* has a core structure of {-4-D-GalNAcS-β-1,3-D-GlcA-β-1-}, and mono-L-Fuc was linked to the each GlcA via α-1,3 linkage as the branch [15]. However, other researchers proposed that the Fuc branches also existed as a di- or tri-saccharide, and L-Fuc branches linked to GalNAc of backbone via α-1,4 or α-1,6 linkage [4,13,16].

Fucan sulfate (FS) is another type of sulfated polysaccharide from the body wall of sea cucumber. It was first reported in 1969, and it only comprises FucS [18]. Compared with fucoidans from brown alga, most FS from echinoderm consists of repeating structural units, thus their structures are relatively more regular [19–22]. Factually, there are great differences among the structures of FS from various sea cucumbers, due to the diversity in chain lengths of repeating units, glycosidic linkages and/or sulfation patterns [5,22–24]. It is reported that FS also has multiple bioactivities, such as anti-thrombosis, antivirus, antitumor, anti-inflammation and anticoagulant activity [25–28]. It is generally considered that FS showed weaker anticoagulant activities, compared with FG, according to the previous studies [28,29]. However, the structure-activity relationship for anticoagulant activity of FS remains unclear, such as the effects of glycosidic linkages and sulfated patterns on its bioactivities.

Apart from FG and FS, a neutral glycan (NG) was also discovered from some sea cucumbers. It showed no significant anticoagulant activity, compared with the sulfated polysaccharides [29].

In this work, three types of polysaccharides, a fucosylated glycosaminoglycan (PmFG), a fucan sulfate (PmFS) and glycogen-like neutral glycans (PmNG-1 & PmNG-2) were isolated and purified from *Pattalus mollis*. For structure and activity analysis, PmFG was depolymerized by H_2O_2 treatment and dPmFG-I – -III were fractioned from the depolymerized products. Composition analysis of PmFG and spectral analysis of dPmFG indicated that PmFG comprised a CS-E-like backbone and the branches of L-FucS (including Fuc_{2S4S}, Fuc_{3S4S} and Fuc_{4S} with a molar ratio of 2:2.5:1) which linked to the GlcA of the backbone as side chain via α-1,3 glycosidic bonds.

1D/2D NMR spectra of PmFS showed that it had a backbone consisting of repetitively linked {-4-L-Fuc_{2S}-α1-}, which was similar to the FS from *Thelenota ananas* [5], while has unique sulfated Fuc branches linked to the backbone via α-1,3 glycosidic bonds. The weight-average molecular mass (Mw, 6.12 kDa) of PmFS was much lower than Mw (61.2 kDa) of the FS from *T. ananas*. In addition, the structures of two neutral glycans, PmNG-1 & -2, were similar to animal glycogen consisting of D-Glc residues which linked via α-1,4 (major) and α-1,6 (minor, branching) glycosidic bonds [29].

Moreover, the anticoagulant activity of PmFG and PmFS was investigated and their structure-activity relationships were discussed. Both of them exhibited potent activity in APTT prolongation and FXase inhibition. Interestingly, compared with some FS from other species of sea cucumber, PmFS showed relatively potent anticoagulant and anti-FXase activities, which might be due to its distinct structure of FucS branches.

2. Results and Discussion

2.1. Isolation and Purification of Polysaccharides from P. mollis

Crude polysaccharides were isolated from *P. mollis* by ethanol precipitation after papain enzymolysis, as described in literature [29–31]. The crude polysaccharides were then fractioned into two fractions, Fraction-1 and Fraction-2, by the addition of ethanol at the final concentration of 40% and 60% (*v/v*), respectively. PmFG, PmNG-1 and PmNG-2 were further isolated from Fraction-1 by ethanol fractionated precipitation (at the presence of 0.5 M KOAc) and strong anion-exchange (FPA98) chromatography. PmFS was obtained from Fraction-2 by strong anion-exchange (FPA98) chromatography and Sephadex G-100 (1.5 cm × 150 cm) chromatography. The purities of these samples were detected by the high-performance gel permeation chromatography (HPGPC) using an Agilent technologies 1200 series apparatus (Agilent Co., USA) equipped with a Shodex OH-pak SB-804 HQ column (8 mm × 300 mm) and RID and DAD detectors, as described previously [10,30]. The single symmetric peak of each sample in the HPGPC profile (Figure 1) indicated that each sample was a homogenous polysaccharide. Additionally, no absorption observed at 280 or 260 nm indicated the absence of protein or nucleic acids.

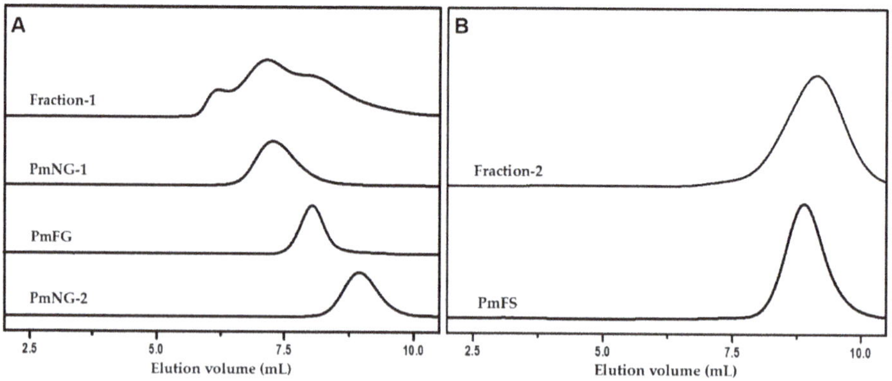

Figure 1. HPGPC profiles of Fraction-1, PmNG-1, PmNG-2 and PmFG (**A**); Fraction-2 and PmFS (**B**). The samples were analyzed on an Agilent Technologies 1200 series equipped with a Shodex OH-pak SB-804 HQ column and eluted with 0.1 M NaCl solution at a flow rate of 0.5 mL/min.

2.2. Physicochemical Analysis

The monosaccharide compositions of polysaccharides were analyzed by reverse-phase HPLC according to PMP derivatization procedures [30,32]. The results showed that PmFG was composed of three monosaccharides, GlcA, GalNAc and Fuc (Figure 2), while PmFS contained only Fuc, and PmNG-1 and PmNG-2 contained only the monosaccharide of Glc.

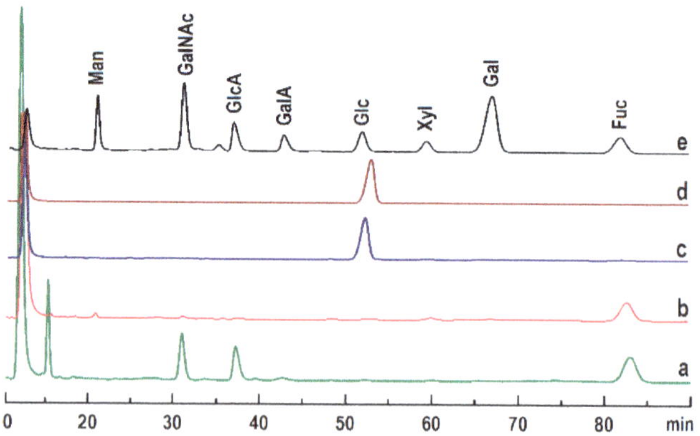

Figure 2. HPLC profiles of monosaccharide-PMP derivates of PmFG (**a**), PmFS (**b**), PmNG-2 (**c**), PmNG-1 (**d**) and standard monosaccharides (**e**).

The acidic groups in PmFG and PmFS were determined by a conductimetric method [30]. Data for the SO_3^- and COO^- determinations are shown in Figure 3 and Table 1. In the titration curve of PmFG, two inflection points V_1 and V_2 indicated it contained two types of acidic groups, which was consistent with that of other FG reported previously [28–30]. While in the titration curve of PmFS, only one inflection point V_3 was detected, in accordance with that it contained the only kind of acidic group, sulfate. The contents of the sulfate groups of PmFG and PmFS were both 30.4%. The SO_3^-/COO^- molar ratio in PmFG was estimated to be 3.2, and the sulfate/Fuc molar ratio in PmFS was about 0.91.

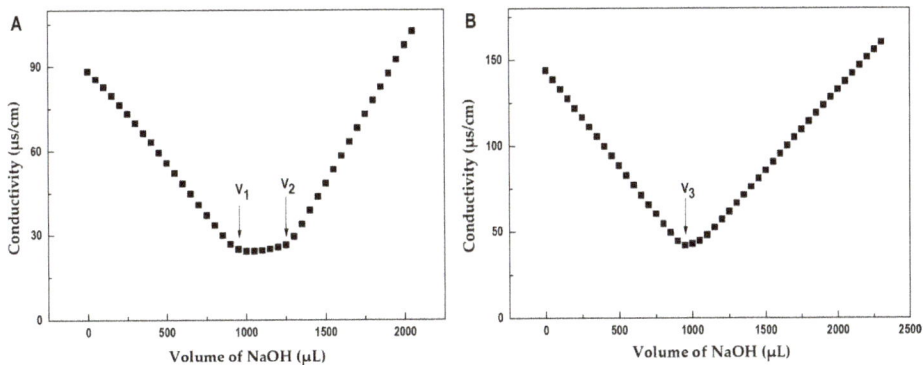

Figure 3. Conductimetric titration curves of PmFG (**A**) and PmFS (**B**).

Table 1. Chemical compositions and physicochemical properties of the polysaccharides from *P. mollis*.

	Monosaccharide Compositions				SO_3^-/COO^- (Molar Ratios)	SO_3^-/Fuc (Molar Ratios)	Mw (kDa)	Specific Rotations
	GlcA	GalNAc	Fuc	Glc				
PmFG	+	+	+	-	3.2	/	60.3	−75.8°
PmFS	-	-	+	-	/	0.9	6.12	−115.2°
PmNG-1	-	-	-	+	/	/	275.6	+172.4°
PmNG-2	-	-	-	+	/	/	22.5	+140.3

The optical rotation of these polysaccharides was detected and is shown in Table 1. Under certain wavelength and temperature conditions, the optical phenomenon of an optically active substance reflects the specific structure and specific rotation along with the structure changes. The specific rotations of PmFG (−75.8°) and PmFS (−115.2°) were both levorotatory, which was compatible with the residues of α-L-Fuc [33], while the specific rotations of PmNG-1 (+172.4°) and PmNG-2 (+140.3°) were both dextrorotatory, which was consistent with α-D-glucose [29].

Moreover, the Mw values of these native polysaccharides were determined by HPGPC using a Shodex 804-HQ column (Table 1). The Mw of PmFG was 60.3 kDa, which was similar to that of FG from other sea cucumbers [8,28–30]. Notably, the Mw of PmFS (6.12 kDa) was obviously lower than that of the FS from other species, which varied from tens to hundreds of kDa [5,24,28,31]. Additionally, the Mws of the two NGs were estimated to be 275.6 kDa (PmNG-1) and 22.5 kDa (PmNG-2), respectively, which were consistent with the chromatographic behavior in their HPGPC profiles.

The functional groups of these polysaccharides were analyzed by IR spectra (Figure 4). In the four spectra, the broad signals at 3250–3750 cm^{-1} and 2975 cm^{-1} were from the stretching vibrations of O-H and C-H, respectively [32,34]. The signals at 1020–1070 cm^{-1} were assigned to the stretching vibration of C-O-C in the polysaccharide skeleton [28]. The signal peaks of 1255 and 850 cm^{-1} in both PmFG and PmFS spectra were derived from the stretching vibrations of S=O and C-O-S in sulfate esters, indicating that the two polysaccharides were substituted by sulfate groups [29]. Additionally, the strong signal peak of PmFG at 1645 cm^{-1} was generated by the stretching vibration of C=O in GalNAc and GlcA. The band at 1420 cm^{-1} came from the symmetric stretch vibration of COO$^-$ in GlcA [10,28,34]. The results showed that different kinds of polysaccharides had their own characteristic signals in FT-IR spectra.

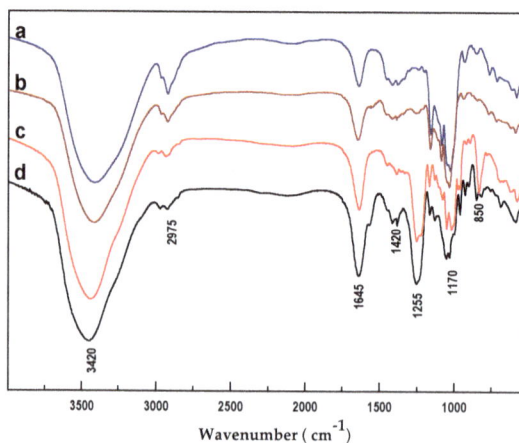

Figure 4. FT-IR spectra of PmNG-1 (**a**), PmNG-2 (**b**), PmFS (**c**) and PmFG (**d**).

2.3. NMR Analysis

The structural features of the sulfated polysaccharides were further elucidated by NMR spectral analysis. For PmFG, in the ^{1}H NMR spectra (Figure 5A), the signals observed in the region approximating 5.2–5.7 ppm could be assigned to anomeric protons of α-L-Fuc residues with different sulfation patterns, including 2,4-di-O-sulfated (Fuc$_{2S4S}$, 5.61 ppm), 3,4-di-O-sulfated (Fuc$_{3S4S}$, 5.26 ppm) and 4-O-sulfated (Fuc$_{4S}$, 5.32 ppm) with a molar ratio of 2:2.5:1, according to previous studies [11,28]. The upfield signals at ~1.25 and 1.97 ppm were assigned to the distinctive methyl protons of Fuc and GalNAc, respectively. The integral ratio of the two signals was approximately 1:1, indicating that Fuc and GalNAc are equal in mole content [10]. Apart from these characteristic signal peaks, others especially in the region of 3.40–4.80 ppm were broad and overlapped, thus hindering the elucidation of the precise structure of PmFG.

To further study the precise structure, its depolymerized product, dPmFG, was prepared by H_2O_2 in the presence of cupric ion as catalyst. The dPmFG was further fractioned to three fractions, dPmFG-I – -III, by GPC using Sephadex G-100 column, among which, dPmFG-II was subjected to spectra analysis to obtain the structural data of PmFG. Its signals in ^{1}H NMR spectrum were similar with that of PmFG but obviously more explicit (Figure 5A,B). Its ^{13}C NMR (Figure 5C) and 2D NMR (^{1}H-^{1}H COSY/TOCSY/ROESY and ^{1}H-^{13}C HSQC/HMBC) were also recorded (Figure 6). In the ^{1}H NMR spectrum of dPmFG-II, the signals at ~1.25 and 1.98 ppm could also be readily assigned to the methyl protons of Fuc residues (-CH$_3$) (Figure 5B), and the signals at 5.61 ppm, 5.27 ppm and 5.32 ppm were ascribed to the anomeric protons of three types of α-L-Fuc residues [11,28]. From these signals, the intra-residue signals in the three types of α-L-Fuc were determined from the ^{1}H-^{1}H COSY and TOCSY spectra (Figure 6A,D). The downfield shifts at 4.42/77.9 ppm and 4.80/84.1 ppm, 4.45/78.4 ppm and 4.96/82.4 ppm and 4.70/83.7 ppm indicated that the sulfate substitutions were at 2,4-, 3,4- and 4-positions, respectively [28]. Additionally, the spin-spin coupling systems from GlcA (U) and GalNAc (A) were also observed based on the COSY and TOCSY spectra. Moreover, the carbon signals were assigned based on the resonance signals of protons in ^{1}H-^{13}C HSQC spectrum (Figure 6B). The signals at 4.73/79.1 ppm and 4.27 & 4.10/70.2 ppm in the residue GalNAc indicated that *O-4* and *O-6* were both substituted by sulfate esters [11].

The sequence and linkages of these residues were confirmed by the signal correlations in the ^{1}H-^{13}C HMBC and ^{1}H-^{1}H ROESY spectra (Figure 6C,D). Specifically, GlcA and GalNAc residues were linked with alternating β-1,3 and β-1,4 bonds according to the cross-peak of 3.97 ppm (H-3, GalNAc) and 4.40 ppm (H-1, GlcA), the correlation of 3.86 ppm (H-4, GlcA) and 4.48 ppm (H-1, GalNAc) in the ROESY spectrum [10]. The linkages were reconfirmed by the correlations of H-1 (GalNAc) and C-4

(79.2 ppm, GlcA), and H-1 (GlcA) and C-3 (76.7 ppm, GalNAc) in the HMBC spectrum. Additionally, three types of α-L-Fuc residues were linked to O-3 of GlcA as side chains according to the correlations of H/C-1 (Fuc) and H/C-3 (GlcA) in the ROESY and HMBC spectra [28,30].

Based on the above analysis, the structure of dPmFG-II was deduced. The chemical shift assignments were shown in Table 2. Its backbone sequence was {-4-D-GlcA-β-1,3-D-GalNAc$_{4S6S}$-β-1-}, the same as that of CS-E. The mono-L-Fuc side chains including three types (Fuc$_{2S4S}$, Fuc$_{3S4S}$ and Fuc$_{4S}$) were linked to GlcA via α-1,3 glycosidic bonds. Finally, the structure of native PmFG was proposed to be {-[L-Fuc$_R$-α-1,3]-D-GlcA-β-1,3-D-GalNAc$_{4S6S}$-β-1,4-}$_n$, in which R was 2S4S: 3S4S: 4S with a molar ratio of 2:2.5:1.

The structure of PmFS was also elucidated by the detailed analysis of its 1D/2D NMR spectra (Figures 7 and 8). In the ^{1}H NMR spectrum (Figure 7A), the signals at 1.18–1.35 ppm could be readily assigned to the methyl protons (-CH$_3$) of Fuc residues [5,31]. Five signals observed in the downfield 5.0–5.5 ppm region were attributed to the anomeric protons of α-L-Fuc residues. Starting from the resonances, five spin-spin coupling systems (marked as residue A, B, C, D and D′, respectively) were assigned according to the ^{1}H-^{1}H COSY and TOCSY spectra (Figure 8A). The chemical shifts of corresponding carbon resonances in the five intra-residues were assigned based on the ^{13}C and ^{1}H-^{13}C HSQC spectra (Figures 7B and 8B). The signals at 95–100 ppm were unambiguously ascribed to the anomeric carbons [5].

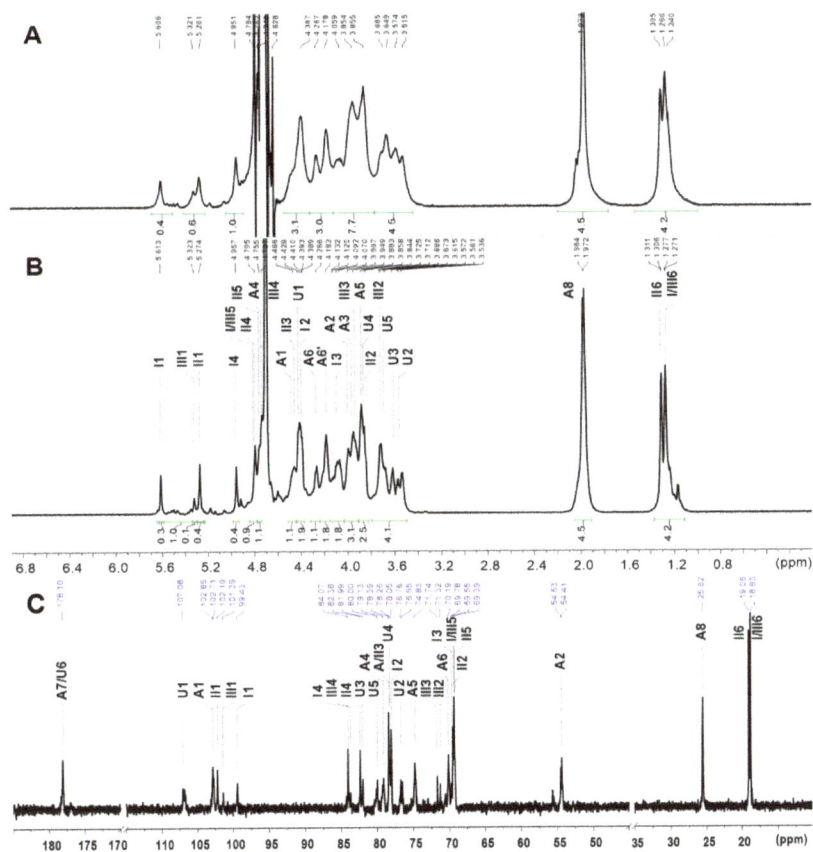

Figure 5. ^{1}H (**A,B**) and ^{13}C (**C**) NMR spectra of PmFG (**A**) and dPmFG-II (**B,C**) and signal assignments. I, Fuc$_{2S4S}$; II, Fuc$_{3S4S}$; III, Fuc$_{4S}$; U, GlcA; A, GalNAc.

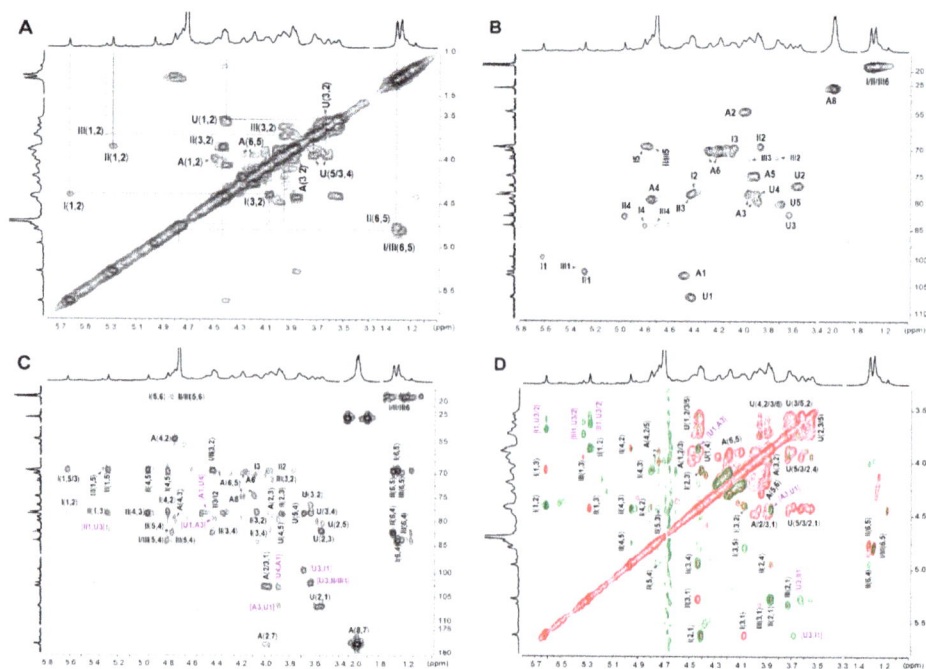

Figure 6. ^{1}H-^{1}H COSY (**A**), ^{1}H-^{13}C HSQC (**B**)/HMBC (**C**), and superimposed ^{1}H-^{1}H TOCSY (red)/ROESY (green) (**D**) and signal assignments (purple: the correlation signals of glycosidic bonds). I, Fuc$_{2S4S}$; II, Fuc$_{3S4S}$; III, Fuc$_{4S}$; U, GlcA; A, GalNAc.

Table 2. ^{1}H/^{13}C NMR chemical shift assignments of dPmFG-II.

Sugar Residues		Chemical Shifts [a]							
		1	2	3	4	5	6	7	8
U	H	4.40	3.56	3.69	3.86	3.60	–		
-4)-β-D-GlcA-(1-	C	107.1	78.2	80.0	79.2	82.0	178.1		
A	H	4.48	4.00	3.97	4.73	3.88	4.27/4.18	–	1.98
-3)-β-D-GalNAc$_{4S6S}$-(1-	C	102.8	54.5	76.7	79.1	74.8	70.2	178.1	25.6
I	H	5.61	4.42	4.09	4.80	4.81	1.27		
α-L-Fuc$_{2S4S}$-(1-	C	99.4	77.9	69.6	84.1	69.4	18.8		
II	H	5.27	3.84	4.45	4.96	4.76	1.30		
α-L-Fuc$_{3S4S}$-(1-	C	102.2	69.4	78.4	82.4	69.6	19.1		
III	H	5.32	3.72	3.94	4.70	4.81	1.27		
α-L-Fuc$_{4S}$-(1-	C	101.4	71.3	71.7	83.7	69.4	18.8		

[a] Data were recorded at 298 K in D$_2$O with a Bruker Avance spectrometer of 800 MHz; chemical shifts are given in ppm with reference to D$_2$O.

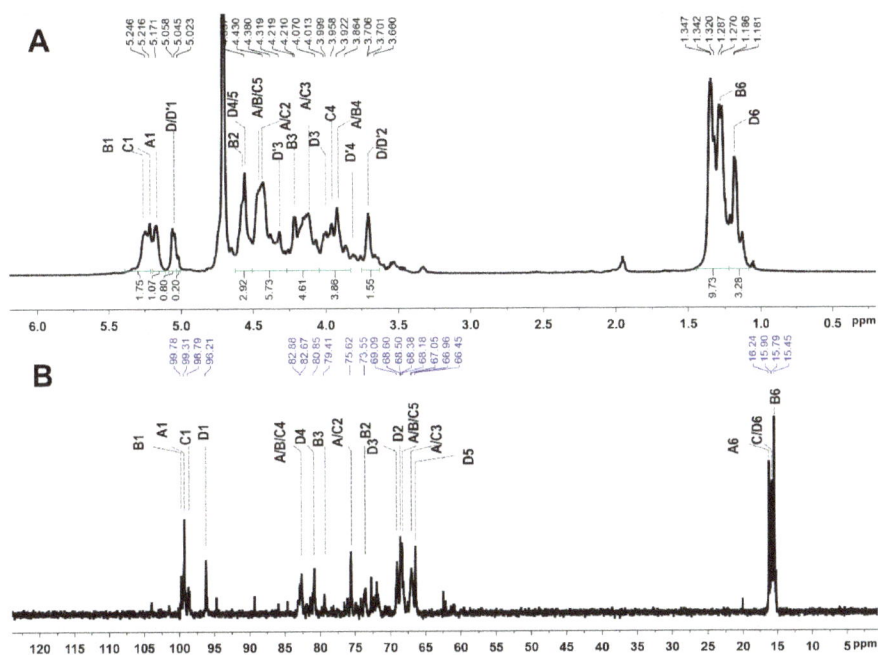

Figure 7. ^{1}H (**A**) and ^{13}C (**B**) NMR spectra of PmFS and signal assignments.

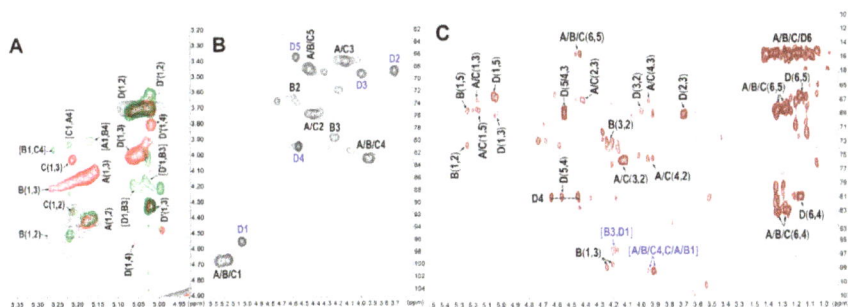

Figure 8. Superimposed ^{1}H-^{1}H COSY (gray) -TOCSY (red) -ROESY (green) (**A**), ^{1}H-^{13}C HSQC (**B**) and ^{1}H-^{13}C HMBC (**C**) spectra of PmFS.

The H-2 shift values of residues A, B and C at 4.4–4.5 ppm were obviously shifted downfield compared with those of non-sulfated Fuc residues, indicating the sulfation substitution at *O*-2 of these residues [24]. These sulfated patterns were reconfirmed by the C-2 shift values at 73–75 ppm. Likewise, the ^{1}H/^{13}C shift values of residues D/D′ indicated that they possessed 4-/3-*O*-sulfated substitutions. Furthermore, the linkages of these residues were proved by the correlation peaks in its ^{1}H-^{1}H ROESY and ^{1}H-^{13}C HMBC spectra (Figure 8A,C). The correlations between H-1 and H-4 of residues A, B and C indicated the presence of α-1,3 glycosidic bonds between them. These linkages were reconfirmed by the correlations of H-4 (residues A, B and C) and C-1 (residues C, A and B). The linkage positions were in agreement with the downfield shifts of C-4 [5,28,31]. Additionally, residues D/D′ were linked to *O*-3 of residue B from the ROESY and HMBC NMR data, with a molar ratio of 4:1, according to the anomeric proton integrals of D and D′. Taken together, the structure of PmFS was determined to be {-L-Fuc$_{2S}$-α-1,4-[L-Fuc$_R$-α-1,3]-L-Fuc$_{2S}$-α-1,4-L-Fuc$_{2S}$-α-1,4-}$_n$, where R was 4S: 3S with a molar ratio of 4:1. The chemical shift assignments are shown in Table 3.

Table 3. ^{1}H/^{13}C NMR chemical shift assignments of the PmFS.

Sugar Residues		Chemical Shifts [a]					
		1	2	3	4	5	6
A	H	5.17	4.43	4.14	3.92	4.44	1.33
	C	99.3	75.6	67.1	82.7	68.5	16.2
B	H	5.25	4.58	4.22	3.92	4.46	1.28
	C	99.8	73.6	79.4	82.9	68.2	15.5
C	H	5.22	4.43	4.16	3.96	4.38	1.35
	C	98.8	75.6	67.0	82.7	68.4	15.9
D	H	5.05	3.70	4.00	4.56	4.56	1.18
	C	96.2	68.6	69.1	80.9	66.5	15.8
D'	H	5.02	3.66	4.32	3.81	–	–
	C	96.2	68.6	69.1	80.9	66.5	15.8

[a] Data were recorded at 298 K in D$_2$O with a Bruker Avance spectrometer of 800 MHz; chemical shifts were given in ppm with reference to D$_2$O.

The structure of PmFG and PmFS is shown in Figure 9A,B, respectively.

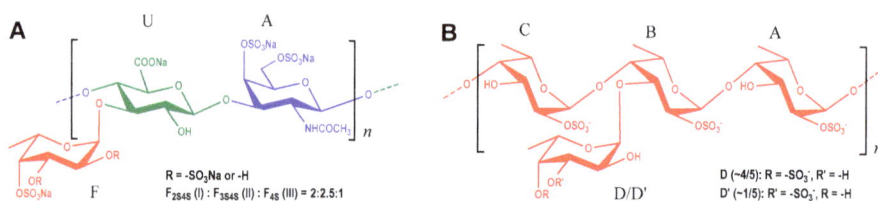

Figure 9. Proposed chemical structures of PmFG (**A**) and PmFS (**B**).

Interestingly, FS is always reported as a linear polysaccharide with different repeated unit numbers [5,24,31]. Previously, our group also obtained an FS from sea cucumber *T. ananas* with a high regular structure of {-4-L-Fuc$_{2S}$-α-1-}. Compared the two FSs, they have the same backbone of {-4-L-Fuc$_{2S}$-α-1-}, while PmFS is unique in its Fuc branches.

2.4. Anticoagulant Activity Evaluation

To assess the anticoagulant activities of the polysaccharides from *P. mollis*, their effects on APTT, PT and TT of normal human plasma were detected compared with LMWH (Table 4).

The results showed that PmFG and PmFS had no significant effect on PT at the concentration up to 128 µg/mL, indicating that they had no effect on the extrinsic coagulation pathway. In the TT assays, PmFG exhibited comparable activity to that of LMWH (the concentration required to double TT were 10.7 µg/mL and 6.06 µg/mL for PmFG and LMWH, respectively), while all the other compounds exhibited no obvious effect on TT at the concentration up to 128 µg/mL [10,29].

The APTT prolonging activity of PmFG was much stronger than that of LMWH (the concentration required to double APTT was 3.50 µg/mL for PmFG and 11.6 µg/mL for LMWH). The concentrations of dPmFG-I – -III required to double APTT were increased from 6.24 µg/mL to 19.3 µg/mL along with the decrease of the molecular weight from 12.8 kDa to 3.71 kDa. This indicated that PmFG and dPmFGs exhibited intrinsic coagulation pathway inhibition activity, and the potency was related to their molecular weight.

The concentrations of PmFS and PmFS-I – -III required to double APTT were 24.3 µg/mL, 22.7 µg/mL, 21.2 µg/mL and 22.5 µg/mL, respectively. Although their APTT prolonging activity was weaker than that of PmFG and dPmFGs, they also had significant anticoagulant activity (their concentrations required for 2APTT were about 2-fold of that of LMWH). Moreover, the activities of PmFSs were similar to TaFS from *T. ananas* (21.7 µg/mL for 2APTT) [5]. Notably, PmFS had the similar backbone to TaFS, but branched with a sulfated α-L-Fuc, and its Mw (6.12 kDa) was only 1/10 of that of TaFS (61.2 kDa). Additionally, the Mw of PmFS-III (5.06 kDa) was approximate to dTaFS (5.14 kDa), while the APTT prolonging activity of PmFS-III was about 3-fold of that of dTaFS (the concentration required for 2APTT was 22.5 µg/mL for PmFS-III and 79.5 µg/mL for dTaFS, respectively) [5]. Compared with some other FS [5,28,31], PmFSs also showed relatively stronger anticoagulant activity.

Table 4. APTT prolongation and anti-FXase activities of polysaccharides.

Sample	Molecular Weight	APTT		Anti-FXase (IC$_{50}$)	
	(kDa)	(µg/mL)	(µM)	(ng/mL)	(nM)
PmFG	60.3	3.50	0.0580	13.7	0.227
dPmFG-I	12.8	6.24	0.488	14.0	1.09
dPmFG-II	6.97	7.97	1.14	17.6	2.53
dPmFG-III	3.71	19.3	5.20	126	34.0
PmFS	6.12	24.3	3.97	74.0	12.1
PmFS-I	8.64	22.7	2.63	87.9	10.2
PmFS-II	6.23	21.2	3.40	109	17.5
PmFS-III	5.06	22.5	4.45	99.2	19.6
TaFS [a]	61.2	21.7	–	197	–
dTaFS [a]	5.14	79.5	–	745	–
LMWH	3.50~5.50	11.6	2.11~3.31	59.0	10.7~16.9

[a] Data cited from Shang, F.N. et al., 2018 [5].

To further study the anticoagulant mechanism of these polysaccharides, anti-factor IIa and anti-factor Xa activities in the presence of antithrombin (AT) and intrinsic FXase inhibition activity were detected. These sulfated polysaccharides exhibited no significant anti-factor IIa and anti-factor Xa activities in the presence of AT compared with LMWH, suggesting that their anticoagulant targets may be different from the heparin-like compounds [8,10].

Particularly, PmFG displayed potent anti-FXase activity (IC$_{50}$, 13.7 ng/mL), similar to the FG from other sea cucumbers. [10,11,28]. The IC$_{50}$ values of dPmFG-I, dPmFG-II and dPmFG-III for FXase inhibition were 14.0 ng/mL, 17.6 ng/mL and 126 ng/mL, respectively, indicating the decrease of activity with the reduction of the chain length. By contrast, the effect of PmFS (IC$_{50}$, 74.0 ng/mL) was much weaker than PmFG (IC$_{50}$, 13.7 ng/mL) while comparable to LMWH (IC$_{50}$, 59.0 ng/mL). The similar activities of PmFS-I – -III (IC$_{50}$ were 87.9 ng/mL, 109 ng/mL and 99.2 ng/mL, respectively) indicated their activity-chain length relationship may be different from dPmFGs. Interestingly, compared the anti-FXase activity of PmFS-III and dTaFG which have the approximate molecular weight, the former was about 7.5-fold stronger than the latter.

According to the chemical structure, PmFS had a similar backbone to dTaFS, while it is uniquely branched with mono-α-L-Fuc linked via α-1,3 glycocidic bond. Intriguingly, PmFG also contained such Fuc branches, and the FG removal of side chains had no significant anticoagulant activity [35]. Besides, the backbone of PmFS was different from PmFG, and the sulfation pattern and distribution of Fuc branches in PmFG and PmFS were also different. PmFG was branched with a sulfated α-L-Fuc in every disaccharide unit, while PmFS possessed a sulfated α-L-Fuc in every trisaccharide unit; and the branch substitutes of PmFG were mainly di-O-sulfated α-L-Fuc, while those of PmFS were mono-O-sulfated α-L-Fuc. The distinctive branch structure of PmFS might contribute to its relatively more potent anticoagulant action compared with FS from other sea cucumbers, and the study of the structure-activity relationship of PmFG and PmFS could provide valuable data to further develop the novel FXase inhibitors.

3. Materials and Methods

3.1. Materials

Dried sea cucumber *P. mollis* was purchased from Guangzhou, China. Amberlite FPA98 anion-exchange resin was obtained from the Rohm and Haas Company (St. Louis, MO, USA). Deuterium oxide (D$_2$O, 99.9% Atom D) was obtained from Sigma-Aldrich (Shanghai, China). LMWH (Enoxaparin, 0.4 mL × 4000 AXaIU) was obtained from Sanofi-Aventis (Paris, France). The activated partial thromboplastin time (APTT), prothrombin time (PT) and thrombin time (TT) reagents, and standard human plasma were obtained from Teco Medical (Neufahrn N.B., Germany). Both Biophen FVIII: C kit and Biophen Heparin Anti-IIa/Anti-Xa kits were obtained from Hyphen Biomed (Paris, France). Human factor VIII was from Bayer HealthCare LLC (Berlin, Germany). All other chemicals were of reagent grade and are commercially available.

3.2. Isolation and Purification of Polysaccharides

Crude polysaccharides were extracted from the body wall of the sea cucumber *P. mollis* according to the method described previously [24,29,30]. Briefly, 300 g dried body wall of *P. mollis* was treated with papain (EC 3.4.22.2), followed by treatment with 0.5 M sodium hydroxide. After neutralization, the mixture was centrifuged at 4000 rpm × 15 min to remove the residues. The supernatant was precipitated by addition of ethanol [final concentration of 40% and 60% (*v*/*v*)] and centrifuged. The two precipitates obtained were designated as Fraction-1 and Fraction-2.

Fraction-1 was decolorized with 3% H$_2$O$_2$ at 45 °C for 2 h (pH 10) according to our previous method [30,31]. The solution was then treated with ethanol at a final concentration of 40% in the presence of KOAc (0.5 M), followed by centrifugation. The precipitate (A) and supernatant (B) were collected. The precipitate (A) was further purified with strong FPA98 ion-exchange chromatography and sequentially eluted with H$_2$O, 0.5 M, 1.0 M, 1.5 M, 2.0 M and 3.0 M NaCl aqueous solution. The 1.5 M NaCl eluate was dialyzed by ultrafiltration with a 3 kDa molecular weight cut-off membrane (Spectrum Laboratories Inc., Piscataway, NJ, USA) and lyophilized to yielded PmFG. The fraction eluted with H$_2$O was collected and further purified by ethanol precipitation (40%, *v*/*v*) in the presence of KOAc (0.5 M). After centrifugation, the supernatant was dialyzed and lyophilized to furnish PmNG-1. Additionally, the supernatant (B) was purified by ethanol precipitation with a final concentration 60%. After centrifugation, the precipitate was lyophilized to give PmNG-2.

Fraction-2 was decolorized using the same method mentioned above. The mixture was also treated with a final concentration of 60% ethanol and followed by centrifugation. The precipitate was collected and further purified by FPA98 ion-exchange chromatography eluted using H$_2$O, 0.5 M, 1.0 M, 1.5 M, 2.0 M and 3.0 M NaCl aqueous solution as eluents. The 2.0 M NaCl fraction was dialyzed by ultrafiltration with a 3 kDa molecular weight cut-off membrane and lyophilized. The ^{1}H NMR spectrum of this fraction showed that it contained some trace amino sugars. Thus, it was further purified by ion-exchange chromatography using a DE-52 column (3.0 cm × 18 cm, GE Healthcare, Uppsala, Sweden) to yield PmFS.

The purity of these polysaccharides was checked by the HPGPC using an Agilent technologies 1200 or 1260 series apparatus (Agilent Co., Santa Clara, CA, USA) equipped with a Shodex OH-pak SB-804 HQ column (8 mm × 300 mm) and RID and DAD. Chromatographic conditions and procedures were performed according to the established method [10,29].

3.3. Analysis of Physicochemical Properties

The optical rotation was measured on the autopol VI, Rudolph research analytical, USA. The sulfate/carboxyl ratio or sulfate group content of PmFG and PmFS was determined by a classic conductimetric method [29].

The Mw values of these polysaccharides were estimated by HPGPC using a Shodex OH-pak SB-804 HQ column (8 mm × 300 mm). Chromatographic conditions and procedures were performed according to the previous method [29]. A standard curve was established by standard D-series Dextrans (D 2–8) and corrected by five reference FG (low molecular weight FG with Mw 27.76 kDa, 13.92 kDa, 8.238 kDa, 5.279 kDa and 3.118 kDa) or by an FS with known molecular weight of 2.5 kDa. Molecular weight calculations were performed by a GPC software, version B01.01 (Agilent Co., Santa Clara, CA, USA).

Monosaccharide compositions of PmFG, PmFS, PmNG-1 and PmNG-2 were determined by HPLC after strong acid hydrolysis and derivatization with PMP according to the procedures in our previous reports [30,32]. Each polysaccharide (2 mg) was dissolved in 2 M trifluoroacetic acid (TFA), then the vessel was sealed and incubated at 110 °C for 4 h in a heating block. Each reaction mixture was then evaporated to remove residual TFA with methanol five times, after which, the samples were dissolved in 500 μL H_2O. Then, 100 μL of each sample solution, 200 μL of 0.5 M PMP in methanol and 100 μL of 0.6M NaOH were mixed and left to react at 70 °C for 30 min. After neutralization, 1 mL of $CHCl_3$ was added to remove the residual PMP (repeated four times). The top aqueous layer was collected for HPLC analysis.

3.4. FT-IR and NMR Spectroscopic Analysis

The FI-IR spectra (KBr pellets) of PmFG, PmFS, PmNG-1 and PmNG-2 (~1 mg) was recorded by Nicolet iS10 (Thermo Fisher, Waltham, MA, USA) in a range of 400–4000 cm^{-1}.

NMR spectra were obtained at 298K in deuterium oxide (D_2O, 99.9% D) by Bruker Avance spectrometer of 600 or 800 MHz, equipped with the $^1H/^{13}C$ dual probe in FT mode as described previously [11]. All samples were dissolved in D_2O and lyophilized three times to replace exchangeable protons with D_2O and then were dissolved in 0.5 mL of 99.9% D_2O at a concentration of 10–20 g/L. The NMR data were analyzed using MestReNova software version 8.0.

3.5. Preparation of dPmFG-I – -III and PmFS-I – -III

As a polysaccharide with a high Mw, PmFG showed broad and overlapped signals in the ^1H NMR spectrum. To further elucidate its structure and study the structure-activity relationship in detail, its depolymerized product, dPmFG, was prepared by H_2O_2 depolymerization according to our previous methods with minor modifications [28,30,36]. PmFG (290 mg) and 2 mg of copper acetate were dissolved in 10.6 mL H_2O. 3.3 mL 10% H_2O_2 solution was added and the mixture was allowed to react at 35 °C for 3 h. Residual H_2O_2 was removed by ethanol precipitation (80%, *v/v*) and the precipitate was collected by centrifugation (4000 rpm × 10 min) three times to give dPmFG. Then, dPmFG was fractionated by Sephadex G-100 column (1.5 cm × 150 cm) to three fractions, designated as dPmFG-I, II and III, according to the molecular weight difference. When compared with FS, which possesses linear structures as reported in previous literature [5,24,31], PmFS was branched by α-L-Fuc monosaccharide in every trifucose unit. To further study its structure-activity relationship in detail, PmFS was also fractionated by Sephadex G-50 (1.5 cm × 150 cm) chromatography to yield PmFS-I, II and III. Each fraction had a different molecular weight and showed a narrower molecular weight distribution than PmFS.

3.6. Anticoagulant Activity Assays

The anticoagulant activity was detected using APTT, PT and TT reagents and standard human plasma on a coagulometer (TECO MC-4000, Neufahrn N.B., Germany) as previously described [10,29].

According to our previous method [5,10], the inhibition of intrinsic FXase was measured using the BIOPHEN FVIII: C kits and recombinant human FVIII. The anti-FIIa and anti-FXa activities in the presence of AT were determined using BIOPHEN Heparin Anti-FIIa kits and Heparin Anti-FXa kits, respectively.

4. Conclusions

In this work, two types of sulfated polysaccharides, PmFG and PmFS, were purified from *P. mollis*. Their physicochemical properties and chemical structures were analyzed and characterized. PmFG comprised a CS-like backbone and monosaccharide branches of sulfated L-Fuc (including Fuc_{2S4S},

Fuc$_{3S4S}$ and Fuc$_{4S}$ with a molar ratio of 2:2.5:1) linked to the GlcA of the backbone via α-1,3 glycosidic bonds. Particularly, PmFS is structurally distinct from some FS from other sea cucumbers. It has a backbone consisting of repetitively linked {-4-L-Fuc$_{2S}$-α-1-} and unique sulfated Fuc branches (Fuc$_{4S}$ or Fuc$_{3S}$ with a molar ratio of 4:1) linked to the backbone also via α-1,3 glycosidic bonds.

Anticoagulant assays indicated that both PmFG and PmFS possessed strong APTT prolonging activity and intrinsic FXase inhibitory activity. Interestingly, when compared with the FS from other sea cucumbers reported previously, PmFS showed relatively potent anti-FXase activity, which might be attributed to its distinct structure of sulfated Fuc branches. The structures and anti-FXase activity of PmFS and PmFG were compared to further clarify their structure-activity relationship.

Author Contributions: W.Z. performed the experiment and wrote the draft. L.Z. (Lutan Zhou) and H.S. assayed the anticoagulant activities. R.Y., Y.C. and N.G. and L.Z. (Longyan Zhao) guided the purification and depolymerization. R.Y., L.Z. (Lutan Zhou) and L.L. revised the manuscript. L.Z. (Longyan Zhao) provided the sea cucumber. J.Z. was the supervisor, designed the experiment and revised the manuscript.

Funding: This research was funded by the National Natural Science Foundation of China (Nos. 81773737, 81703374 and 31600649).

Acknowledgments: We thank Xiaohuo Shi and Jianchao Chen (Kunming Institute of Botany, Chinese Academy of Sciences) for performing the NMR experiments.

Conflicts of Interest: The authors declare no conflict of interest.

References

1. Bordbar, S.; Anwar, F.; Saari, N. High-value components and bioactivities from sea cucumbers for functional foods-A review. *Mar. Drugs* **2011**, *9*, 1761–1805. [CrossRef] [PubMed]
2. Pomin, V.H. Holothurian fucosylated chondroitin sulfate. *Mar. Drugs* **2014**, *12*, 232–254. [CrossRef] [PubMed]
3. Chen, S.G.; Xue, C.H.; Yin, L.; Tang, Q.J.; Yu, G.L.; Chai, W.G. Comparison of structures and anticoagulant activities of fucosylated chondroitin sulfates from different sea cucumbers. *Carbohydr. Polym.* **2011**, *83*, 688–696. [CrossRef]
4. Yang, J.; Wang, Y.H.; Jiang, T.F.; Lv, Z.H. Novel branch patterns and anticoagulant activity of glycosaminoglycan from sea cucumber *Apostichopus japonicus*. *Int. J. Biol. Macromol.* **2015**, *72*, 911–918. [CrossRef]
5. Shang, F.N.; Mou, R.R.; Zhang, Z.D.; Gao, N.; Lin, L.S.; Li, Z.; Wu, M.Y.; Zhao, J.H. Structural analysis and anticoagulant activities of three highly regular fucan sulfates as novel intrinsic factor Xase inhibitors. *Carbohydr. Polym.* **2018**, *195*, 257–266. [CrossRef]
6. Kariya, Y.; Mulloy, B.; Imai, K.; Tominaga, A.; Kaneko, T.; Asari, A.; Suzuki, K.; Masuda, H.; Kyogashima, M.; Ishii, T. Isolation and partial characterization of fucan sulfates from the body wall of sea cucumber *Stichopus japonicus* and their ability to inhibit osteoclastogenesis. *Carbohydr. Res.* **2004**, *339*, 1339–1346. [CrossRef]
7. Huang, N.; Wu, M.Y.; Zheng, C.B.; Zhu, L.; Zhao, J.H.; Zheng, Y.T. The depolymerized fucosylated chondroitin sulfate from sea cucumber potently inhibits HIV replication via interfering with virus entry. *Carbohydr. Res.* **2013**, *380*, 64–69. [CrossRef] [PubMed]
8. Wu, M.Y.; Wen, D.D.; Gao, N.; Xiao, C.; Yang, L.; Xu, L.; Lian, W.; Peng, W.L.; Jiang, J.M.; Zhao, J.H. Anticoagulant and antithrombotic evaluation of native fucosylated chondroitin sulfates and their derivatives as selective inhibitors of intrinsic factor Xase. *Eur. J. Med. Chem.* **2015**, *92*, 257–269. [CrossRef]
9. Borsig, L.; Wang, L.; Cavalcante, M.C.; Cardilo-Reis, L.; Ferreira, P.L.; Mourão, P.A.; Esko, J.D.; Pavão, M.S. Selectin blocking activity of a fucosylated chondroitin sulfate glycosaminoglycan from sea cucumber. Effect on tumor metastasis and neutrophil recruitment. *J. Biol. Chem.* **2007**, *282*, 14984–14991. [CrossRef]
10. Zhao, L.Y.; Wu, M.Y.; Xiao, C.; Yang, L.; Zhou, L.T.; Gao, N.; Li, Z.; Chen, J.; Chen, J.C.; Liu, J.K.; et al. Discovery of an intrinsic tenase complex inhibitor: Pure nonasaccharide from fucosylated glycosaminoglycan. *Proc. Natl. Acad. Sci. USA* **2015**, *112*, 8284–8289. [CrossRef]
11. Yin, R.H.; Zhou, L.T.; Gao, N.; Li, Z.; Zhao, L.Y.; Shang, F.N.; Wu, M.Y.; Zhao, J.H. Oligosaccharides from depolymerized fucosylated glycosaminoglycan: Structures and minimum size for intrinsic factor Xase complex inhibition. *J. Biol. Chem.* **2018**, *293*, 14089–14099. [CrossRef]

12. Mourão, P.A.; Bastos, I.G. Highly acidic glycans from sea cucumbers. Isolation and fractionation of fucose-rich sulfated polysaccharides from the body wall of *Ludwigothurea grisea*. *Eur. J. Biochem.* **1987**, *166*, 639–645. [CrossRef] [PubMed]

13. Kariya, Y.; Watabe, S.; Hashimoto, K.; Yoshida, K. Occurrence of chondroitin sulfate E in glycosaminoglycan isolated from the body wall of sea cucumber *Stichopus japonicus*. *J Biol. Chem.* **1990**, *265*, 5081–5085. [PubMed]

14. Vieira, R.P.; Pedrosa, C.; Mourão, P.A. Extensive heterogeneity of proteoglycans bearing fucose-branched chondroitin sulfate extracted from the connective tissue of sea cucumber. *Biochemistry* **1993**, *32*, 2254–2262. [CrossRef] [PubMed]

15. Yoshida, K.I.; Minami, Y.; Nemoto, H.; Numata, K.; Yamanaka, E. Structure of DHG, a depolymerized glycosaminoglycan from sea cucumber, *Stichopus japonicus*. *Tetrahedron Lett.* **1992**, *33*, 4959–4962. [CrossRef]

16. Kariya, Y.; Watabe, S.; Kyogashima, M.; Ishihara, M.; Ishii, T. Structure of fucose branches in the glycosaminoglycan from the body wall of the sea cucumber *Stichopus japonicus*. *Carbohydr. Res.* **1997**, *297*, 273–279. [CrossRef]

17. Kariya, Y.; Watanabe, S.; Ochiai, Y.; Murata, K. Glycosaminoglycan from the body wall of the sea cucumber *Stichopus japonicas*. *Comp. Biochem. Physiol. B Biochem. Mol. Biol.* **1990**, *95*, 387–392. [CrossRef]

18. Katzman, R.L.; Jeanloz, R.W. Acid polysaccharides from invertebrate connective tissue: phylogenetic aspects. *Science* **1969**, *166*, 758–759. [CrossRef] [PubMed]

19. Holtkamp, A.D.; Kelly, S.; Ulber, R.; Lang, S. Fucoidans and fucoidanases-focus on techniques for molecular structure elucidation and modification of marine polysaccharides. *Appl. Microbiol. Biotechnol.* **2009**, *82*, 1–11. [CrossRef]

20. Pomin, V.H.; Mourão, P.A.S. Structure, biology, evolution, and medical importance of sulfated fucans and galactans. *Glycobiology* **2008**, *18*, 1016–1027. [CrossRef]

21. Chevolot, L.; Mulloy, B.; Ratiskol, J.; Foucault, A.; Colliec-Jouault, S. A disaccharide repeat unit is the major structure in fucoidans from two species of brown algae. *Carbohydr. Res.* **2001**, *330*, 529–535. [CrossRef]

22. Pereira, M.S.; Mulloy, B.; Mourão, P.A.S. Structure and anticoagulant activity of sulfated fucans: comparison between the regular, repetitive and linear fucans from echinoderms with the more heterogeneous and branched polymers from brown algae. *J. Biol. Chem.* **1999**, *274*, 7656–7667. [CrossRef] [PubMed]

23. Yu, L.; Ge, L.; Xue, C.; Chang, Y.; Zhang, C.; Xu, X.; Wang, Y. Structural study of fucoidan from sea cucumber *Acaudina molpadioides*: a fucoidan containing novel tetra-fucose repeating unit. *Food Chem.* **2014**, *142*, 197–200. [CrossRef] [PubMed]

24. Wu, M.Y.; Xu, L.; Zhao, L.Y.; Xiao, C.; Gao, N.; Luo, L.; Yang, L.; Li, Z.; Chen, L.Y.; Zhao, J.H. Structural analysis and anticoagulant activities of the novel sulfated fucan possessing a regular well-defined repeating unit from sea cucumber. *Mar. Drugs* **2015**, *13*, 2063–2084. [CrossRef] [PubMed]

25. Berteau, O.; Mulloy, B. Sulfated fucans, fresh perspectives: structures, functions, and biological properties of sulfated fucans and an overview of enzymes active toward this class of polysaccharide. *Glycobiology* **2003**, *13*, 29R–40R. [CrossRef] [PubMed]

26. Pomin, V.H. Review: An overview about the structure-function relationship of marine sulfated homopolysaccharides with regular chemical structures. *Biopolymers* **2009**, *91*, 601–609. [CrossRef] [PubMed]

27. Pomin, V.H. Sulfated glycans in inflammation. *Eur. J. Med. Chem.* **2015**, *92*, 353–369. [CrossRef]

28. Yang, W.J.; Cai, Y.; Yin, R.H.; Lin, L.S.; Li, Z.; Wu, M.Y.; Zhao, J.H. Structural analysis and anticoagulant activities of two sulfated polysaccharides from the sea cucumber *Holothuria coluber*. *Int. J. Biol. Macromol.* **2018**, *115*, 1055–1062. [CrossRef]

29. Luo, L.; Wu, M.Y.; Xu, L.; Lian, W.; Xiang, J.Y.; Lu, F.; Gao, N.; Xiao, C.; Wang, S.M.; Zhao, J.H. Comparison of physicochemical characteristics and anticoagulant activities of polysaccharides from three sea cucumbers. *Mar. Drugs* **2013**, *11*, 399–417. [CrossRef]

30. Li, X.M.; Luo, L.; Cai, Y.; Yang, W.J.; Lin, L.S.; Li, Z.; Gao, N.; Purcell, S.W.; Wu, M.Y.; Zhao, J.H. Structural elucidation and biological activity of a highly regular fucosylated glycosaminoglycan from the edible sea cucumber *Stichopus herrmanni*. *J. Agric. Food Chem.* **2017**, *65*, 9315–9323. [CrossRef]

31. Cai, Y.; Yang, W.J.; Yin, R.H.; Zhou, L.T.; Li, Z.; Wu, M.Y.; Zhao, J.H. An anticoagulant fucan sulfate with hexasaccharide repeating units from the sea cucumber *Holothuria albiventer*. *Carbohydr. Res.* **2018**, *464*, 12–18. [CrossRef] [PubMed]

32. Liu, J.; Zhou, L.T.; He, Z.C.; Gao, N.; Shang, F.N.; Xu, J.P.; Li, Z.; Yang, Z.M.; Wu, M.Y.; Zhao, J.H. Structural analysis and biological activity of a highly regular glycosaminoglycan from *Achatina fulica*. *Carbohydr. Polym.* **2018**, *181*, 433–441. [CrossRef] [PubMed]

33. Vieira, R.P.; Mulloy, B.; Mourão, P.A.S. Structure of a fucose-branched chondroitin sulfate from sea cucumber. *J. Biol. Chem.* **1991**, *266*, 13530–13536. [PubMed]

34. Shang, F.N.; Gao, N.; Yin, R.H.; Lin, L.S.; Xiao, C.; Zhou, L.T.; Li, Z.; Purcell, S.W.; Wu, M.Y.; Zhao, J.H. Precise structures of fucosylated glycosaminoglycan and its oligosaccharides as novel intrinsic factor Xase inhibitors. *Eur. J. Med. Chem.* **2018**, *148*, 423–435. [CrossRef] [PubMed]

35. Wu, M.Y.; Huang, R.; Wen, D.D.; Gao, N.; He, J.B.; Li, Z.; Zhao, J.H. Structure and effect of sulfated fucose branches on anticoagulant activity of the fucosylated chondroitin sulfate from sea cucumber *Thelenata ananas*. *Carbohydr. Polym.* **2012**, *87*, 862–868. [CrossRef]

36. Wu, M.Y.; Xu, S.M.; Zhao, J.H.; Kang, H.; Ding, H. Physicochemical characteristics and anticoagulant activities of low molecular weight fractions by free-radical depolymerization of a fucosylated chondroitin sulphate from sea cucumber *Thelenata ananas*. *Food Chem.* **2010**, *122*, 716–723. [CrossRef]

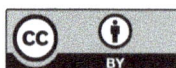

marine drugs

MDPI

Article

The Sialic Acid-Dependent Nematocyst Discharge Process in Relation to Its Physical-Chemical Properties Is a Role Model for Nanomedical Diagnostic and Therapeutic Tools

Ruiyan Zhang [1,*], Li Jin [1], Ning Zhang [1,2], Athanasios K. Petridis [3], Thomas Eckert [4,5,6], Georgios Scheiner-Bobis [4], Martin Bergmann [7], Axel Scheidig [8], Roland Schauer [9], Mingdi Yan [10], Samurdhi A. Wijesundera [10], Bengt Nordén [11], Barun K. Chatterjee [12] and Hans-Christian Siebert [2,*]

[1] Institute of BioPharmaceutical Research, Liaocheng University, Liaocheng 252059, China
[2] RI-B-NT—Research Institute of Bioinformatics and Nanotechnology, Schauenburgerstr. 116, 24118 Kiel, Germany
[3] Neurochirurgische Klinik, Universität Düsseldorf, Geb. 11.54, Moorenstraße 5, 40255 Düsseldorf, Germany
[4] Institut für Veterinärphysiolgie und-Biochemie, Fachbereich Veterinärmedizin, Justus-Liebig-Universität Gießen, Frankfurter Str. 100, 35392 Gießen, Germany
[5] Department of Chemistry and Biology, University of Applied Sciences Fresenius, Limburger Str. 2, 65510 Idstein, Germany
[6] RISCC—Research Institute for Scientific Computing and Consulting, Ludwig-Schunk-Str. 15, 65510 Heuchelheim, Germany
[7] Institut für Veterinäranatomie, Histologie und Embryologie, Fachbereich Veterinärmedizin, Justus-Liebig-Universität Gießen, Frankfurter Str. 98, 35392 Giessen, Germany
[8] Zoologisches Institut-Strukturbiologie, Zentrum für Biochemie und Molekularbiologie, Christian-Albrechts-Universität, Am Botanischen Garten 19, 24118 Kiel, Germany
[9] Biochemisches Institut, Christian-Albrechts Universität Kiel, Olshausenstrasse 40, 24098 Kiel, Germany
[10] Department of Chemistry, University of Massachusetts Lowell, 1 University Avenue, Lowell, MA 01854, USA
[11] Department of Chemical and Biological Engineering, Chalmers University of Technology, SE-41296 Gothenburg, Sweden
[12] Department of Physics, Bose Institute, 93/1, A P C Road, Kolkata 700009, India
* Correspondence: zry147896@163.com (R.Z.); hcsiebert@aol.com (H.C.S.)

Received: 1 June 2019; Accepted: 6 August 2019; Published: 12 August 2019

check for updates

Abstract: Formulas derived from theoretical physics provide important insights about the nematocyst discharge process of Cnidaria (Hydra, jellyfishes, box-jellyfishes and sea-anemones). Our model description of the fastest process in living nature raises and answers questions related to the material properties of the cell- and tubule-walls of nematocysts including their polysialic acid (polySia) dependent target function. Since a number of tumor-cells, especially brain-tumor cells such as neuroblastoma tissues carry the polysaccharide chain polySia in similar concentration as fish eggs or fish skin, it makes sense to use these findings for new diagnostic and therapeutic approaches in the field of nanomedicine. Therefore, the nematocyst discharge process can be considered as a bionic blue-print for future nanomedical devices in cancer diagnostics and therapies. This approach is promising because the physical background of this process can be described in a sufficient way with formulas presented here. Additionally, we discuss biophysical and biochemical experiments which will allow us to define proper boundary conditions in order to support our theoretical model approach. PolySia glycans occur in a similar density on malignant tumor cells than on the cell surfaces of Cnidarian predators and preys. The knowledge of the polySia-dependent initiation of the nematocyst discharge process in an intact nematocyte is an essential prerequisite regarding the further development of target-directed nanomedical devices for diagnostic and therapeutic purposes. The theoretical description as well as the computationally and experimentally derived results about the biophysical and biochemical parameters can contribute to a proper design of anti-tumor drug ejecting vessels which use a stylet-tubule system. Especially, the role of nematogalectins is of interest because these bridging proteins contribute as well as special collagen fibers to the elastic band properties. The basic concepts of the nematocyst discharge process inside the tubule cell walls of nematocysts were studied in jellyfishes and in Hydra which are ideal model organisms. Hydra has already been chosen by Alan Turing in order to figure out how the chemical basis of morphogenesis can be described in a fundamental way. This encouraged us to discuss the action of nematocysts in relation to morphological aspects and material requirements. Using these insights, it is now possible to discuss natural and artificial nematocyst-like vessels with optimized properties for a diagnostic and therapeutic use, e.g., in neurooncology. We show here that crucial physical parameters such as pressure thresholds and elasticity properties during the nematocyst discharge process can be described in a consistent and satisfactory way with an impact on the construction of new nanomedical devices.

Keywords: nematocyst discharge process; theoretical model; polysialic acid (polySia); nematogalectin; nanomedical devices

---

1. Introduction

The structural development of Hydras can be discussed under the general aspects of morphology generation as it has been published by Alan Turing in his pioneering paper already in the year 1952 [1]. Hydra is an ideal organism to study morphogenetic models directly derived from the laws of mathematics, theoretical physics and biophysical chemistry. We focus on different Cnidaria species as model organisms in general because their biological principles, especially the nematocyst discharge processes are not too complex for descriptions which originate from mathematics and theoretical physics. This is therefore a proper example which shows that complex processes in living nature can be described with such methods [1–9]. These model descriptions have to be combined with data from structural biology and biochemistry. The nematocyst capsule is filled with γ-glutamate polymers, which binds a 2 M concentration of cations, thereby generating a high osmotic internal pressure of more than 15 MPa [10,11]. A sialic acid dependent chemical-mechanic trigger initiates exocytosis in a living model organism [12,13].

The nematocyst ejects a stylet with a highly elastic tubule under the pressure of nearly 7 GPa and a velocity of over 15 m/s [14]. This punches a hole into the prey's integument and toxins are injected. In this case, one can identify nearly identical surface signatures on the cells of preys or predators and on malignant tumor cells a nematocyst-like device could be the bionic blue-print of a new nanomedical approach in cancer diagnostic and therapy. Since the nematocyst has a mechanic-chemical receptor on its surface which interacts with polysialic acid (polySia) fragments and protein-like contact-molecules in a specific way, the corresponding glycan moieties are proper candidates. PolySia occurs on the cell surfaces of cnidarians preys and predators as well as on many tumor cells. We have chosen nematocysts from Hydra and tissue materials from certain jellyfishes in order to start our theoretical and experimental analysis. Hydra and other cnidarian organisms have proven that these organisms are feasible objects to study biological phenomena such as immunological principles and stem cell maintenance [15–21]. Carbohydrate-protein interactions play an important role in interaction processes on cell surfaces [22–29]. When the nematocyst discharge process is studied on a molecular level, carbohydrate-protein interactions are of central importance. It has been proven by Alan Turing on a fundamental morphological level that differential equations describe the time-dependence of activator and inhibitor concentrations in Hydra. Such equations can be solved and used for computational simulations which are in accordance with the Gierer-Meinhardt model [3–5,30]. The nematocyst discharge process itself is often characterized as a kind of Coulomb explosion which has recently been discussed for a different phenomenon in anorganic chemistry, analytic chemistry and material sciences [31–33]. We argue here that the central effect of the nematocyst discharge process, the expulsion of the stylet is only loosely related to the Coulomb explosions described in the literature cited above. The nematocyst discharge process is initiated by Coulombic stress due to the buildup of charge inside the nematocyst and at some threshold values of this stress the stylet is ejected explosively (suddenly and with large acceleration). It is therefore obvious that the nematocyst discharge process should be described successfully with formulas from theoretical physics. Further insights concerning the boundary conditions of the discharge process in respect to material requirements and surrounding conditions are provided by biophysical experiments such as QCM (Quartz Crystal Microbalance) methods, EM - Electron Microscopy (especially TEM—Transmission Electron Microscopy), AFM—Atomic Force Microscopy, SPR—Surface Plasmon Resonance, MS—Mass Spectrometry and NMR—Nuclear Magnetic Resonance techniques. Furthermore, X-ray crystallographic structure models from the protein data bank are essential to construct nematogalectin architectures which show the bridging activity of these molecules with proteoglycan fragments in the tubule cell wall. The nano-architecture in which mini-collagens, proteoglycans and nematogalectins are involved is responsible for the physical properties of the nematocyst membrane and the tubule system to which the stylet is connected [21].

The main components of the capsule wall of nematocysts, the explosive organelles of Hydra, jellyfish, corals and other Cnidaria, are collagens which are termed mini-collagens because of their shortest known collagen-like sequence of Gly-Xaa-Yaa repeats. Mini-collagens are the major components of the Hydra nematocysts capsule wall where they form a tight three-dimensional network by disulfide reassembling of their terminal cysteine-rich domains. Mini-collagens contain a short collagen triple helix flanked by polyproline stretches and terminal cysteine-rich domains. These N- and C-terminal proline- and cystine-rich domains of mini-collagen-1 are relatively short peptides (23 and 24 residues, respectively) containing 6 cysteine residues in an identical sequence pattern. The related synthetic peptides were found to refold in an oxidation process almost quantitatively into one topoisomer. Surprisingly, the two refolded domains exhibit different cystine frameworks despite their identical cysteine pattern and a high sequence homology. Therefore, the structural elements responsible for their distinct structures were analyzed to gain possible information about the mechanisms of mini-collagen disulfide rearrangement in their assembly into polymeric fibers. With better information on this process, mini-collagens containing functional domains of type I and IV collagens could be used for the preparation of mechanically highly resistant frameworks for cell adhesion and thus constitute promising innovative biomaterials [34]. However, their architecture is also of interest when nematocyts in various intact nematocytes are tested concerning its diagnostic feasibility when coming into contact with sialic acid coated surfaces. It is possible to reference the corresponding molecular concentration and density with tailor-made sialic acid-coated nanoparticles as outlined later. Sialic acids trigger the initiation of the Coulomb repulsion inside the nematocyst in an intact nematocyte. In this initiation process sialic acid mediated protein–carbohydrate interactions on the surfaces of nematocysts play a crucial role. It is our aim to figure out whether such bionic concepts provide guidelines for nanomedical and nanopharmaceutical devices in order to improve cancer diagnostic and therapies. The chemical and mechanical properties of the nanomedical tools from cnidarian origin can be studied in an ideal way when using first the well described Hydra nematocysts as blueprints. We show here that classical physics in combination with structural biology and theoretic biochemistry [1,2,7–9,24,35–41] is essential for an accelerated biophysical development of new diagnostic strategies analyzing the spread of highly-malignant tumor cells. It has to be emphasized here that this is only possible with in intact nematocytes. The corresponding vessels in a living nematocyte must have a robust consistence which enable them to resist the forces of a nematocyst discharge process. As outlined by 't Hooft [9]: "Instruments of atomic dimensions could be used for any purpose imaginable, but particularly in medical sciences. Remote controlled robots could be sent to any part of the human body to resolve problems. Less advanced, passive robots could be attached to capsules containing medications; the capsules would be injected into the body, with the robots ensuring administration of the medication in the right dosages for weeks or even years." Our approach discussed here emphasizes that blueprints of bionic robot systems already exist in form of Cnidaria nematocysts which can be used due to their molecular interaction specificity, as nanomedical tools. This is extremely promising because of their polySia-directed target function as diagnostic and therapeutic devices in order to identify tumor tissues, especially, polysialic acid rich cancer cells coated in a highly characteristic way which often remain in the tumor-hole after a neurosurgical intervention due to its location in close proximity to crucial regions of the brain.

2. Results

The morphologies and consistencies of the drug-containing vessels (Figure 1) and their potential targets (Figure 2) were analyzed in detail using electron microscopy (EM), especially, transmission electron microscopy. The structural parameters obtained from Figure 1 are essential to define the boundary conditions of our theoretical model which is described below. When analyzing potential target structures for the drug-containing vessels, it turned out that malignant neuroblasts from a neuroblastoma cell line show peculiar bubble-like morphologies in the electron microscopical pictures (see arrows in Figure 2). This argues in favor of an alteration in the surface consistency of the corresponding cell membranes and the existence of peculiar topologies of special target regions. Besides the occurrence of polySia moieties on the tumor cells, such topological and morphological data are of highest importance to identify the Achilles heel of cancer cells. Furthermore, an extremely robust but also elastic consistency of the targeting cells is essential for our nanomedical devices. Under special consideration are here the nematocyte wall and the stylet-connected tubule system. The stylets of the nematocysts are ejected by a specific biological signal (sialic acids, especially polySia) which is present on fish eggs but also on various tumor cells [42,43]. The consistence of the collagen strands and of the nematogalectins which occur in the tubule walls [44,45] have to be studied on a sub-molecular level. This is also the case for the proteoglycans [36] in the nematocyst's cell wall and the collagens in the exumbrella tissue of jellyfishes after their extraction. It turned out that biophysical methods which are based on QCM (Quartz Crystal Microbalance) techniques are feasible and helpful tools (Table 1) for testing the state of the extracted collagen-strands of jellyfish exumbrella tissues (Table 1).

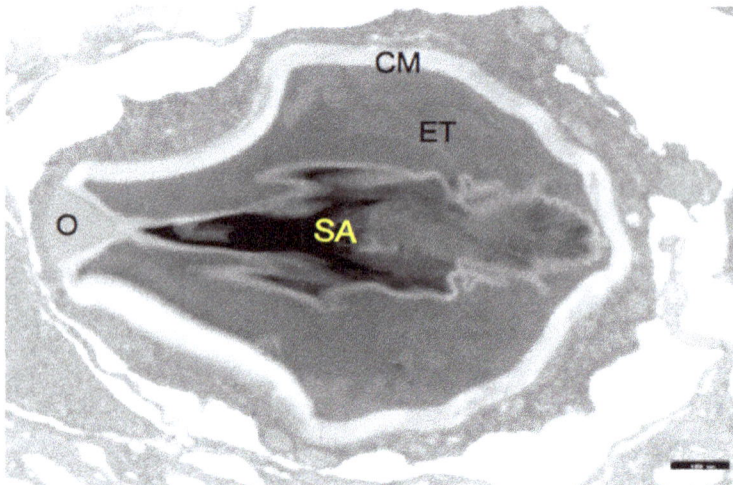

Figure 1. Structure of a Hydra nematocyst: Stylet apparatus with large and small spines (SA), external tubule (ET), capsule membrane (CM), operculum (O). The black scale bar in the lower right corner corresponds to 1 μm.

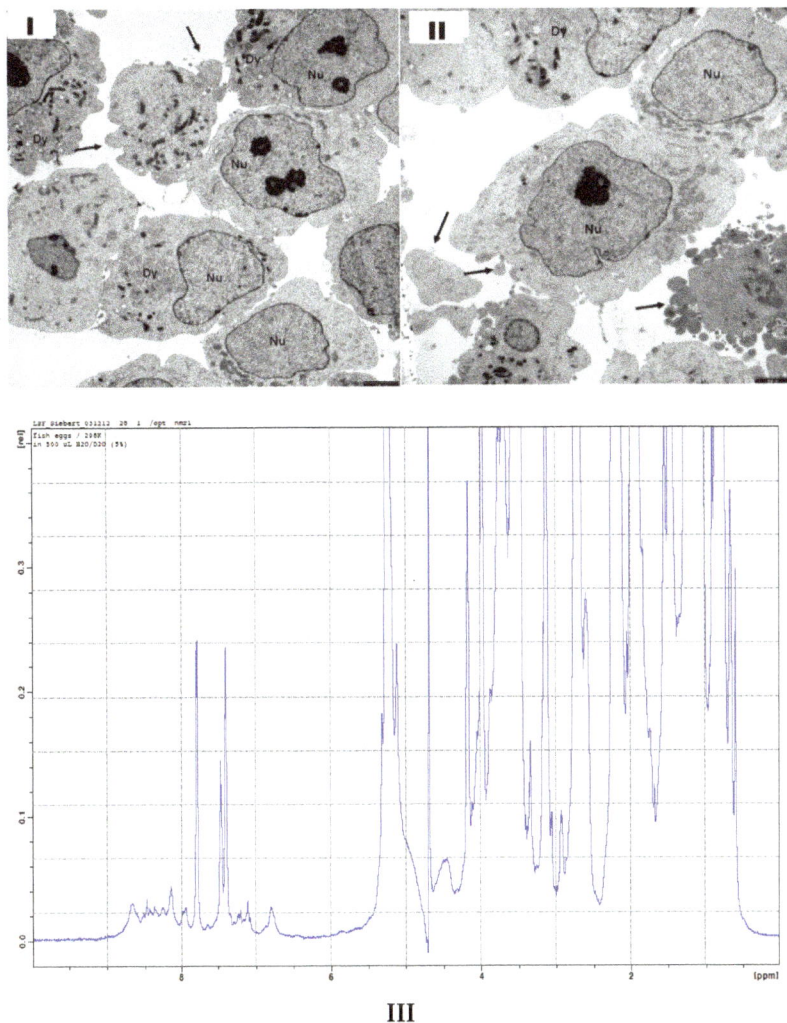

Figure 2. Structures of (**I,II**) neuroblastoma cells from a cell-line as revealed by transmission electron microscopy (TEM). Neuroblastoma cells show differences in their plasticity which could be of importance for an attack with a nanomedical device. (**III**) 1D proton NMR spectrum of broken fish eggs after their destruction in a nematocyst discharge process. A comparison with a 1D proton NMR spectrum of intact fish eggs is shown in Supplementary Materials.

A theoretical model which is discussed under Section 2.1 can be used to analyze experimental data in a more sophisticated way. As documented in Figure 1; Figure 2 nematocyst cells from Hydra and brain-tumor cells with a high concentration of polySia molecules on their surface as well as fish-eggs with a comparable polySia density are available for complementary biophysical and biochemical experiments. The theoretical model provides a clear standard description in which certain physical parameters are addressed. NMR experiments in which fish-eggs are used [46] as suited model targets, e.g., (Figure 2III), can be designed in a better way when the theoretical model description is applied in a suited way. Furthermore, the influence of certain ions on the nematocyst discharge process can be studied in the framework of certain NMR experiments in order to shed light on questions which are related to neurological diseases and mental disorders [47]. In full agreement with Alan Turing's vision, it is indeed possible to use the partial simplicity of cnidarian organisms to answer basic questions with tools from applied mathematics and theoretical physics.

2.1. Theoretical Model

We describe the discharge of the nematocyst as a five-stage process. The first stage comprises the triggering of the cnidocil, where an external chemical-mechanical signal provides the key-signal for the Coulomb explosion. After the process has been started by the external signal, it is translated to an internal Ca^{2+} signal initiating the next stage of the discharge process. In the second stage, a chemical trigger initiates proteolysis in the poly-γ-glutamic acid (PGGA) resulting in an increase of the H^+ concentration in the nematocyst. Since the diffusion constant of H^+ in water is large, ambipolar diffusion of H^+ through the semipermeable wall of the nematocyst leaves behind a negatively charged matrix. The electrostatic potential developed between the centre of the nematocyst and the surface, is termed the Donnan potential. The charge density distribution in the nematocyst would be ideally governed by the expression:

$$\nabla^2 \ln\left(1 + \frac{\rho}{en_0}\right) = \frac{\mu\rho}{\varepsilon D} \tag{1}$$

where n_0 is the initial concentration of H^+ ions, μ is the mobility and D is the diffusion constant of H^+ ions through the membrane and ε is the dielectric constant.

In the third stage, the charge density of the negatively charged matrix would give rise to a high pressure which would be governed by

$$p = -\frac{\partial U}{\partial V} \tag{2}$$

where V is the volume of the nematocyst and U is the internal energy (electrostatic potential energy). The internal energy is given as:

$$U = \frac{1}{2}\int \rho(\vec{r})\int \frac{\rho(\vec{r'})}{4\pi\varepsilon|\vec{r}-\vec{r'}|}dV'dV \tag{3}$$

where ρ is the charge density. When the pressure exceeds a threshold value, the operculum opens up and after a second threshold the stylet, which is held back by a tough collagen bottle-neck, overcomes the restraint and is ejected at an immense speed. This stage could be termed as the Coulomb explosion stage as the movements take place at nanosecond time scales. Subsequently it gives rise to accelerations in the range of few million times that due to gravity and this explosive process is initiated by Coulomb repulsion, which is very much like a Coulomb explosion.

In the fourth stage, the opercular chamber is distended by the proteolysis of the matrix in the opercular chamber and loss of H^+ ion from it. This further pushes out the stylet thereby locking it with barbs in the victim or in some cases disposes off the outer sheath of the stylet. In the fifth stage, the tubule everts (i.e., turns inside out) through the hollow stylet and itself, exposing the poisonous barbs into its victim.

Here, assuming a homogeneous and spherical nematocyst we get

$$\frac{1}{r^2}\frac{\partial}{\partial r}r^2\frac{\partial}{\partial r}\ln\left(1 + \frac{\rho}{en_0}\right) = \frac{\mu\rho}{\varepsilon D} \tag{4}$$

which can be scaled to a dimensionless form with $\lambda = \sqrt{\frac{\mu e n_0}{\varepsilon D}}$, $x = \lambda r$ and $y = \frac{\rho}{en_0} = y(x)$, as,

$$\frac{1}{x^2}\frac{d}{dx}x^2\frac{d}{dx}\ln(1+y) = y \tag{5}$$

Here n_0 is the initial number density of $[H^+]$, $\rho = -e(n_0 - n)$ is the charge density, μ and D are the mobility and diffusion constant of $[H^+]$ through the semipermeable membrane, ε is the dielectric constant of water and e is the charge of the electron.

The boundary conditions $y(\infty) = 0$ and $y'(\infty) = 0$ does not aid in the solution of this nonlinear equation and does not reflect the spherical shape of the nematocyst. Since the charge buildup would be mostly near the inner surface of the nematocyst, a simple linear model is used, which would be valid near the surface $u = R - r$ of the nematocyst and also assuming that $\rho \ll en_0$ one can write

$$\frac{d^2}{du^2}\rho = \lambda^2\rho \tag{6}$$

which can be solved to give $\rho = -en_0\exp(-\lambda(R-r)) = \rho_0\exp(-\lambda(R-r))$, assuming that at $r = R$ all H^+ has diffused out.

This gives the Coulombic self-potential energy as U as

$$U = \frac{2\pi\rho_0^2}{\lambda^5\varepsilon}\left\{\left(X^3 - \frac{7}{2}X^2 + \frac{11}{2}X - \frac{11}{4}\right) - 4(X-1)\exp(-X) - \frac{5}{4}\exp(-2X)\right\} \tag{7}$$

where $X = \lambda R$ and a Donnan potential

$$\varphi = \frac{\rho_0}{\lambda^2\varepsilon}\{(X-1) + \exp(-X)\} \tag{8}$$

This gives rise to the Coulombic pressure $(p = -\frac{\partial U}{\partial V})$ which gives

$$p = \frac{\rho_0^2}{2\varepsilon\lambda^2 X^2}\left\{\begin{array}{c}-\left(3X^2 - 7X + \frac{11}{2} + 4(X-2)\exp(-X) + \frac{5}{2}\exp(-2X)\right) \\ +\frac{4(X-1+\exp(-X))\left[\left(X^3 - \frac{7}{2}X^2 + \frac{11}{2}X - \frac{11}{4}\right) - 4(X-1)\exp(-X) - \frac{5}{4}\exp(-2X)\right]}{(X^2-2X+2-2\exp(-2X))}\end{array}\right\} \tag{9}$$

One easily observes that in the limit $\lambda \to 0$ (a homogeneously charged sphere) this reduces to the usual

$$p = \frac{\rho_0^2 R^2}{15\varepsilon} \tag{10}$$

with a Donnan potential $\varphi = \frac{\rho_0 R^2}{2\varepsilon}$, and, in the limit $\lambda \to \infty$ (a thin spherical shell of charge, with surface density $\sigma = \rho_0/\lambda$) this reduces to the usual

$$p = \frac{\sigma^2}{2\varepsilon} \tag{11}$$

with a Donnan potential $\varphi = \frac{\sigma R}{\varepsilon}$.

The stylet emission is governed by the equation of a static balance of forces

$$\pi\beta^2 p = \left(-\frac{\partial\beta}{\partial\xi}\right)_{\xi>\xi_1} \frac{2\pi\alpha Y(\beta - \beta_0)}{\beta_0} \tag{12}$$

where the term on the left is the force on the stylet due to the Coulomb pressure, while the term on the right hand side is the restoring force on the stylet due to elastic materials (the elasticity of the nematocyst wall and the escape orifice is provided by minicollagen fibrils) restraining the emission of the stylet. The elastic material restraining the stylet is forced to be extended to the radius $\beta(p)$ from the unstretched radius β_0 due to the pressure p. The radius (β) of the stylet is assumed to be a function of the axial position (ξ) and that the maximum radius of the stylet occurs at ξ_1. The Young's modulus of the elastic material surrounding the stylet is Y and is of a cross section α.

Assuming that the shape of the stylus is governed by the equation

$$\beta = \frac{a\xi(1-\xi)}{d+\xi}$$ (13)

where β is the radius at the axial position ξ, with slopes of al/d and $-al/(d+l)$ at $\xi = 0$ and l, and a maximum radius $\beta_x = a\left(1 + 2d - 2\sqrt{d(1+d)}\right)$ at $\xi_1 = \sqrt{d(1+d)}$. For certain values of a, l and d, it looks like a carrot (e.g., $a = 0.2$, $l = 1$ and $d = 0.01$) as in Figure 3.

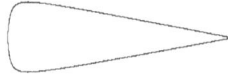

Figure 3. The shape of the stylet for $a = 0.2, l = 1$ and $d = 0.01$ as given by Equation (12), please see theoretical part.

The displacement

$$\delta = \frac{\beta(0) - \beta(P)}{2a} + \sqrt{\left(\frac{l}{2} - \frac{\beta(P)}{2a}\right)^2 - \frac{d\beta(P)}{a}} - \sqrt{\left(\frac{l}{2} - \frac{\beta(0)}{2a}\right)^2 - \frac{d\beta(0)}{a}}$$ (14)

increases nonlinearly with the pressure P (Figure 4), till at a certain threshold pressure $\beta(P_{thres}) = \beta$ the displacement diverges, and the stylet is ejected. The threshold pressure varies as

$$P_{thres} \approx \frac{(1-d)Ya\alpha}{2r_0^2}$$ (15)

where P_{thres} and Y have the same dimensions, and all the lengths are scaled by the length l of the stylus.

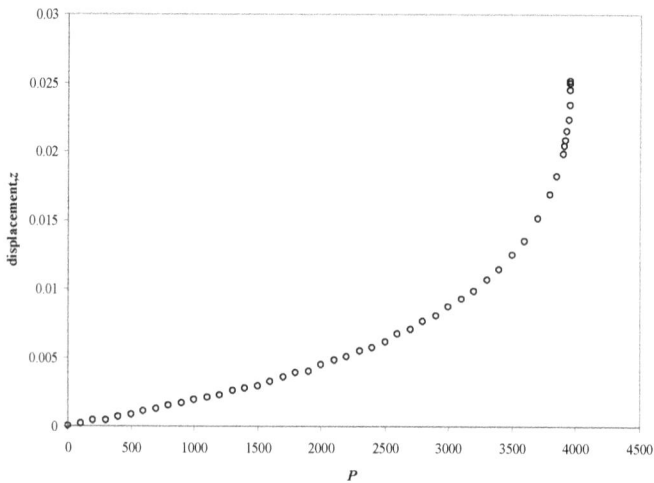

Figure 4. The displacement of the stylet ($a = 0.2, l = 1$, and $d = 0.01$) as a function of the applied pressure (in units of Y). The threshold pressure is about 3960 and all lengths are in units of the length of the stylet, please see theoretical part.

The stylet can only accelerate after the pressure exceeds the threshold pressure and the acceleration of the stylus is then $\pi R^2 P_{thres}/m$. The maximum acceleration (f_{max}) of the stylus will be given by

$$f_{max} = \frac{P_{thres} \pi R_x^2}{m} \qquad (16)$$

With R_x is the maximum radius and m is the mass of the stylet. In terms of the parameters described above, one may represent this acceleration as,

$$f_{max} = \frac{Y a \pi a^3 (1-d)}{2(1.18 + 7d) m r_0^2} \qquad (17)$$

and can be very large for small values of r_0. Here we see that very large accelerations are possible if the radius of the exit orifice (r_0) is small, and if the shape parameter (a) is large. The threshold pressure is proportional to the elastic modulus (Y) of the capsule and hence the exit orifice. Now these findings have to be correlated with experimental settings. In order to do this, biophysical, biochemical and cell-biological approaches have to be combined in a proper way. In this context it is of highest importance that *in silico* molecular modelling calculations support these approaches in an appropriate way. For a successful application of the theoretical model, it is of importance to know further details of the materials/molecules which constitute the corresponding parts in a cnidarian organism. This is outlined in the following paragraph.

2.2. Biophysical Experiments

Two major things have to be taken into consideration before a nematocyst-like device can be used as nanomedical diagnostic tool for a target directed tumor cell-attack and as promising source for the design of innovative therapeutic tools in cancer therapy. Firstly, PolySia specific targeting by lectins, especially, mini-lectins which mimic the receptors on the nematocyst surface must be defined in detail [25,38,39,48]. Secondly, the interactions between the molecules in the nematocyst's cell wall (mini-collagens as well as nematogalectins) and in its stylet-connected tubule system have to be described in detail on a sub-molecular level in a consistent way (Figure 5a,b and Figure 6a–c). Figure 5 shows two identical conformations at two different orientations. On the left side orientation a is shown and on the right side orientation b. For comparison, it is also of importance to analyze the collagen strands in the exumbrella tissue of jellyfishes with Quartz Crystal Microbalance (QCM) techniques.

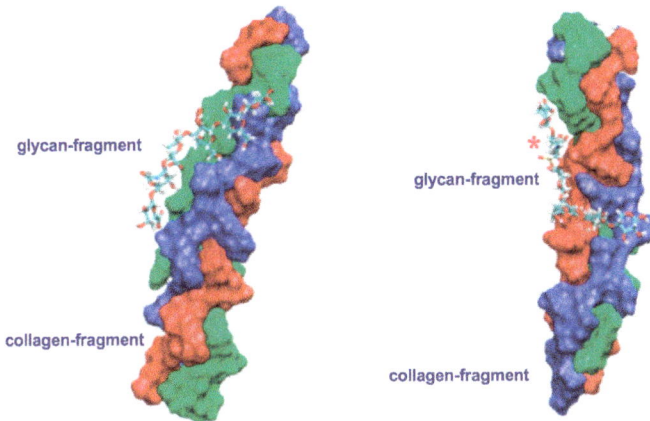

Figure 5. Triple-helical collagen strands in complex with non-sulfated (left side, orientation **a**) and sulfated (right side, orientation **b**) glycan-fragments. These models represent typical interaction state out of a great variety of other collagen- proteoglycan complexes. Sulfur-groups are highlighted by a red asterisk (*). Our results are in full agreement with AFM (Atomic Force Microscopy) and *in silico* studies on collagen strands interacting with proteoglycans [36].

2.3. QCM Analysis of Collagen Fragments from Cnidaria

It is essential to combine our theoretical results with data obtained by biophysical experiments. The correlation of theoretical and experimental data provides sophisticated information how nematocyst discharge processes could be used as nanomedical tools in cancer diagnostic and therapy. In this context the special consistence of the nematocyst cell wall is of highest interest. When testing various collagen hydrolysates in respect to their molecular composition it is instructive to carry out Quartz Crystal Microbalance (QCM) measurements [49] as complementary technique to NMR, AFM, SPR an MS [24,29,37,50]. QCM measurements allow the discrimination between triple helical and non-triple helical collagen fragments (Table 1). The results shown in Table 1 indicate that the triple helical collagen strands in mixtures of collagen fragments from jellyfishes exist and can be analyzed by QCM techniques. The raw material from cnidarian organisms (prepared according to Hoyer [51] and Sewing [52] degrade and dissociate above 45 °C in an irreversible way. It has to be emphasized that the source (e.g., fish or jellyfish) is not important for the occurrence of larger fragments but for the special production process. The upper section of Table 1 documents the results of measurements carried out over a total time period of 7000 s and a temperature limit up to 45 °C which is reached for the first time after 1500 s. When the temperature limit is 45 °C one can observe by the frequency alterations that the collagen strands are denatured and not reversible anymore. After 2500 s a low temperature region of 15 °C is reached again but the triple helical strands are denatured and did not renaturate anymore. A new increase of the temperature leads to a different profile of the Δv values. When altering the temperature between 15 °C and 37 °C only the frequency pattern, which is detectable, indicates a completely reversible processes in respect to the cnidarian collagen strands under study (as documented in the lower section of Table 1). The collagen strands remain triple-stranded and are proper target-structures for the proteoglycan saccharide chains as shown in Figure 5. Therefore, this method is beside NMR, SPR and AFM experiments in combination with molecular modelling calculations [24,36,37] a valuable supporting technique when nematocyst-like medical devices have to be improved.

Table 1. Measurements on triple and non-triple helical collagen fragments from exumbrellatissue from the jellyfish species *Rhopilema esculentum* [36,37,51,52] have been performed on the Quartz Crystal Microbalance system QCM 200 SRS. The differences of the detected frequencies are given by Δv in Hz. The experimental temperature is T in °C and the experimental time is t in s. In the table on the top 45 °C has been chosen as highest temperature which leads to a denaturation of the collagen strands. In the case 37 °C is the highest temperature (table on the bottom) no denaturation of the same material is detected.

Δv, Hz	0	300	250	300	−300	300	0	−300	−100	150
T, °C	15	30	45	40	15	45	30	15	15	15
t, sec	0	1000	1500	2000	2500	4000	4500	5000	5500	6000
Δv, Hz	0	700	300	100	700	300	100	700	300	100
T, °C	15	37	25	15	37	25	15	37	25	15
t, sec	0	1500	2000	2500	3500	4000	4500	6000	6500	7000

2.4. Molecules Constituting the Nematocyst Membrane

To explain the nematocyst discharge process in a physically consistent way one has to consider the morphology and the constitution of the nematocyst cell membrane in which proteins and carbohydrates are interacting with each other in order to generate the elastic properties enabling the high pressure and velocity values during the Coulomb repulsion process. According to our theoretical model, this is much more important in the upper part of the nematocyst than in the lower part. Using this model description, morphological alterations of nematocysts which occur in Hydra, jellyfishes and sea-anemones can be handled using theoretically derived parameters in combination with experimentally obtained data. Triple-stranded collagen strands in the nematocyst cell wall which are associated with cysteine-rich mini-collagens interact with proteoglycans and nematogalectins and are therefore the building blocks for nematocyst-like nanomedical devices. Unspecific interactions between parts from the carbohydrate chains of proteoglycans with collagen strands (Figure 5) as well as highly specific interactions between certain moieties of proteoglycan carbohydrate chains with certain lectins (especially nematogalectins, [44,45,53]) (Figure 6a–c) have to be taken into account when the origin of the flexibility properties in the stylet-connected nematocyst's tubule system is analyzed in molecular detail. Due to homology modelling, the nematogalectin structure could be constructed using the Swiss-model tool [54]: http://swissmodel.expasy.org/.

The rhamnose binding lectin [55] CSL3 (pdb-entry: 2ZX2.pdb) has been identified as the most suited template. The model structures are shown in Figure 6a–c. As described in the literature, the proteoglycan carbohydrate chains stabilize the cell-wall structure of the nematocyst in an essential way [56]. Model structures of the glycan and protein parts of proteoglycans are available [36]. Own molecular modelling calculations have shown that protein parts of proteoglycans, i.e., the leucine-rich biglycan [57–59] interact with other proteins in a highly specific way (Figure 7a,b). This is of importance when interactions with CD14 are in the focus [57–59], however, the interplay of such leucine rich molecules are also crucial players when the regeneration of the head region of Hydras is studied. In respect to the nematocyst membrane properties (Table 1) the glycan chains are of highest interest. Therefore, we have studied various proteoglycan fragments with molecular modelling methods concerning their interactions with collagen fragments and nematogalectins (Figure 5, Figure 6a–c, Figure 8a–f). All structural data sets concerning the key-molecules which constitute the nematocyst membrane and the wall of the stylet-connected tubule systems are considered in our molecular modelling studies. Molecular Dynamics (MD) simulations of collagen molecules [24] which are comparable to mini-collagen structures [60–62] in Cnidarian mini-collagens have a triple-helical core. This provides insights into the corresponding molecular organization processes in respect to their potential to interact with proteoglycans or collagen-binding proteins [23,36,37]. The corresponding interactions are mainly dominated by polar hydrogen bonds. Additional ionic interactions have to be considered. Unspecific associations of carbohydrate moieties from proteoglycans with collagen (Figure 5) as well as specific carbohydrate protein interactions mediated by nematogalectin (Figure 6a–c) were studied with molecular modelling method in the same way as described in the literature for receptor interactions with sialic acids and sulfated carbohydrate chains [24,25,27,38]. These data are used to test the reliability of the theoretical nematocyst model including all essential physical parameters. Our electron-microscopical (EM) analysis on nematocyst geometry has shown that the shape can be characterized as a combination of spherical and conical geometries (Figure 2). This is of importance for testing the predictions in relation to the theoretical five-stage model. Since the nematocyst discharge process is triggered by a mechanic-chemical signal which is initiated by sialic acid/polysialic acid molecules [63] on the skin of Cnidaria's enemies and preys sialic acid coated nano-particles are extremely supportive artificial analytical tools beside naturally occurring sialic acid pattern on tumor cells [25,39]. In this context sialic acid conjugated Fluorescent Silica Nano Particles (FSNP-Sia) and functionalization of Semiconductor Quantum Dots (SQDs) with sialic acid are extremely helpful analytic tools (this will be outlined in a follow-up publication). Furthermore, additional NMR control-experiments have been designed. These control experiments were performed (this will also be discussed in a follow-up publication) using fish eggs [42] and analyzed by NMR with a similar setting as described for living eukaryotic cells [64]. The results of the one-dimensional NMR experiment will be shown in a follow-up publication because the first promising results suggest extended experimental series with various fish-eggs and nematocytes/nematocysts from different cidarian species. This experimental setting can be applied to nematocytes/nematocysts (Figure 1) but also to numerous tumor cells (Figure 2). Echinodermata, which are predators of Cnidaria, have developed sialic acids in evolution half a billion years ago. A number of special sialic acid molecules can be found in starfishes [65]. Therefore, it is instructive and intriguing to test various sialic acids as initiating molecules of the nematocyst discharge process. Our knowledge about the architecture of the nematocyst [66–68] including the consistence of its cell-wall and the stylet-connected tubule system allows us to discuss the question of in which way the presence or the absence of sulfate groups on the proteoglycan carbohydrate chains have any impact on the material characteristics. Although, in principle, sulfated proteoglycan fragments are able to interact with triple helical collagen fragments (Figure 5). We finally conclude that the absence or the presence of a sulfate group has a kind of sign-function because of the impact on the orbitals of the corresponding carbohydrate residue [36]. The knowledge concerning the evolution of Cnidaria and Echinodermata [69–72] enables us to discuss potential clinical applications in diagnostic and therapy under a nano-bionic aspect. Exploding nematocysts and their effect on tumor cells can be controlled by NMR as it has been shown for fish-eggs before and after their destruction. Artificial nematocyst-like devices could be used as powerful nanomedical tool which is able to attack polySia-rich tumor cells [43].

a

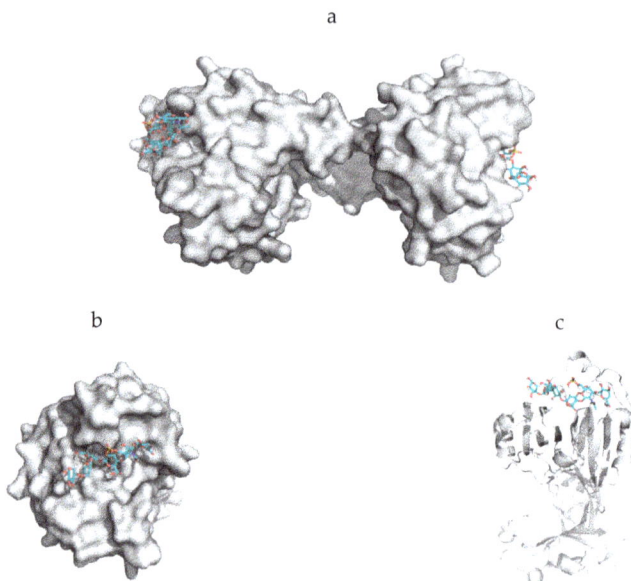

b

c

Figure 6. Model presentations of nematogalectin, a lectin which occurs in the capsule membrane (CM) of nematocysts. Interactions exist between parts from the carbohydrate chains of proteoglycans with collagen strands (Figure 5c) as well as highly specific interactions between certain moieties of the proteoglycan non-sulfated carbohydrate chains and the lectin are responsible for the cell membrane (CM) properties. Our calculations show that sulfated carbohydrates are also tolerated. The best template structure in the protein data bank is 2ZX2.pdb from the rhamnose binding lectin CSL3 [71]. (a) Surface presentation of the nematogalectin—showing its function as bridging molecule with two proteoglycan fragments in a stick structure. (b) Surface presentation—direct view on the binding pocket. (c) Ribbon structure of one part of the nematogalectin in complex with a proteoglycan fragment in a stick structure.

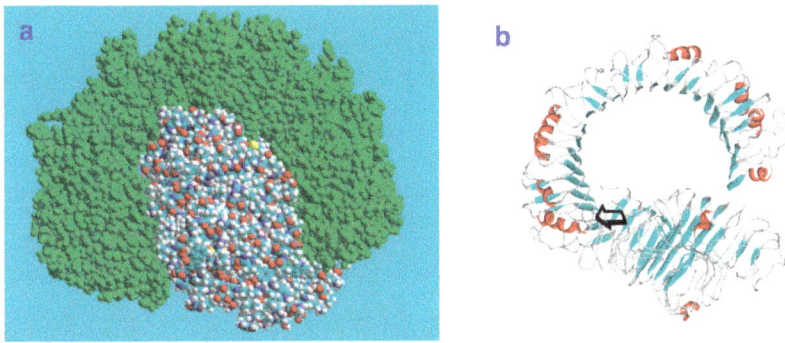

Figure 7. (**a**): CD14 (colored) and biglycan (green) in their space-filling states associate at a preferred contact region in order to establish a stable complex. (**b**): The initial contact point is marked by an arrow. The matrix component biglycan is proinflammatory and signals through Toll-like receptors 4 and 2 in macrophages [57–59].

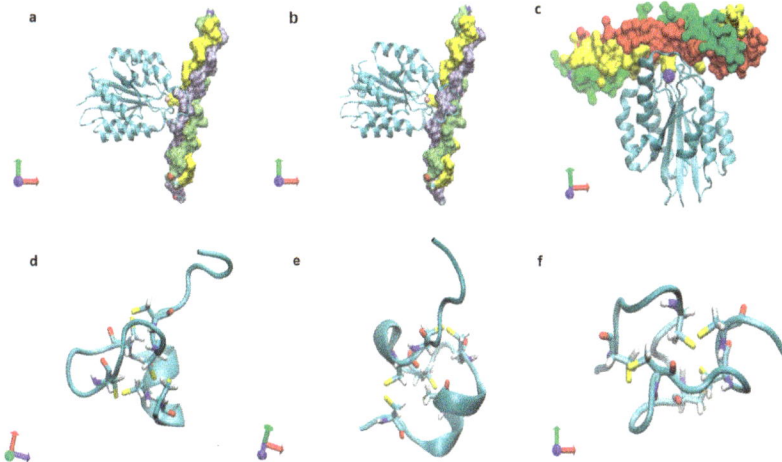

Figure 8. Triple-helical collagen in complex with integrins (**a–c**, in which a and b with pdb entery: 2m32.pdb, c with PDB entry: 1dzi.pdb, and mini-collagens (**d–f**, in which d with PDB entry: 1sop.pdb, c with PDB (Protein Data Bank) entry: 1sp7.pdb, f with PDB entry: 1zpx.pdb).

3. Discussions

In order to understand the nematocyst discharge process on a basic physical level, we combined approaches from applied and theoretical physics. When analyzing this process, a satisfactory model description allows deeper insights into basic physical details. Our theoretical model permits a discussion of the nematocyst discharge process in the dependence of key-parameters such as vessel morphologies, pressure values, forces and ejection velocities. With this model, we are able to depict the major effects leading to the stylet emission in an adequate way independent from structural deviations between the nematocysts of various species (Hydra, jellyfishes, box-jellyfishes and sea-anemones). The elastic properties of the materials surrounding the stylet near the operculum require a special molecular arrangement. It is necessary that the cell-wall sections in that region have a higher elasticity because they have to endure higher stresses than the rest of the cell membrane. Experimental data, including the parameters of various boundary conditions can be determined by a strategic combination of suited biophysical methods such as Surface Plasmon Resonance (SPR) [28], Atomic Force Microscopy

(AFM) [24,37,48,73,74], nano-particle analysis supported by confocal laser scanning microscopy [75–79], Electron Microscopy (EM) (Figures 1 and 2), NMR spectroscopy [37], Quartz Crystal Microbalance (QCM) techniques [49] (Table 1) and molecular modelling [25,36,38–41] (Figures 5–8) provide essential biophysical data about the morphological and material characteristics of nematocysts. It is therefore possible to use these data as a first concept in a feasibility study for the construction of nematocyst-like nanomedical diagnostic devices, i.e., tailor-made nematocysts which contain therapeutic drugs. These nanomedical devices have to be effective and specific in respect to various carbohydrate signatures in the glycocalyx of tumor-cells. For this purpose, it is essential to understand the target-directed nematocyst discharge process in all aspects of the fundamental physical laws. The biochemical properties which are correlated with these laws can be modified accordingly when nematocyst-like nanomedical devices are constructed.

Physical Properties of Nematocysts and Their Potential Targets

In non-equlibrium thermodynamics [80] one has to describe the intact nematocyst in its metastable state first. This state will be reached after a contact of the intact nematocyte with sialic acids. The mechanic-chemical contact to the sialic acid sensitive receptor is therefore responsible for non-reproducible fluctuations. If the stationary state of the process is metastable, then non-reproducible fluctuations involve local transient decreases of entropy. The reproducible response of the system increases the entropy back to its maximum by irreversible processes: the fluctuation cannot be reproduced with a significant level of probability. Fluctuations about stable stationary states are extremely small except near critical points [80]. The information which we derived by methods from applied and theoretical physics are sufficient to describe the complete nematocyst discharge process in its five stages. Furthermore, the initial release mechanism triggered by an interaction of cell-surface exposed receptor with sialic acid molecules can be studied in detail using biophysical methods in combination with suited model systems [25,38,41,42]. NMR experiments, molecular dynamics (MD) simulations and microscopic studies provide complementary information to our theoretical five-stage model description. These results are the basis for a follow-up NMR study on fish-eggs, nematocysts, tumor cells and sialic acid coated nanoparticles [75–77] which are a prerequisite for the corresponding clinical studies. Cancer cells have distinct morphological parameters and a special signature of carbohydrate chains on their cell surface in which sialic acids play a prominent role. Polysialic acid (building block: Neu5Ac-alpha2-8-Neu5Ac) in high concentration on the surface of cells (e.g., fish eggs [42] or tumor cells [25,38,43] can initiate the nematocyst discharge process. However, in some cases, it is necessary to increase the sialic acid concentration in the vicinity of the nematocysts to support the discharge processes. It is an advantage for our strategy that the physical properties of cancer cells in respect to their plasticity differ in a significant way from normal cells as it turned out after TEM (transmission electron microscopy) studies on neuroblastoma (Figure 2I,II) but also on glioblastoma (own observation) cells. The cancer cells under study are much weaker and show a higher degree of protrusions than normal tissue cells. These findings are of importance since neuroblastoma and glioblastoma cells which carry the polySia molecules on their surfaces are suited targets for modified nematocysts which are able to attack cancer cells in a specific way. Our five-stage theoretical model which describes the different phases of the nematocyst discharge process is a first step aiming in a complete adaption of such a concept for diagnostic and therapeutic applications which focus on a target-directed destruction of cancer cells.

With the five-stage model, we can explain the basic physical properties of the nematocyst discharge process providing the force and the energy for the ejection of the toxic stylets when Cnidaria are defending the attacks from their predators. Molecular dynamics (MD) simulations of collagen fragments [24] and of crucial parts of the proteoglycan carbohydrate chains [36] (Figure 5) which are forming the structures of nematocyst cell membrane as well as electron microscopical studies on the shape variations of nematocysts (Figure 1) deliver the boundary conditions for the five-stage model, such as elasticity, pressure and other material-dependent parameters, e.g., Figure 4 and Table 1. Values for the conical and spherical geometries of the nematocyst vessels and the shape variations of their stylets (Figures 1 and 3) are also of importance. The number of the nematocyst discharge processes strongly depends on the concentration of polySia molecules in the environment of the cells (own observation) and will be analyzed in more detail in a follow-up study with labeled neuraminic acid molecules [75–79]. The chain lengths of polySia seem to play only a minor role (Figure 5) as revealed by microscopy and NMR spectroscopy [38,48]. The spider lectin SHL-1 [23] other small lectin-like structures have to be considered as proper polySia interacting peptides [38,39,48] on nematocyst-like nanomedical devices. The amino acid sequence of the effector domain of the myristoylated alanine-rich kinase C substrate (MARCKS-ED) is such a candidate. The amino acid sequence indicates by its composition that arginine and aromatic amino acid residues play a crucial role for a specific polySia binding. This is also the case for the spider lectin SHL-1 [38,39]. In particular, the role of aromatic amino acid residues is underlined by amino acid sequence of the MARCKS-ED control peptide [38] which has no binding specificity for polySia. The phenylalanines that were changed to alanines in the control peptide support polySia binding of MARCKS-ED but the alanine residues in the control peptide are not. As a first test for the effect of exploding nematocysts suited cells are necessary. In our case we have chosen fish eggs which have polySia in high concentration on their surface in a similar way than various tumor cells [42,43]. The state of the fish egg before and after its destruction can be documented by 1D NMR spectra (Figure 2II and Supplementary Materials). Besides microscopic studies, it is therefore also possible with NMR experiments [64] to figure out in which way an increased concentration of sialic acids and polySia fragments are able to support the initiation of the nematocyst discharge process. Of special interest are polySia glycomimetics, e.g., Tegaserod [38,81,82], which are also interacting partners of sialic acid receptors. It has to be emphasized that the polysaccharide polySia in which the sialic acid Neu5Ac building-blocks are linked by an α2-8 bond to each other are the natural triggers which are responsible for the inition of a nematocyst discharge event. Beside sialic acid binding other specific carbohydrate—protein interactions play a crucial role in this study and concern nematogalectins. Galectins [83–87] are galactose binding animal lectins which have various biological functions. In respect to nematogalectins, it is of importance to clearly identify the corresponding contact region of this cnidarian lectin (Figure 6a–c). Also, in this case, the benefit of molecular modelling *in silico* calculations under special consideration of *ab initio* calculations is obvious [24,25,36,38–41,88,89], since this theoretical approach shows under which prerequisites nematocyst-like nanomedical devices can be constructed; in detail: which material requirements are necessary [90–100]. Fast-growing tumor cells typically have more permeable membranes than healthy cells, allowing the leakage of marked sialic acid molecules into their cell body. Moreover, tumor cells lack an effective lymphatic drainage system, which leads to subsequent accumulation of these particles. Since sialic acids (especially Neu5Ac) initiate the nematocyst discharge process labeled Neu5Ac molecules, even free in solution could be used to trigger the nematocyst discharge process and will also be helpful markers inside the nematocyst. Therefore, sialic acid coated nanoparticles are suited tools to improve the efficiency of our approach [75–79]. Besides a target-directed attack against tumor cells, nano-bionic nematocyst-like devices from cnidarian origin could in principle be applied for therapies which support neuronal regeneration because the state of neuronal de- and re-differentiation depends also on the polySia concentration on the nerve cell surfaces ([25,38] and literature cited within). Additionally, in the case of treatments against certain pathogens (viruses and bacteria) [39–41] the use of sialic acid sensitive nematocyst-like vesicles has to be considered as promising diagnostic and therapeutic option, especially, when multiresistent pathogens have to be taken into account. Our approach in which nematocysts are used as bionic blueprints has therefore multiple benefits in the fields of nanomedicine and nanopharmacology. Especially, the theoretical model described here enables us to modify the nematocyst architecture and adapt it for diagnostic and therapeutic clinical applications. It is essential in this context to understand the role of nematogalectin as a component of the tubule system and its interactions with mini-collagen strands and proteoglycans. As outlined here, corresponding experiments on triple helical collagen fragments can be performed by a combination of QCM techniques (Table 1) and molecular modelling methods (Figure 5, Figure 6a–d). These results have to be combined with NMR data from cellular test-systems. Such suited cellular test systems are fish-eggs which carry polySia on their cell surfaces. The high tumbling rate of the surface exposed bio-macromolecules lead to broad signals of the one-dimensional proton NMR spectrum (not shown). After the destruction of the fish eggs, highly resolved signals from the inside of the cell can be detected. This is also the case when sialic acid coated nanoparticles are studied.

4. Materials and Methods

4.1. Tumor Cells: Neuroblastoma Cells

Cell line SK-N-AS corresponding to neural bone marrow metastasis cells from a human source were purchased from American Type Culture Collection (Manassas, VA, USA). Glioblastoma cells: Cells were taken from a glioblastoma multiforme (WHO stage four).

4.2. Hydra Culture

Experiments were carried out using *Hydra vulgaris* strain AEP. Animals were cultured according to standard procedures [101].

4.3. Proteoglycans, Algae Polysaccharides and Collagen Fragments from Marine Organisms and Bacteria

Fish cartilage [102], green algae [39,103] and Cnidaria (*Rhopilema esculentum*) [36,37,51,52] are our sources for proteoglycans, polysaccharides and collagen-fragments. Polysialic acid (polySia): Polisialic acid fragments of various chain lengths are derived from colominic acid of *E. coli*.

4.4. Electron Microscopy

Specimen were fixed in 6% glutaraldehyde in 0.1 M Na-cacodylate buffer overnight, rinsed three times for 10 min in 0.1 m Na-cacodylate buffer, and postfixed in 1% osmiumtetroxide (OsO4) for one hour. Samples were dehydrated in a series of alcohol (50%, 70%, 80%, and 96% ethanol for 15 min, 100% ethanol for 1 h), and embedded in Epon. Semithin sections (1 µm) were stained with methylene blue. Ultrathin sections (100 Å) were contrasted with lead citrate (2%) and uranylacetate (0.5%) and examined in a Zeiss 109 electron microscope.

4.5. Measurements with a QCM System

The quartz crystal microbalance system QCM 200 SRS (Stanford Research Systems, 1290-D Reamwood Ave, Sunnyvale, CA 94089, USA) was used to analyze jellyfish collagen and collagen hydrolysate samples under various temperature conditions.

4.6. Molecular Modelling

The conformational analysis and energy optimization of sulfated and non-sulfated glycans was carried out with Hyperchem 8.0 Prof. (using the CHARMM27 force field, Chemistry at HARvard Macromolecular Mechanics, Cambridge (Massachusetts) USA) and Gaussian16 (B3LYP/6-31G*). Glycan-protein docking was performed with the Molegro 5.0 trial version. For protein-protein docking calculations the Webserver Haddock 2.2 version was used. MD-simulations were carried out with YASARA v.19.4.29 using the YASARA force field under physiological conditions [36,104–106] and additional references in Supplementary Materials.

4.7. Preparation of FSNP-Sia

FSNP-Sia was synthesized using fluorescein-doped silica nanoparticles (FSNP) and the photocoupling strategy to conjugate Sia on FSNP, following previously developed protocols [75–79,107].

4.7.1. Synthesis of Fluorescent Silica Nanoparticles (FSNP)

Fluorescein 5-isothiocyanate (39 mg) was dissolved in anhydrous ethanol (16 mL) and (3-aminopropyl) trimethoxysilane (17 µL) was added while stirring. The mixture was stirred overnight at 42 °C to produce the precursor solution. For the synthesis of fluorescein isothiocynate (FITC)-doped silica nanoparticles, 5.0 mL of the precursor solution was added to anhydrous ethanol (34 mL) while stirring followed by the addition of tetraethyl orthosilicate (1.7 mL) and aqueous ammonia (1.4 mL, 25% v/v). The mixture was stirred for 48 hours to give the FSNP solution.

4.7.2. Synthesis of Perfluorophenyl Azide (PFPA)-functionalized Fluorescent Silica Nanoparticles (FSNP-PFPA)

FSNP-PFPA was synthesized by adding a solution of silane-derivatized PFPA in toluene (7.0 mL, 10 mg/mL) into the FSNP solution and stirring at room temperature for 24 h. The product was purified by repeated washing and centrifugation in acetone (12,000 rpm, 30 min), and was re-suspended in 10 mL of acetone to give FSNP-PFPA.

4.7.3. Synthesis of Sialic Acid-Conjugated FSNP (FSNP-Sia)

To 1 mL of FSNP-PFPA in acetone, an aqueous solution of sialic acid (1.0 mL, 3.6 mg/mL) was added. The glass jar containing the mixture was covered with a 280 nm long-path optical filter and was subsequently irradiated with a 450 W medium-pressure mercury lamp for 40 minutes. The resulting FSNP-Sia was purified by repeated washing in Milli-Q water and centrifugation (12000 rpm, 30 min). The final product was re-suspended in water.

5. Conclusions

The nematocyst discharge process is initiated by a mechanic-chemical interaction when an object is in contact with the surface of a nematocyte carrying an intact nematocyst. Furthermore, sialic acids or polySia molecules have to be involved. Data about the molecular details of this procedure obtained from theoretical approaches in combination experimentally derived results enables us to consider the possibilities of nematocysts as blueprints for nanomedical devices in tumor cell diagnostic and cancer therapy. The chemical reactions related to the nematocyst discharge mechanisms mainly depend on the de-protonation and the swelling process of γ-polyglutamate. In the case of a nematocyst discharge, which is caused by sialic acids, the chemical and physical-mechanic data can be separated [1]. As described in our five-stage model, one has to take into account that the sialic acids do not occur in Cnidaria. Using our theoretical model, it is possible to consider nematocysts of various species with different morphologies for further studies. Sialic acid molecules which play also a crucial role in developmental processes [90,91] were invented during the evolution in Echinodermata (e.g., starfishes). Therefore, Cnidaria (e.g., Hydra, sea-anemones, jellyfishes) have developed a strategy to protect themselves against the attacks of these enemies, at first Echinodermata, by a diffusion-dependent polySia sensitive defense system (related to the concentration of sialic acid molecules and their density on the cell-surfaces). The monosaccharide sialic acid which forms the alpha2-8 linked polysialic acid (polySia) has been identified as key-molecule which identifies a predator. A potential application in nanomedicine is possible since polySia occurs also in high concentration in the glycocalyx of tumor cells and are responsible for their degree of malignancy. When the experimental methods applied here are supported by approaches from theoretical physics it is feasible to invent new diagnostic and therapeutic concepts flanked by encapsulation and target strategies. In detail, similar cell surface signatures which induce the nematocyst discharges are also specific target structures on highly malignant cells [92,93]. These carbohydrate target structures undergo specific interactions with lectins [22,38,78,94] but possibly also with carbohydrate chains [95–97]. Besides encapsulation and targeting of potent anti-tumor drugs, its identification [98–100] also plays a crucial role. Polysaccharides from marine organisms [39,102,103] provide homogenous encapsulation materials. In combination with specially prepared collagen fragments [29,50] it is possible to construct nano-bionic medical devices [107–110] for which nematocysts are the blueprints. In summary, our investigated theoretical model describes a nematocyst discharge process which is initiated by a contact with sialic acids [111] causing a Coulomb repulsion [112] which leads to the ejection of a toxic stylet [113]. This nano-bionic model has inspired us to analyze such processes under various boundary conditions aiming at new diagnostic and therapeutic approaches with innovative nanomedical devices. Besides the shape of the nematocyst, the consistence of the nematocyst membrane and the stylet-connected tubule system are important to figure out how the sialic acid dependent triggering of the nematocyst discharge process in an intact nematocyte can be used for cellular targeting. Our theoretical and experimental approaches enable us to decide which are the most promising nanomedical blueprints for our endeavor to establish a target-directed tumor cell attack, e.g., in the field of neuro-oncology. Since highly malignant brain tumor cells are coated on their surfaces with polysialic acid (polySia) molecules similar like fish-eggs we use these insights for a strike against the Achilles heel of cancer cells. Therefore, we have to identify the most effective toxin which is able to block the growth and the spreading of brain tumor cells such as glioblastomas. These toxins have to be encapsulated in a nanomatrix which consists of liposomes/micelles, polysaccharide- and collagen-fragments (especially mini-collagens, Figure 8d–f) in a similar composition as found in nematocysts. The target-directed intervention of the toxin-loaded nanoparticles in the dependence of the polySia rich contact structures on the brain tumor cells is performed by polySia binding mini-lectins on the surfaces of nematocyst-like nanoparticles.

Supplementary Materials: The following are available online at http://www.mdpi.com/1660-3397/17/8/469/s1, Comparison between a 1D proton NMR spectrum of intact fish-eggs with a 1D proton-NMR spectrum of the same fish-eggs which are destroyed in a nematocyst discharge event.

Author Contributions: R.Z.: conceptualization and investigation; L.J. and N.Z.: methodology and resources; T.E.: software and molecular modelling; A.K.P. and G.S.-B.: resources and methodology; M.B. and A.S.: resources and methodology; R.S. and B.N.: data curation; M.Y. and S.A.W.: resources and methodology; B.K.C.: conceptualization and investigation, especially, the development of the Theoretical Model. H.-C.S.: conceptualization, investigation and writing the manuscript.

Funding: This work was supported in part by Open Project of Shandong Collaborative Innovation Center for Antibody Drugs (No. CIC-AD1829, No. CIC-AD1834 and No. CIC-AD1839), Doctoral Foundation of Liaocheng University (No. 318051738 and No. 318051827), and Key R&D project of Shandong Province (No. 2018YYSP008). We indicate that the free publication quota granted by the Editorial Office has been used for this publication.

Acknowledgments: We thank Fabian Siebert, trainee at the Clinic of Obstetrics, Gynecology and Andrology for Small and Large Animals, Justus-Liebig University Giessen for taking care of the Hydra population and Susanne Schubert-Porth, Institute of Veterinary Anatomy, -Histology, and -Embryology for skillful technical assistance for electron microscopy. We are indebted to H. Maximilian Mehdorn (Department of Neurosurgery, Universitätsklinikum Schleswig-Holstein Campus Kiel, Kiel, Germany) and Gerald 't Hooft (Institute for Theoretical Physics Utrecht University and Spinoza Institute Utrecht, The Netherlands) for fruitful and valuable discussions concerning clinical aspects and theoretical physics related to nematocyst discharge processes. We also thank H. Wienk and R. Boelens (Utrecht Facility for High-resolution NMR Bijvoetcenter for Biomolecular Research, University Utrecht, The Netherlands) for their support in respect of the NMR experiments (European Commission's Framework Program 7 Bio-NMR; project number 261863) as well as Philipp Siebert (RI-B-NT) for technical assistance.

Conflicts of Interest: The authors declare no conflict of interest.

References

1. Turing, A.M. The chemical basis of morphogenesis. *Bull. Math. Biol.* **1990**, *52*, 153–197; discussion 119–152. [CrossRef]

2. Von Neumann, J.; Burks, A.W. *Theory of Self-Reproducing Automata*; University of Illinois Press: Champagne, IL, USA, 1966; pp. 64–87.

3. Gierer, A.; Berking, S.; Bode, H.; David, C.N.; Flick, K.; Hansmann, G.; Schaller, H.; Trenkner, E. Regeneration of Hydra from reaggregated cells. *Nat. New Biol.* **1972**, *239*, 98–101. [CrossRef] [PubMed]

4. Gierer, A.; Meinhardt, H. A theory of biological pattern formation. *Kybernetik* **1972**, *12*, 30–39. [CrossRef] [PubMed]

5. Meinhardt, H. Turing's theory of morphogenesis of 1952 and the subsequent discovery of the crucial role of local self-enhancement and long-range inhibition. *Interface Focus* **2012**, *2*, 407–416. [CrossRef] [PubMed]

6. Maini, P.K.; Woolley, T.E.; Baker, R.E.; Gaffney, E.A.; Lee, S.S. Turing's model for biological pattern formation and the robustness problem. *Interface Focus* **2012**, *2*, 487–496. [CrossRef] [PubMed]

7. Kauffman, S. Answering Descartes: Beyond Turing. In *The Once and Future Turing: Computing the World*; Cooper, S.B., Hodges, A., Eds.; Cambridge University Press: Cambridge, UK, 2012.

8. 't Hooft, G. Can the ultimate laws of nature be found? Under the spell of the gauge principle. In *Advanced Series in Mathematical Physics*; World Scientific Publishing Company: Calgary, AB, Canada, 1994; pp. 666–676.

9. 't Hooft, G. Playing with Planets. *World Scientific News*, October 2008.

10. Holstein, T.W.; Benoit, M.; Herder, G.V.; David, C.N.; Wanner, G.; Gaub, H.E. Fibrous minicollagens in Hydra nematocysts. *Science* **1994**, *265*, 402–404. [CrossRef] [PubMed]

11. Weber, J. Nematocysts (stinging capsules of Cnidaria) as Donnan-potential-dominated osmotic systems. *Eur. J. Biochem.* **1989**, *184*, 465–476. [CrossRef] [PubMed]

12. Morabito, R.; Marino, A.; Dossena, S.; La Spada, G. Nematocyst discharge in *Pelagia noctiluca* (Cnidaria, Scyphozoa) oral arms can be affected by lidocaine, ethanol, ammonia and acetic acid. *Toxicon* **2014**, *83*, 52–58. [CrossRef] [PubMed]

13. Todaro, D.; Watson, G.M. Force-dependent discharge of nematocysts in the sea anemone Haliplanella luciae (Verrill). *Biol. Open* **2012**, *1*, 582–587. [CrossRef]

14. Nuchter, T.; Benoit, M.; Engel, U.; Özbek, S.; Holstein, T.W. Nanosecond-scale kinetics of nematocyst discharge. *Curr. Biol.* **2006**, *16*, R316–R318. [CrossRef] [PubMed]

15. Holstein, T.W.; Hobmayer, E.; Technau, U. Cnidarians: An evolutionarily conserved model system for regeneration? *Dev. Dyn.* **2003**, *226*, 257–267. [CrossRef] [PubMed]

16. Bosch, T.C.G. Why polyps regenerate and we don't: Towards a cellular and molecular framework for Hydra regeneration. *Dev. Biol.* **2007**, *303*, 421–433. [CrossRef] [PubMed]

17. Bosch, T.C.G.; Augustin, R.; Anton-Erxleben, F.; Fraune, S.; Hemmrich, G.; Zill, H.; Rosenstiel, P.; Jacobs, G.; Schreiber, S.; Leippe, M.; et al. Uncovering the evolutionary history of innate immunity: The simple metazoan Hydra uses epithelial cells for host defence. *Dev. Comp. Immunol.* **2009**, *33*, 559–569. [CrossRef] [PubMed]

18. Fraune, S.; Augustin, R.; Anton-Erxleben, F.; Wittlieb, J.; Gelhaus, C.; Klimovich, V.B.; Samoilovich, M.P.; Bosch, T.C.G. In an early branching metazoan, bacterial colonization of the embryo is controlled by maternal antimicrobial peptides. *Proc. Natl. Acad. Sci. USA* **2010**, *107*, 18067–18072. [CrossRef] [PubMed]

19. Boehm, A.M.; Khalturin, K.; Anton-Erxleben, F.; Hemmrich, G.; Klostermeier, U.C.; Lopez-Quintero, J.A.; Oberg, H.H.; Puchert, M.; Rosenstiel, P.; Wittlieb, J.; et al. FoxO is a critical regulator of stem cell maintenance in immortal Hydra. *Proc. Natl. Acad. Sci. USA* **2012**, *109*, 19697–19702. [CrossRef] [PubMed]

20. Augustin, R.; Fraune, S.; Franzenburg, S.; Bosch, T.C.G. Where simplicity meets complexity: Hydra, a model for host-microbe interactions. *Adv. Exp. Med. Biol.* **2012**, *710*, 71–81. [PubMed]

21. Chapman, J.A.; Kirkness, E.F.; Simakov, O.; Hampson, S.E.; Mitros, T.; Weinmaier, T.; Rattei, T.; Balasubramanian, P.G.; Borman, J.; Busam, D.; et al. The dynamic genome of Hydra. *Nature* **2010**, *464*, 592–596. [CrossRef]

22. Gabius, H.-J.; Siebert, H.-C.; André, S.; Jiménez-Barbero, J.; Rüdiger, H. Chemical biology of the sugar code. *ChemBioChem* **2004**, *5*, 740–764. [CrossRef]

23. Siebert, H.-C.; Lu, S.Y.; Wechselberger, R.; Born, K.; Eckert, T.; Liang, S.; von der Lieth, C.-W.; Jiménez-Barbero, J.; Schauer, R.; Vliegenthart, J.F.G.; et al. A lectin from the Chinese bird-hunting spider binds sialic acids. *Carbohydr. Res.* **2009**, *344*, 1515–1525. [CrossRef]

24. Siebert, H.-C.; Burg-Roderfeld, M.; Eckert, T.; Stötzel, S.; Kirch, U.; Diercks, T.; Humphries, M.J.; Frank, M.; Wechselberger, R.; Tajkhorshid, E.; et al. Interaction of the alpha 2A domain of integrin with small collagen fragments. *Protein Cell* **2010**, *1*, 393–405. [CrossRef] [PubMed]

25. Siebert, H.-C.; Scheidig, A.; Eckert, T.; Wienk, H.; Boelens, R.; Mahvash, M.; Petridis, A.K.; Schauer, R. Interaction studies of sialic acids with model receptors contribute to nanomedical therapies. *J. Neurol. Disord.* **2015**, *3*, 1–6. [CrossRef]

26. Simon, P.; Baumner, S.; Busch, O.; Rohrich, R.; Kaese, M.; Richterich, P.; Wehrend, A.; Muller, K.; Gerardy-Schahn, R.; Muhlenhoff, M.; et al. Polysialic acid is present in mammalian semen as a post-translational modification of the neural cell adhesion molecule NCAM and the polysialyltransferase ST8SiaII. *J. Biol. Chem.* **2013**, *288*, 18825–18833. [CrossRef] [PubMed]

27. Bhunia, A.; Vivekanandan, S.; Eckert, T.; Burg-Roderfeld, M.; Wechselberger, R.; Romanuka, J.; Bächle, D.; Kornilov, A.V.; von der Lieth, C.-W.; Jiménez-Barbero, J.; et al. Why structurally different cyclic peptides can be glycomimetics of the HNK-1 carbohydrate antigen. *J. Am. Chem. Soc.* **2010**, *132*, 96–105. [CrossRef] [PubMed]

28. Tsvetkov, Y.E.; Burg-Roderfeld, M.; Loers, G.; Arda, A.; Sukhova, E.V.; Khatuntseva, E.A.; Grachev, A.A.; Chizhov, A.O.; Siebert, H.-C.; Schachner, M.; et al. Synthesis and molecular recognition studies of the HNK-1 trisaccharide and related oligosaccharides. The specificity of monoclonal anti-HNK-1 antibodies as assessed by surface plasmon resonance and NMR. *J. Am. Chem. Soc.* **2012**, *134*, 426–435. [CrossRef] [PubMed]

29. Schadow, S.; Siebert, H.-C.; Lochnit, G.; Kordelle, J.; Rickert, M.; Steinmeyer, J. Collagen metabolism of human osteoarthritic articular cartilage as modulated by bovine collagen hydrolysates. *PLoS ONE* **2013**, *8*, 1–9. [CrossRef] [PubMed]

30. Meinhardt, H.; Gierer, A. Generation and regeneration of sequence of structures during morphogenesis. *J. Theor. Biol.* **1980**, *85*, 429–450. [CrossRef]

31. Mason, P.E.; Uhlig, F.; Vanek, V.; Buttersack, T.; Bauerecker, S.; Jungwirth, P. Coulomb explosion during the early stages of the reaction of alkali metals with water. *Nat. Chem.* **2015**, *7*, 250–254. [CrossRef]

32. Banerjee, S.; Mazumdar, S. Electrospray ionization mass spectrometry: A technique to access the information beyond the molecular weight of the analyte. *Int. J. Anal. Chem.* **2012**, *2012*, 1–40. [CrossRef]

33. Lin, X.H.; Chen, H.Q.; Jiang, S.Y.; Zhang, C.B. A Coulomb explosion theoretical model of femtosecond laser ablation materials. *Sci. China Technol. Sci.* **2012**, *55*, 694–701. [CrossRef]

34. Tursch, A.; Mercadante, D.; Tennigkeit, J.; Grater, F.; Özbek, S. Minicollagen cysteine-rich domains encode distinct modes of polymerization to form stable nematocyst capsules. *Sci. Rep.* **2016**, *6*, 1–11. [CrossRef] [PubMed]

35. Feynman, R. Plenty of room at the bottom. *Am. Phys. Soc. Pasadena* **1959**. [CrossRef]

36. Eckert, T.; Stötzel, S.; Burg-Roderfeld, M.; Sewing, J.; Lütteke, T.; Nifantiev, N.E.; Vliegenthart, J.F.G.; Siebert, H.-C. In silico study on sulfated and non-sulfated carbohydrate chains from proteoglycans in cnidaria and interaction with collagen. *Open J. Phys. Chem.* **2012**, *2*, 123–133. [CrossRef]

37. Stötzel, S.; Schurink, M.; Wienk, H.; Siebler, U.; Burg-Roderfeld, M.; Eckert, T.; Kulik, B.; Wechselberger, R.; Sewing, J.; Steinmeyer, J.; et al. Molecular organization of various collagen fragments as revealed by atomic force microscopy and diffusion-ordered NMR spectroscopy. *ChemPhysChem* **2012**, *13*, 3117–3125. [CrossRef] [PubMed]

38. Zhang, R.; Eckert, T.; Lütteke, T.; Hanstein, S.; Scheidig, A.J.; Bonvin, A.M.; Nifantiev, N.E.; Kožár, T.; Schauer, R.; Enani, M.A.; et al. Structure-function relationships of antimicrobial peptides and proteins with respect to contact molecules on pathogen surfaces. *Curr. Top. Med. Chem.* **2016**, *16*, 89–98. [CrossRef] [PubMed]

39. Zhang, R.; Loers, G.; Schachner, M.; Boelens, R.; Wienk, H.; Siebert, S.; Eckert, T.; Kraan, S.; Rojas-Macias, M.A.; Lütteke, T.; et al. Molecular basis of the receptor interactions of polysialic acid (polySia), polySia mimetics, and sulfated polysaccharides. *ChemMedChem* **2016**, *11*, 990–1002. [CrossRef] [PubMed]

40. Zhang, R.; Wu, L.; Eckert, T.; Burg-Roderfeld, M.; Rojas-Macias, M.A.; Lütteke, T.; Krylov, V.B.; Argunov, D.A.; Datta, A.; Markart, P.; et al. Lysozyme's lectin-like characteristics facilitates its immune defense function. *Q. Rev. Biophys.* **2017**, *50*, e9. [CrossRef] [PubMed]

41. Zhang, R.; Zhang, N.; Mohri, M.; Wu, L.; Eckert, T.; Krylov, V.B.; Antosova, A.; Ponikova, S.; Bednarikova, Z.; Markart, P.; et al. Nanomedical relevance of the intermolecular interaction dynamics-Examples from lysozymes and insulins. *ACS Omega* **2019**, *4*, 4206–4220. [CrossRef] [PubMed]

42. Sato, C.; Kitajima, K.; Tazawa, I.; Inoue, Y.; Inoue, S.; Troy, F.A. Structural diversity in the alpha 2->8-linked polysialic acid chains in salmonid fish egg glycoproteins. Occurrence of poly(Neu5Ac), poly(Neu5Gc), poly(Neu5Ac, Neu5Gc), poly(KDN), and their partially acetylated forms. *J. Biol. Chem.* **1993**, *268*, 23675–23684.

43. Rawnaq, T.; Quaas, A.; Zander, H.; Gros, S.J.; Reichelt, U.; Blessmann, M.; Wilzcak, W.; Schachner, M.; Sauter, G.; Izbicki, J.R.; et al. L1 is highly expressed in tumors of the nervous system: A study of over 8000 human tissues. *J. Surg. Res.* **2012**, *173*, 314–319. [CrossRef]

44. Shpirer, E.; Chang, E.S.; Diamant, A.; Rubinstein, N.; Cartwright, P.; Huchon, D. Diversity and evolution of myxozoan minicollagens and nematogalectins. *BMC Evol. Biol.* **2014**, *14*, 1–12. [CrossRef] [PubMed]

45. Beckmann, A.; Xiao, S.; Muller, J.P.; Mercadante, D.; Nuchter, T.; Kroger, N.; Langhojer, F.; Petrich, W.; Holstein, T.W.; Benoit, M.; et al. A fast recoiling silk-like elastomer facilitates nanosecond nematocyst discharge. *BMC Biol.* **2015**, *13*, 1–15. [CrossRef] [PubMed]

46. Cai, H.; Chen, Y.; Cui, X.; Cai, S.; Chen, Z. High-resolution ¹H NMR spectroscopy of fish muscle, eggs and small whole fish via Hadamard-encoded intermolecular multiple-quantum coherence. *PLoS ONE* **2014**, *9*, e86422. [CrossRef] [PubMed]

47. Fisher, M.P.A. Are we quantum computers, or merely clever robots? *Int. J. Mod. Phys. B* **2017**, *31*, 1743001. [CrossRef]

48. Theis, T.; Mishra, B.; von der Ohe, M.; Loers, G.; Prondzynski, M.; Pless, O.; Blackshear, P.J.; Schachner, M.; Kleene, R. Functional role of the interaction between polysialic acid and myristoylated alanine-rich C kinase substrate at the plasma membrane. *J. Biol. Chem.* **2013**, *288*, 6726–6742. [CrossRef] [PubMed]

49. Dixon, M.C. Quartz crystal microbalance with dissipation monitoring: Enabling real-time characterization of biological materials and their interactions. *J. Biomol. Tech.* **2008**, *19*, 151–158. [PubMed]

50. Schadow, S.; Simons, V.S.; Lochnit, G.; Kordelle, J.; Gazova, Z.; Siebert, H.-C.; Steinmeyer, J. Metabolic response of human osteoarthritic cartilage to biochemically characterized collagen hydrolysates. *Int. J. Mol. Sci.* **2017**, *18*, 207. [CrossRef] [PubMed]

51. Hoyer, B.; Bernhardt, A.; Lode, A.; Heinemann, S.; Sewing, J.; Klinger, M.; Notbohm, H.; Gelinsky, M. Jellyfish collagen scaffolds for cartilage tissue engineering. *Acta Biomater.* **2014**, *10*, 883–892. [CrossRef]

52. Sewing, J.; Klinger, M.; Notbohm, H. Jellyfish collagen matrices conserve the chondrogenic phenotype in two- and three-dimensional collagen matrices. *J. Tissue Eng. Regen. Med.* **2015**, *11*, 916–925. [CrossRef]

53. Hwang, J.S.; Takaku, Y.; Momose, T.; Adamczyk, P.; Özbek, S.; Ikeo, K.; Khalturin, K.; Hemmrich, G.; Bosch, T.C.G.; Holstein, T.W.; et al. Nematogalectin, a nematocyst protein with GlyXY and galectin domains, demonstrates nematocyte-specific alternative splicing in Hydra. *Proc. Natl. Acad. Sci. USA* **2010**, *107*, 18539–18544. [CrossRef]

54. Benkert, P.; Biasini, M.; Schwede, T. Toward the estimation of the absolute quality of individual protein structure models. *Bioinformatics* **2011**, *27*, 343–350. [CrossRef] [PubMed]

55. Shirai, T.; Watanabe, Y.; Lee, M.S.; Ogawa, T.; Muramoto, K. Structure of rhamnose-binding lectin CSL3: Unique pseudo-tetrameric architecture of a pattern recognition protein. *J. Mol. Biol.* **2009**, *391*, 390–403. [CrossRef] [PubMed]

56. Adamczyk, P.; Zenkert, C.; Balasubramanian, P.G.; Yamada, S.; Murakoshi, S.; Sugahara, K.; Hwang, J.S.; Gojobori, T.; Holstein, T.W.; Özbek, S. A non-sulfated chondroitin stabilizes membrane tubulation in cnidarian organelles. *J. Biol. Chem.* **2010**, *285*, 25613–25623. [CrossRef] [PubMed]

57. Schaefer, L.; Beck, K.F.; Raslik, I.; Walpen, S.; Mihalik, D.; Micegova, M.; Macakova, K.; Schonherr, E.; Seidler, D.G.; Varga, G.; et al. Biglycan, a nitric oxide-regulated gene, affects adhesion, growth, and survival of mesangial cells. *J. Biol. Chem.* **2003**, *278*, 26227–26237. [CrossRef] [PubMed]

58. Schaefer, L.; Babelova, A.; Kiss, E.; Hausser, H.J.; Baliova, M.; Krzyzankova, M.; Marsche, G.; Young, M.F.; Mihalik, D.; Gotte, M.; et al. The matrix component biglycan is proinflammatory and signals through Toll-like receptors 4 and 2 in macrophages. *J. Clin. Investig.* **2005**, *115*, 2223–2233. [CrossRef] [PubMed]

59. Roedig, H.; Nastase, M.V.; Frey, H.; Moreth, K.; Zeng-Brouwers, J.; Poluzzi, C.; Tzung-Harn Hsieh, L.; Brandts, C.; Fulda, S.; Wygrecka, M.; et al. Biglycan is a new high-affinity ligand for CD14 in macrophages. *Matrix Biol.* **2019**, *77*, 4–22. [CrossRef] [PubMed]

60. Engel, U.; Pertz, O.; Fauser, C.; Engel, J.; David, C.N.; Holstein, T.W. A switch in disulfide linkage during minicollagen assembly in Hydra nematocysts. *EMBO J.* **2001**, *20*, 3063–3073. [CrossRef] [PubMed]

61. Engel, U.; Özbek, S.; Engel, R.; Petri, B.; Lottspeich, F.; Holstein, T.W. Nowa, a novel protein with minicollagen Cys-rich domains, is involved in nematocyst formation in Hydra. *J. Cell Sci.* **2002**, *115*, 3923–3934. [CrossRef] [PubMed]

62. Pokidysheva, E.; Milbradt, A.G.; Meier, S.; Renner, C.; Haussinger, D.; Bachinger, H.P.; Moroder, L.; Grzesiek, S.; Holstein, T.W.; Özbek, S.; et al. The structure of the Cys-rich terminal domain of Hydra minicollagen, which is involved in disulfide networks of the nematocyst wall. *J. Biol. Chem.* **2004**, *279*, 30395–30401. [CrossRef]

63. Ozacmak, V.H.; Thorington, G.U.; Fletcher, W.H.; Hessinger, D.A. N-acetylneuraminic acid (NANA) stimulates in situ cyclic AMP production in tentacles of sea anemone (Aiptasia pallida): Possible role in chemosensitization of nematocyst discharge. *J. Exp. Biol.* **2001**, *204*, 2011–2020.

64. Charlton, L.M.; Pielak, G.J. Peeking into living eukaryotic cells with high-resolution NMR. *Proc. Natl. Acad. Sci. USA* **2006**, *103*, 11817–11818. [CrossRef] [PubMed]

65. Muralikrishna, G.; Reuter, G.; Peter-Katalinic, J.; Egge, H.; Hanisch, F.G.; Siebert, H.-C.; Schauer, R. Identification of a new ganglioside from the starfish Asterias rubens. *Carbohydr. Res.* **1992**, *236*, 321–326. [CrossRef]

66. Zenkert, C.; Takahashi, T.; Diesner, M.O.; Özbek, S. Morphological and molecular analysis of the Nematostella vectensis cnidom. *PLoS ONE* **2011**, *6*, e22725. [CrossRef] [PubMed]

67. Petersen, H.O.; Höger, S.K.; Looso, M.; Lengfeld, T.; Kuhn, A.; Warnken, U.; Nishimiya-Fujisawa, C.; Schnölzer, M.; Krüger, M.; Özbek, S.; et al. A comprehensive transcriptomic and proteomic analysis of Hydra head regeneration. *Mol. Biol. Evol.* **2015**, *32*, 1928–1947. [CrossRef] [PubMed]

68. Berking, S.; Herrmann, K. Formation and discharge of nematocysts is controlled by a proton gradient across the cyst membrane. *Helgol. Mar. Res.* **2006**, *60*, 180–188. [CrossRef]

69. Ogawa, T.; Watanabe, M.; Naganuma, T.; Muramoto, K. Diversified carbohydrate-binding lectins from marine resources. *J. Amino Acids* **2011**, *2011*, 838–914. [CrossRef] [PubMed]

70. Datta, D.; Talapatra, S.N.; Swarnakar, S. An overview of lectins from freshwater and marine macroinvertebrates. *World Sci. News* **2016**, *46*, 77–87.

71. Technau, U.; Steele, R.E. Evolutionary crossroads in developmental biology: Cnidaria. *Development* **2011**, *138*, 1447–1458. [CrossRef] [PubMed]

72. Steele, R.E.; David, C.N.; Technau, U. A genomic view of 500 million years of cnidarian evolution. *Trends Genet.* **2011**, *27*, 7–13. [CrossRef]

73. Raspanti, M.; Congiu, T.; Alessandrini, A.; Gobbi, P.; Ruggeri, A. Different patterns of collagen-proteoglycan interaction: A scanning electron microscopy and atomic force microscopy study. *Eur. J. Histochem.* **2000**, *44*, 335–343.

74. Kar, R.K.; Gazova, Z.; Bednarikova, Z.; Mroue, K.H.; Ghosh, A.; Zhang, R.; Ulicna, K.; Siebert, H.-C.; Nifantiev, N.E.; Bhunia, A. Evidence for Inhibition of lysozyme amyloid fibrillization by peptide fragments from human lysozyme: A combined spectroscopy, microscopy, and docking study. *Biomacromolecules* **2016**, *17*, 1998–2009. [CrossRef] [PubMed]

75. Jayawardena, H.S.; Jayawardana, K.W.; Chen, X.; Yan, M. Maltoheptaose promotes nanoparticle internalization by Escherichia coli. *Chem. Commun.* **2013**, *49*, 3034–3036. [CrossRef] [PubMed]

76. Chen, X.; Ramstrôm, O.; Yan, M. Glyconanomaterials: Emerging applications in biomedical research. *Nano Res.* **2014**, *7*, 1381–1403. [CrossRef]

77. Sundhoro, M.; Park, J.; Jayawardana, K.W.; Chen, X.; Jayawardena, H.S.N.; Yan, M. Poly(HEMA-co-HEMA-PFPA): Synthesis and preparation of stable micelles encapsulating imaging nanoparticles. *J. Colloid Interface Sci.* **2017**, *500*, 1–8. [CrossRef] [PubMed]

78. Wang, X.; Ramstrôm, O.; Yan, M. Dynamic light scattering as an efficient tool to study glyconanoparticle–lectin interactions. *Analyst* **2011**, *136*, 4174–4178. [CrossRef] [PubMed]

79. Jayawardana, K.W.; Jayawardena, H.S.; Wijesundera, S.A.; De Zoysa, T.; Sundhoro, M.; Yan, M. Selective targeting of Mycobacterium smegmatis with trehalose-functionalized nanoparticles. *Chem. Commun.* **2015**, *51*, 12028–12031. [CrossRef] [PubMed]

80. Kondepudi, D.P.; Prigogine, I. *Modern Thermodynamics: From Heat Engines to Dissipative Structures, Chapter 19.5: Turing Structures and Propagating Waves*; Wiley Chichester: Chichester, UK, 1998; pp. 444–450.

81. Bushman, J.; Mishra, B.; Ezra, M.; Gul, S.; Schulze, C.; Chaudhury, S.; Ripoll, D.; Wallqvist, A.; Kohn, J.; Schachner, M.; et al. Tegaserod mimics the neurostimulatory glycan polysialic acid and promotes nervous system repair. *Neuropharmacology* **2014**, *79*, 456–466. [CrossRef] [PubMed]

82. Loers, G.; Saini, V.; Mishra, B.; Papastefanaki, F.; Lutz, D.; Chaudhury, S.; Ripoll, D.R.; Wallqvist, A.; Gul, S.; Schachner, M.; et al. Nonyloxytryptamine mimics polysialic acid and modulates neuronal and glial functions in cell culture. *J. Neurochem.* **2014**, *128*, 88–100. [CrossRef]

83. Siebert, H.-C.; André, S.; Lu, S.Y.; Frank, M.; Kaltner, H.; van Kuik, J.A.; Korchagina, E.Y.; Bovin, N.; Tajkhorshid, E.; Kaptein, R.; et al. Unique conformer selection of human growth-regulatory lectin galectin-1 for ganglioside GM1 versus bacterial toxins. *Biochemistry* **2003**, *42*, 14762–14773. [CrossRef]

84. Siebert, H.-C.; Born, K.; André, S.; Frank, M.; Kaltner, H.; von der Lieth, C.-W.; Heck, A.J.; Jiménez-Barbero, J.; Kopitz, J.; Gabius, H.-J. Carbohydrate chain of ganglioside GM1 as a ligand: Identification of the binding strategies of three 15 mer peptides and their divergence from the binding modes of growth-regulatory galectin-1 and cholera toxin. *Chem. Eur. J.* **2006**, *12*, 388–402. [CrossRef]
85. André, S.; Kaltner, H.; Lensch, M.; Russwurm, R.; Siebert, H.-C.; Fallsehr, C.; Tajkhorshid, E.; Heck, A.J.; von Knebel Doeberitz, M.; Gabius, H.-J.; et al. Determination of structural and functional overlap/divergence of five proto-type galectins by analysis of the growth-regulatory interaction with ganglioside GM1 in silico and in vitro on human neuroblastoma cells. *Int. J. Cancer* **2005**, *114*, 46–57. [CrossRef] [PubMed]
86. Wu, A.M.; Singh, T.; Liu, J.H.; Krzeminski, M.; Russwurm, R.; Siebert, H.-C.; Bonvin, A.M.; André, S.; Gabius, H.-J. Activity-structure correlations in divergent lectin evolution: Fine specificity of chicken galectin CG-14 and computational analysis of flexible ligand docking for CG-14 and the closely related CG-16. *Glycobiology* **2007**, *17*, 165–184. [CrossRef] [PubMed]
87. Wu, A.M.; Singh, T.; Liu, J.H.; André, S.; Lensch, M.; Siebert, H.-C.; Krzeminski, M.; Bonvin, A.M.; Kaltner, H.; Wu, J.H.; et al. Adhesion/growth-regulatory galectins: Insights into their ligand selectivity using natural glycoproteins and glycotopes. *Adv. Exp. Med. Biol.* **2011**, *705*, 117–141. [PubMed]
88. Siebert, H.-C.; Tajkhorshid, E.; Dabrowski, J. Barrier to rotation around the C-sp(2)-C-sp(2) bond of the ketoaldehyde enol ether MeC(O)CH=CH-OEt as determined by 13C NMR and ab initio calculations. *J. Phys. Chem. A* **2001**, *105*, 8488–8494. [CrossRef]
89. Van Lenthe, J.H.; den Boer, D.H.W.; Havenith, R.W.A.; Schauer, R.; Siebert, H.-C. Ab initio calculations on various sialic acids provide valuable information about sialic acid-specific enzymes. *J. Mol. Struct. THEOCHEM* **2004**, *677*, 29–37. [CrossRef]
90. Schwarzkopf, M.; Knobeloch, K.P.; Rohde, E.; Hinderlich, S.; Wiechens, N.; Lucka, L.; Horak, I.; Reutter, W.; Horstkorte, R. Sialylation is essential for early development in mice. *Proc. Natl. Acad. Sci. USA* **2002**, *99*, 5267–5270. [CrossRef] [PubMed]
91. Watanabe, H.; Fujisawa, T.; Holstein, T.W. Cnidarians and the evolutionary origin of the nervous system. *Dev. Growth Differ.* **2009**, *51*, 167–183. [CrossRef]
92. Siebert, H.-C.; von der Lieth, C.-W.; Dong, X.; Reuter, G.; Schauer, R.; Gabius, H.-J.; Vliegenthart, J.F.G. Molecular dynamics-derived conformation and intramolecular interaction analysis of the N-acetyl-9-O-acetylneuraminic acid-containing ganglioside GD1a and NMR-based analysis of its binding to a human polyclonal immunoglobulin G fraction with selectivity for O-acetylated sialic acids. *Glycobiology* **1996**, *6*, 561–572.
93. Yeh, S.C.; Wang, P.Y.; Lou, Y.W.; Khoo, K.H.; Hsiao, M.; Hsu, T.L.; Wong, C.H. Glycolipid GD3 and GD3 synthase are key drivers for glioblastoma stem cells and tumorigenicity. *Proc. Natl. Acad. Sci. USA* **2016**, *113*, 5592–5597. [CrossRef]
94. Sackmann, E.; Keber, F.; Heinrich, D. Physics of cellular movements. *Annu. Rev. Conden. Matter* **2010**, *1*, 257–276. [CrossRef]
95. Haseley, S.R.; Vermeer, H.J.; Kamerling, J.P.; Vliegenthart, J.F.G. Carbohydrate self-recognition mediates marine sponge cellular adhesion. *Proc. Natl. Acad. Sci. USA* **2001**, *98*, 9419–9424. [CrossRef]
96. Vilanova, E.; Santos, G.R.; Aquino, R.S.; Valle-Delgado, J.J.; Anselmetti, D.; Fernandez-Busquets, X.; Mourao, P.A. Carbohydrate-carbohydrate interactions mediated by sulfate esters and calcium provide the cell adhesion required for the emergence of early metazoans. *J. Biol. Chem.* **2016**, *291*, 9425–9437. [CrossRef]
97. Lai, C.H.; Hutter, J.; Hsu, C.W.; Tanaka, H.; Varela-Aramburu, S.; De Cola, L.; Lepenies, B.; Seeberger, P.H. Analysis of carbohydrate-carbohydrate interactions using sugar-functionalized silicon nanoparticles for cell imaging. *Nano Lett.* **2016**, *16*, 807–811. [CrossRef]
98. Lombardi, G.; Della Puppa, A.; Zustovich, F.; Pambuku, A.; Farina, P.; Fiduccia, P.; Roma, A.; Zagonel, V. The combination of carmustine wafers and fotemustine in recurrent glioblastoma patients: A monoinstitutional experience. *Biomed. Res. Int.* **2014**, *2014*, 1–4. [CrossRef]
99. Rahman, R.; Hempfling, K.; Norden, A.D.; Reardon, D.A.; Nayak, L.; Rinne, M.L.; Beroukhim, R.; Doherty, L.; Ruland, S.; Rai, A.; et al. Retrospective study of carmustine or lomustine with bevacizumab in recurrent glioblastoma patients who have failed prior bevacizumab. *Neuro-Oncology* **2014**, *16*, 1523–1529. [CrossRef]
100. Sieren, J.C.; Quelle, D.; Meyerholz, D.K.; Rogers, C.S. Porcine cancer models for translational oncology. *Mol. Cell. Oncol.* **2014**, *1*, e969626. [CrossRef]

101. Lenhoff, H.M.; Brown, R.D. Mass culture of Hydra: An improved method and its application to other aquatic invertebrates. *Lab. Anim.* **1970**, *4*, 139–154. [CrossRef]

102. Krylov, V.B.; Grachev, A.A.; Ustyuzhanina, N.E.; Ushakova, N.A.; Preobrazhenskaya, M.E.; Kozlova, N.I.; Portsel, M.N.; Konovalova, I.N.; Novikov, V.Y.; Siebert, H.-C.; et al. Preliminary structural characterization, anti-inflammatory and anticoagulant activities of chondroitin sulfates from marine fish cartilage. *Russ. Chem. B* **2011**, *60*, 746–753. [CrossRef]

103. Holdt, S.L.; Kraan, S. Bioactive compounds in seaweed: Functional food applications and legislation. *J. Appl. Phycol.* **2010**, *23*, 543–597. [CrossRef]

104. Van Zundert, G.C.P.; Rodrigues, J.; Trellet, M.; Schmitz, C.; Kastritis, P.L.; Karaca, E.; Melquiond, A.S.J.; van Dijk, M.; de Vries, S.J.; Bonvin, A. The HADDOCK2.2 Web Server: User-Friendly Integrative Modelling of Biomolecular Complexes. *J. Mol. Biol.* **2016**, *428*, 720–725. [CrossRef]

105. Krieger, E.; Vriend, G. YASARA View—molecular graphics for all devices-from smartphones to workstations. *Bioinformatics* **2014**, *30*, 2981–2982. [CrossRef]

106. Krieger, E.; Joo, K.; Lee, J.; Lee, J.; Raman, S.; Thompson, J.; Tyka, M.; Baker, D.; Karplus, K. Improving physical realism, stereochemistry, and side-chain accuracy in homology modelling: Four approaches that performed well in CASP8. *Proteins* **2009**, *77* (Suppl. 9), 114–122. [CrossRef]

107. Jayawardena, H.S.; Wang, X.; Yan, M. Classification of lectins by pattern recognition using glyconanoparticles. *Anal. Chem.* **2013**, *85*, 10277–10281. [CrossRef]

108. Szczepanek, S.; Cikala, M.; David, C.N. Poly-gamma-glutamate synthesis during formation of nematocyst capsules in Hydra. *J. Cell Sci.* **2002**, *115*, 745–751.

109. Soriano, J.; Rudiger, S.; Pullarkat, P.; Ott, A. Mechanogenetic coupling of Hydra symmetry breaking and driven Turing instability model. *Biophys. J.* **2009**, *96*, 1649–1660. [CrossRef]

110. Nobrega, F.L.; Costa, A.R.; Kluskens, L.D.; Azeredo, J. Revisiting phage therapy: New applications for old resources. *Trends Microbiol.* **2015**, *23*, 185–191. [CrossRef]

111. Schauer, R.; Kamerling, J.P. Sialic acids, Part I: Historical background and development, and chemical synthesis. *Adv. Carbohydr. Chem. Biochem.* **2018**, *75*, 1–354.

112. Morabito, R.; Dossena, S.; La Spada, G.; Marino, A. Heavy metals affect nematocysts discharge response and biological activity of crude venom in the jellyfish *Pelagia noctiluca* (Cnidaria, Scyphozoa). *Cell. Physiol. Biochem.* **2014**, *34*, 244–254. [CrossRef]

113. Abdullah, N.S.; Saad, S. Rapid detecion of N-acetylneuraminic acid from false clownfish using HPLC-FLD for symbiosis to host sea anemone. *Asian J. Sci. Technol.* **2015**, *3*, 858–864.

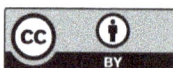

marine drugs

MDPI

Article

Heterologous Expression of a Thermostable β-1,3-Galactosidase and Its Potential in Synthesis of Galactooligosaccharides

Haitao Ding, Lili Zhou, Qian Zeng, Yong Yu and Bo Chen *

SOA Key Laboratory for Polar Science, Polar Research Institute of China, Shanghai 200136, China;
htding@outlook.com (H.D.); lilizhou1199@163.com (L.Z.); zengqianmu@126.com (Q.Z.);
yuyong@pric.org.cn (Y.Y.)
* Correspondence: chenbo@pric.org.cn; Tel.: +86-21-58711026

Received: 16 October 2018; Accepted: 25 October 2018; Published: 30 October 2018

check for
updates

Abstract: A thermostable β-1,3-galactosidase from *Marinomonas* sp. BSi20414 was successfully heterologously expressed in *Escherichia coli* BL21 (DE3), with optimum over-expression conditions as follows: the recombinant cells were induced by adding 0.1 mM of IPTG to the medium when the OD_{600} of the culture reached between 0.6 and 0.9, followed by 22 h incubation at 20 °C. The recombinant enzyme β-1,3-galactosidase (rMaBGA) was further purified to electrophoretic purity by immobilized metal affinity chromatography and size exclusion chromatography. The specific activity of the purified enzyme was 126.4 U mg^{-1} at 37 °C using ONPG (*o*-nitrophenyl-β-galactoside) as a substrate. The optimum temperature and pH of rMaBGA were determined as 60 °C and 6.0, respectively, resembling with its wild-type counterpart, wild type (wt)MaBGA. However, rMaBGA and wtMaBGA displayed different thermal stability and steady-state kinetics, although they share identical primary structures. It is postulated that the stability of the enzyme was altered by heterologous expression with the absence of post-translational modifications such as glycosylation, as well as the steady-state kinetics. To evaluate the potential of the enzyme in synthesis of galactooligosaccharides (GOS), the purified recombinant enzyme was employed to catalyze the transgalactosylation reaction at the lab scale. One of the transgalactosylation products was resolved as 3′-galactosyl-lactose, which had been proven to be a better bifidogenic effector than GOS with β-1,4 linkage and β-1,6 linkages. The results indicated that the recombinant enzyme would be a promising alternative for biosynthesis of GOS mainly with β-1,3 linkage.

Keywords: β-galactosidase; recombinant; thermostable; transglycosylation; galactooligosaccharides; *Marinomonas*

---

1. Introduction

Galactooligosaccharides (GOS) are non-digestible oligosaccharides composed of 3–10 galactosyl groups and a terminal glucose [1]. As an important type of dietary supplement, GOS is difficult to digest by the gastrointestine directly, whereas it can specifically stimulate the growth of the prebiotics inhabited in the intestine, such as *Lactobacillus* and *Bifidobacteria*, rather than maleficent bacteria [2]. It is well known that the growth of probiotics can improve immunity and prevent cancer [3]. As a matter of fact, it is impossible to obtain enough natural GOS from milk to satisfy the increasing demanding due to the low amount of GOS in milk [4].

To provide sufficient GOS for humans, chemical and enzymatic approaches have been developed to synthesis of GOS in practice [5]. However, because of a lack of specificity of the product and the extreme condition for hydrolysis of lactose to generate monosaccharides, chemical methods are not utilized on a large scale. In contrast, enzymatic synthesis of GOS exhibits good stereoselectivity and regioselectivity, with mild reaction conditions [6]. Thus, GOS present in the market are all produced from lactose by employing various β-D-galactosidases (E.C. 3.2.1.23, BGAs) [7].

BGAs could be produced by a great number of organisms, including microorganisms, and animal and plant cells [8]. All BGAs are capable of catalyzing the hydrolysis of the β-glycosylic linkage of lactose to generate glucose and galactose, as well as transferring of the galactose onto the galactose moiety of lactose to yield GOS [6]. Generally, the hydrolytic activity of BGA has been employed to remove lactose from milk for people with lactose intolerance, while the transgalactosylation activity has been developed for the production of diverse functional galactosylated products, especially prebiotics like GOS [9].

BGAs catalyze two forms of transglycosylation reactions, including intramolecular and intermolecular reactions. The former involves the direct transfer of galactosyl groups to glucose to produce lactose isomers, such as allolactose, which formed β-1,6 linkage near the end of the hydrolysis reactions, before the glycosyl molecules diffuse out of the active site. Unlike the intramolecular reaction, the intermolecular reaction can produce disaccharides, trisaccharides, tetrasaccharides, and polysaccharides with a higher degree of polymerization. During the catalytic reaction of β-galactosidase, the synthesized GOS can also serve as a substrate for the hydrolysis reaction, resulting in dynamic changes in the components and amounts of GOS [10].

As a rule of thumb, thermal stability is imperative for the application of enzymes in practice. To obtain quantified BGAs for GOS manufacturing, BGAs from various sources had been extensively studied [11–13]. In our previous study, a novel β-1,3-galactosidase (MaBGA) from *Marinomonas* sp. BSi20414, a strain isolated from the Arctic Ocean, has been purified and characterized [14]. This enzyme showed robust thermal stability and strict substrate specificity toward β-1,3 linkage, providing a competitive candidate for biosynthesis of GOS with β-1,3 linkage. In the present work, the enzyme MaBGA was heterologously expressed in *Escherichia coli* and the purified enzyme was subsequently employed to catalyze the transglycosylated reaction to generate oligosaccharides, for evaluating the potential application of MaBGA in biosynthesis of GOS.

2. Results

2.1. Construction of Recombinant Cells

The gene *mabga* was amplified from *Marinomonas* sp. BSi20414 using the corresponding primer pairs. The purified PCR product was digested with restriction endonucleases *Nde*I and *Xho*I, as well as plasmid pET-22b (+). The digested PCR product and vector were ligated together to construct recombinant plasmid. The recombinant plasmid was transformed into *E. coli* DH5α and the positive clones were picked for sequencing. Subsequently, the verified plasmid with correct insert sequence was transformed into *E. coli* BL21 (DE3) for expression.

2.2. Optimization of the Expression Condition of rMaBGA

To obtain more soluble recombinant protein, one-factor-at-a-time design was implemented for optimization of the expression condition of recombinant MaBGA (rMaBGA), using cell density, concentration of inducer, temperature, and duration for induction as four variables. According to the soluble expression of rMaBGA under different expression conditions (Figure 1), examined by SDS-PAGE (sodium dodecyl sulfate polyacrylamide gel electrophoresis), the optimized expression condition was adopted as follows: the recombinant cells were induced by adding 0.1 mM of IPTG to the medium when the OD_{600} of the culture reached between 0.6 and 0.9, followed by 22 h incubation at 20 °C.

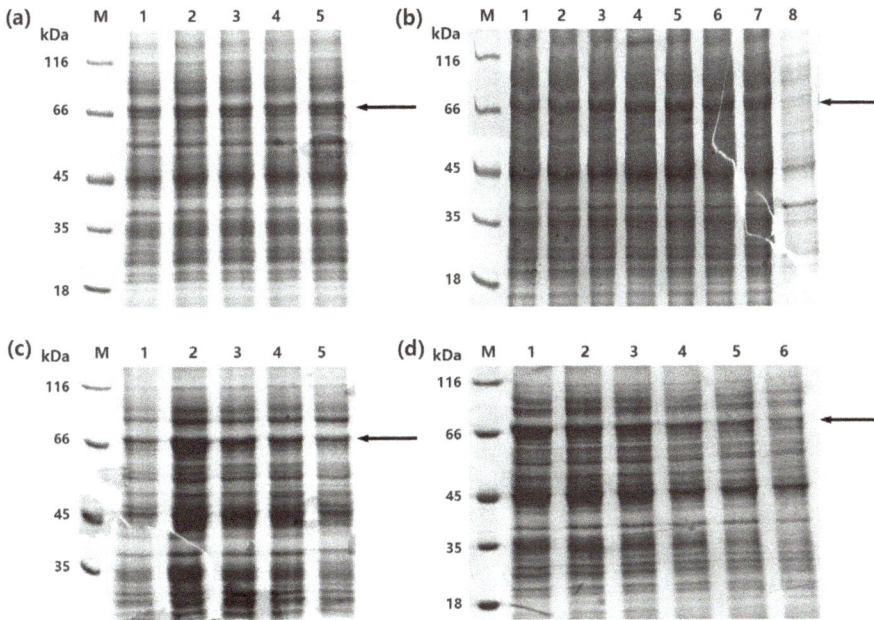

Figure 1. SDS-PAGE (sodium dodecyl sulfate polyacrylamide gel electrophoresis) analysis of the production of the recombinant enzyme β-1,3-galactosidase (rMaBGA) under different expression conditions. (**a**) The supernatant of cell lysates induced at different OD. Lane 1–5: OD reached 0.2, 0.6, 0.7, 0.9, and 1.3, respectively. (**b**) The supernatant of cell lysates induced with different IPTG concentration. Lane 1–8: the IPTG concentration was 0.05, 0.1, 0.3, 0.5, 0.7, 0.9, 1.2, and 0 mM, respectively. (**c**) The supernatant of cell lysates induced at different temperatures. Lane 1–5: the induced temperature was set to 15, 20, 25, 30, and 37 °C, respectively. (**d**) The supernatant of cell lysates induced for different time. Lane 1–6: the induced time was 22, 10, 8, 7, 4, and 2 h, respectively. Lane M: protein molecular weight marker. The location of rMaBGA was marked with black arrows.

2.3. Purification of rMaBGA

In general, most recombinant protein containing 6X His-tag could be easily purified to electrophoretic purity by one-step immobilized metal affinity chromatography (IMAC). However, rMaBGA cannot be purified to a single band after loading onto a column packed with Ni-NTA agarose, as shown on the gel in Figure 2a. Therefore, the elute of IMAC was further purified by size exclusion chromatography (SEC). As expected, the purified enzyme was represented as a homogeneous band corresponding to 66 kDa on the gel (Figure 2b), indicating that rMaBGA had been purified to electrophoretic purity. The specific activity of the purified rMaBGA was 126.4 U mg^{-1} at 37 °C using ONPG (o-nitrophenyl-β-galactoside) as substrate.

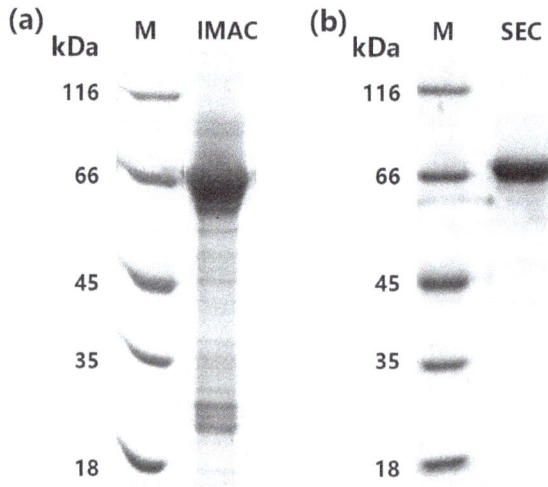

Figure 2. SDS-PAGE analysis of rMaBGA first purified by immobilized metal affinity chromatography (IMAC) (**a**) and then purified by size exclusion chromatography (SEC) (**b**). Lane M: protein molecular weight marker. Lane IMAC: rMaBGA purified by IMAC. Lane SEC: rMaBGA purified by IMAC and SEC, sequentially.

2.4. Enzymatic Characterization of MaBGA

2.4.1. Effect of pH and Temperature on the Activity of rMaBGA

The recombinant MaBGA showed its maximum activity at 60 °C (Figure 3a), as well as the wild type MaBGA (wtMaBGA). Although rMaBGA and wtMaBGA displayed a similar temperature-activity relationship at temperatures below 60 °C, the activity of rMaBGA dropped to 10% of its highest activity at 65 °C, whereas wtMaBGA still retained nearly 80% of its highest activity at the same temperature. The optimum pH of rMaBGA was determined as 6.0 (Figure 3b), resembling wtMaBGA. Moreover, the pH-activity profile of rMaBGA was also similar to that of wtMaBGA.

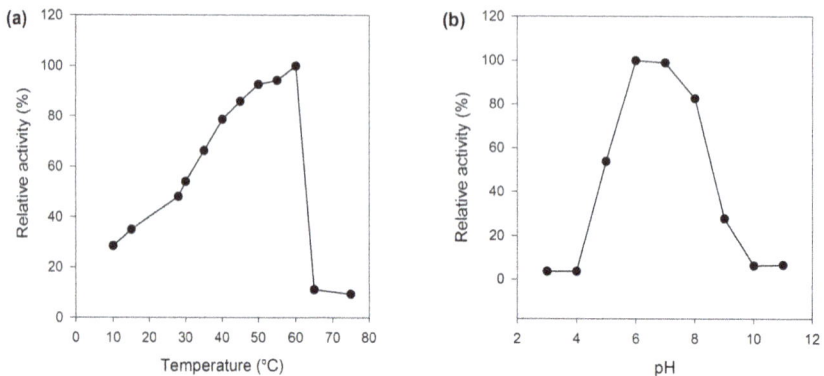

Figure 3. Effects of temperature and pH on the activity of rMaBGA. (**a**) Effect of temperature on the activity of rMaBGA; (**b**) effect of pH on the activity of rMaBGA.

2.4.2. Thermal Denaturation Kinetic of rMaBGA

As shown in Table 1, the half-life at 50 °C and 60 °C of wtMaBGA was 1.66 and 2.42 times more, respectively, than those of rMaBGA, indicating that rMaBGA was less stable than wtMaBGA, also indicated by the values of inactivation enthalpy (ΔH), inactivation free energy (ΔG), and inactivation entropy (ΔS).

Table 1. Thermodynamics of irreversible thermal denaturation of β-1,3-galactosidase (MaBGA). wt—wild type; r—recombinant enzyme.

Enzyme	Temperature (°C)	k_d (h^{-1})	$t_{1/2}$ (h)	ΔH ($KJ\,mol^{-1}$)	ΔG ($KJ\,mol^{-1}$)	ΔS ($J\,mol^{-1}\,K^{-1}$)
wtMaBGA	50	0.0433	16.00	114.03	87.75	81.35
	60	0.1597	4.34	113.94	86.94	81.10
rMaBGA	50	0.0721	9.61	147.75	86.38	189.99
	60	0.3879	1.79	147.66	84.48	189.74

2.4.3. Steady-State Kinetic of rMaBGA

The Michaelis–Menten constant K_m and the maximum reaction velocity V_{max} of rMaBGA were determined as 6.85 mM and 64.13 µM min^{-1} (Table 2), respectively, using a nonlinear fitting plot. However, the values of K_m and V_{max} for the recombinant MaBGA showed a significant difference from those of its wild type counterpart, which were measured as 14.19 mM and 1.05 µM min^{-1}, respectively, in our previous study [14].

Table 2. Kinetic constants of rMaBGA.

Enzyme	K_m (mM)	V_{max} (µM min^{-1})
rMaBGA	6.85	64.13
wtMaBGA	14.19	1.05

2.5. Synthesis of Galactooligosaccharides

2.5.1. Thin-Layer Chromatography Analysis

The reaction mixture was subjected to thin-layer chromatography analysis after removal of the enzyme. It is obvious that the reaction mixture (Figure 4) contained spots corresponding to spots A (galactose), B (glucose), and C (lactose), indicating the occurrence of the hydrolysis reaction. In addition, several blurry spots can be found from Lane 4 at the position below spot C. It is supposed that the substance represented as blurry spots might be the products of transglycosylation reaction catalyzed by rMaBGA.

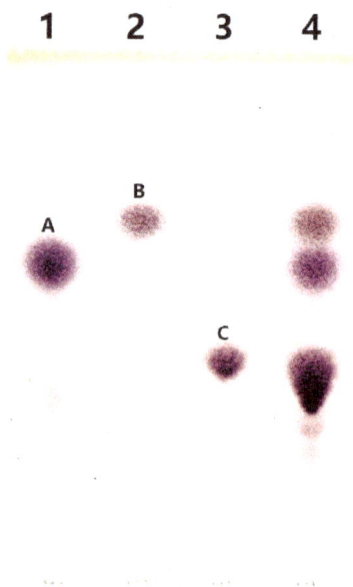

Figure 4. Analysis of transgalactosylation activity of rMaBGA by TLC (thin layer chromatography). Lane 1: galactose (spot A); Lane 2: glucose (spot B); Lane 3: lactose (spot C); Lane 4: the products of lactose catalyzed by rMaBGA.

2.5.2. Characterization of the Products of Transglycosylation

The transglycosylation products were purified and separated into three components, designated as LLZ-01, LLZ-02, and LLZ-03, using gel chromatography and HPLC. Based on the ESI-MS and NMR analyses, component LLZ-01 characterized as a mixture of α-lactose and β-lactose with ratios between 1:7 and 1:8, whereas component LLZ-02 was determined to be the mixture of α-lactose/β-lactose and trisaccharides with a ratio of 1:1. Unfortunately, the low purity of LLZ-03 resulted in complex MS and NMR signals, which was difficult to resolve. Additional purification steps are indispensable for characterization of LLZ-03 in further studies.

In the present study, two-dimensional NMR techniques, ^{1}H-^{1}H COSY and NOESY were adopted to resolve structure of the trisaccharides presented in LLZ-02 (Figure 5), using trisaccharide O-β-D-galactopyranosyl-(1-4)-O-β-D-galactopyranosyl-(1-4)-D-glucopyranose (4′-galactosyl-lactose) as reference in the analysis. All the chemical shifts were tabulated in Table 3 according to the signal of ^{1}H-^{1}H COSY. Clear NOE was detected between H1 of β-galactosyl-A (4.37 ppm) and H4 of α-glucosyl (3.50 ppm)/β-glucosyl (3.46 ppm), as well as between H1 of β-galactosyl-B (4.50 ppm) and H3 of β-glucosyl (3.42 ppm). It is suggested that the linking between β-galactosyl-A and α-glucosyl/β-glucosyl occurred at the 1,4 sites, and the linking between β-galactosyl-B and β-glucosyl occurred at the 1,3 sites. Therefore, the trisaccharide of LLZ-02 was determined as β-D-galactosyl-(1-3)-β-D-galactosyl-(1-4)-D-glucose (3′-galactosyl-lactose, Figure 6).

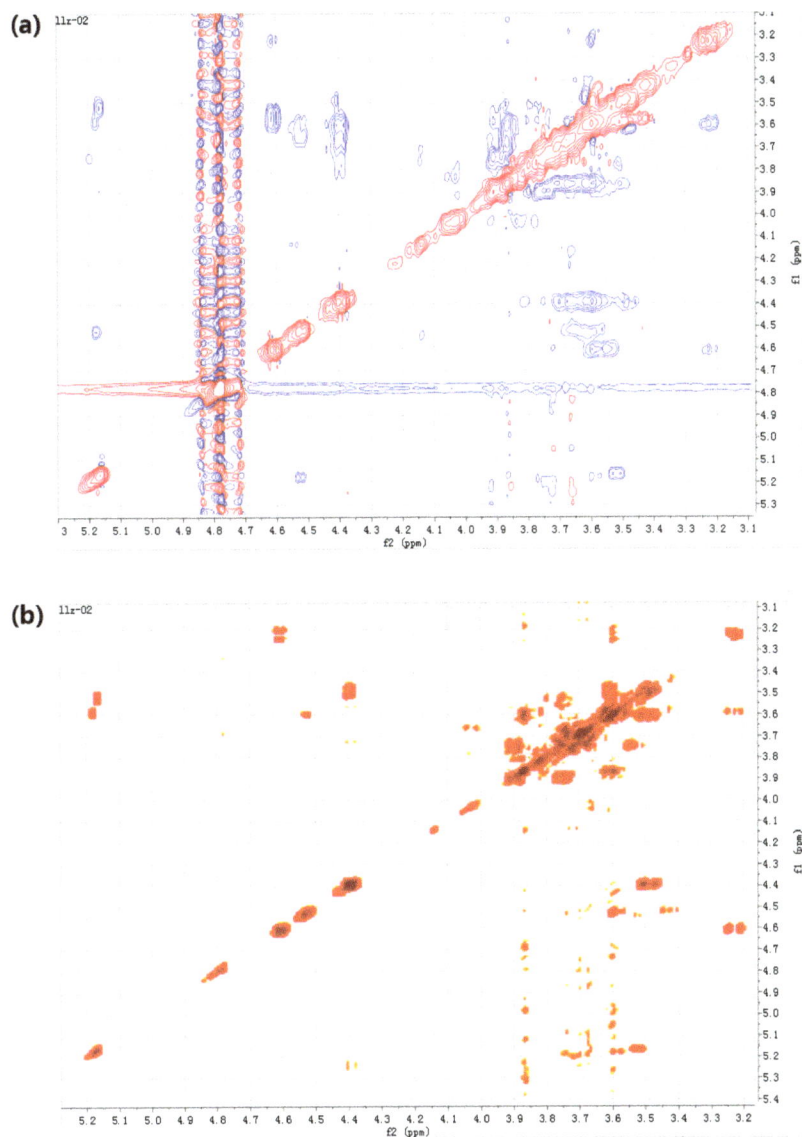

Figure 5. Two-dimensional NMR analysis of LLZ-02. (**a**) ^{1}H-^{1}H COSY spectrum. (**b**) NOESY spectrum.

Table 3. Proton chemical shifts for LLZ-02.

Unit	α-glucosyl	β-glucosyl	β-galactosyl-A	β-galactosyl-B
1	5.14	4.59	4.37	4.50
2	3.52	3.21	3.62	3.62
3	3.79	3.42	3.84	3.70
4	3.50	3.46	4.01	3.86
5	3.85	3.60	3.70	3.67
6	3.75–3.88	3.75–3.88	3.70–3.85	3.70–3.85

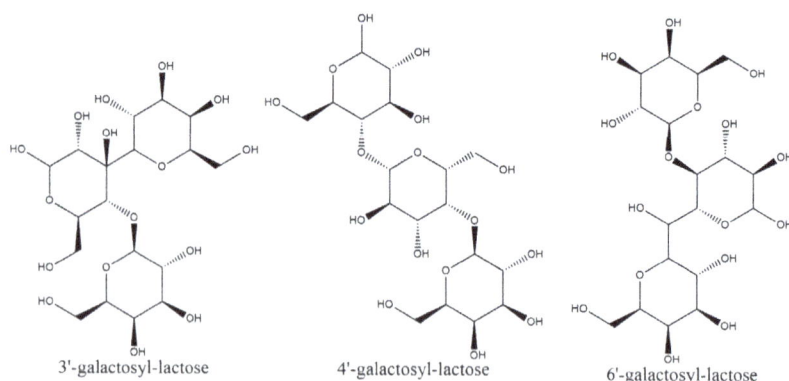

Figure 6. Molecular structures of 3′-galactosyl-lactose, 4′-galactosyl-lactose, and 6′-galactosyl-lactose.

3. Discussion

In this study, a thermostable β-1,3-galactosidase from *Marinomonas* sp. BSi20414 was successfully heterologously expressed in *Escherichia coli* BL21 (DE3), with optimized over-expression conditions. The purified recombinant enzyme was characterized biochemically and employed to the synthesis of GOS, which were further analyzed by ESI-MS and NMR to resolve the molecular structures.

Although rMaBGA displayed similar optimum catalytic pH and temperature to those of its wild-type counterpart, these two-form enzymes, which share an identical primary structure, exhibited different thermal stability and steady-state kinetics. Beyond expectations, the half-life at 50 °C and 60 °C of wtMaBGA were 1.66 and 2.42 times more, respectively, than those of rMaBGA. The decrease in values of ΔH and ΔG of both wtMaBGA and rMaBGA was concomitant with increase in the temperature, suggesting that the conformation of the protein was altered changed by heat treatment. The higher values of ΔG for wtMaBGA than those for rMaBGA indicated that wtMaBGA showed more resistance against thermal denaturation than rMaBGA at the same temperature, also suggested by the increase of entropy of inactivation (ΔS), which is often accompanied by disruption of enzyme structure. As rMaBGA and wtMaBGA share exactly the same amino acid sequences, it is supposed that the difference in stability and kinetics between them might be caused by the post-translational modification (PTM) occurring in the wild-type strain. PTM, such as glycosylation [15], phosphorylation [16], and methylation [17], affects the kinetic, stability, and structural features of proteins through regulating their biophysical characteristics. Several studies reported that the glycosylated proteins exhibited higher stability, which have higher melting temperature and greater free energy than their non-glycosylated wild-type counterpart [18]. Therefore, it is postulated that the stability of the enzyme was altered by heterologous expression with the lack of PTM, as well as the steady-state kinetics. Although the recombinant MaBGA was less stable than its wild-type counterpart, its thermal stability is still qualified for practical application. Every coin has two sides, the recombinant enzyme showed superior catalytic activity than the wild-type form, as the V_{max} of the former was 61-fold higher than that of the latter.

Generally, β-galactosidases from various sources produce diverse GOS mixtures with different degrees of polymerization (DP) and glycosidic linkages. For instance, β-galactosidase from *Bacillus circulans* produces predominantly β-1,4 linked GOS, while β-galactosidase from *Kluyveromyces lactis* mainly forms GOS with β-1,6 linkage [4,19], whereas the dominant transglycosylation product in this study was identified as trisaccharide with β-1,3 linkages. Regardless of the fact that β-1,4 and β-1,6 are common linkages in GOS, β-1,3 linkage is relatively rare [20]; the latter showed stronger prebiotic effect than the former. Previous studies have shown that GOS containing mainly β-1,3 linkage had a better bifidogenic effect than GOS containing mainly β-1,4 and β-1,6 linkages after one week of intake by healthy humans [21]. Therefore, owing to its soluble over-expression, thermal stability, and selectivity toward β-1,3 linkage, the recombinant MaBGA was proven to be a promising alternative for biosynthesis of 3′-galactosyl-lactose, a probiotic with better bifidogenic effect.

4. Materials and Methods

4.1. Expression and Purification of rMaBGA

4.1.1. Strains, Plasmids, and Culture Conditions

Strain *Marinomonas* sp. BSi20414, isolated from the Arctic Ocean [22], was used as the source of β-galactosidase. *Escherichia coli* DH5α and BL21 (DE3), cultivated in Luria–Bertani medium at 37 °C, were used for gene cloning and expression, respectively. Plasmid pET22b (+) was employed to construct recombinant plasmid. All chemicals were of analytical grade.

4.1.2. Construction of Recombinant Strains

The gene encoding for MaBGA was amplified using DNA of *Marinomonas* sp. BSi20414 as a template with the forward primer 5′-GGAATTCCATATGAAGTTAGGTGTATGTTACTACC-3′ and the reverse primer 5′-GTTCGCGCTCGAGGATTTCTTGCCAAATGGC-3′, carrying the cleavage sites of *Nde*I and *Xho*I (underlined), respectively. The PCR product was digested with restriction endonucleases *Nde*I and *Xho*I simultaneously, and ligated with the vector pET-22b (+) digested by the same enzymes. The constructed plasmid was transformed into *E. coli* DH5α competent cells for sequencing. Subsequently, the verified plasmid harboring the desired gene was transformed into *E. coli* BL21 (DE3) competent cells for expression.

4.1.3. Optimization of the Production of rMaBGA

Cells were cultivated in Luria–Bertani broth at 37 °C with 100 $\mu g\,mL^{-1}$ ampicillin added. Subsequently, single-factor experimental design was employed for the optimization of the production of rMaBGA. Soluble expression of rMaBGA was estimated under different cell density, IPTG concentration, incubation temperature, and time adopted for induction.

4.1.4. Expression and Purification of rMaBGA

The expression of the rMaBGA was performed according to the optimization procedure, as follows: the induction of the recombinant cells was started by adding 0.1 mM IPTG to the broth when the OD_{600} of the culture reached between 0.6 and 0.9, followed by 22 h incubation at 20 °C. Cultures were collected by centrifugation at $10,000\times g$ for 10 min. The precipitate was washed and suspended with lysis buffer (50 mM sodium phosphate buffer, 10 mM imidazole, 200 mM NaCl, 0.5% glycerol, pH 7.0). Cells were then lysed by ultrasonication (burst of 5 s followed by intervals of 10 s repeated 90 times). The cell debris was discarded by centrifugation at $10,000\times g$ for 15 min and the crude enzyme was loaded onto a column packed with Ni-NTA resin. The resin was washed with wash buffer (50 mM sodium phosphate buffer, 20 mM imidazole, 200 mM NaCl, 0.5% glycerol, pH 7.0) and subsequently eluted with elution buffer (50 mM sodium phosphate buffer, 250 mM imidazole, 200 mM NaCl, 0.5% glycerol, pH 7.0). The eluted enzyme was concentrated by ultrafiltration and then subjected to a prepacked gel filtration column filled with Surperdex G200 with a flow rate of 0.4 mL min^{-1}. The eluted enzyme was desalted and concentrated by ultrafiltration and stored at −80 °C. All purification steps were implemented at 4 °C. The protein concentration was measured by Bradford method using bovine serum albumin (BSA) as a standard [23].

4.1.5. SDS-PAGE Analysis

The purified rMaBGA was examined by SDS-PAGE running on a 5% stacking gel and an 8% separating gel [24]. Gel was stained with Coomassie Brilliant Blue R-250. The molecular weight of rMaBGA was determined using protein molecular weight marker (MBI) as a reference.

4.2. Enzymatic Characterization of rMaBGA

4.2.1. Enzyme Activity Assay

The enzyme activity was measured by monitoring the absorbance of ONP (*o*-nitrophenyl) at 420 nm in 50 mM PBS buffer (pH 7.0) at 37 °C, with 10 mM of ONPG was used as substrate. The concentration of ONP was obtained from the standard curve. One unit of β-galactosidase activity was defined as the amount of enzyme demanded for catalyzing the formation of 1 μmol ONP per minute.

4.2.2. Effect of pH and Temperature on the Activity of rMaBGA

The optimum pH for rMaBGA was measured by assaying its activity with different pH ranging from 3.0 to 11.0 in Britton–Robinson buffer. The optimum temperature for rMaBGA was measured by assaying its activity at different temperatures from 10 to 70 °C.

4.2.3. Thermal Denaturation Kinetic of rMaBGA

The thermal stability of rMaBGA was evaluated by measuring the remaining activity after incubation of the enzyme at 50 °C and 60 °C for 1 h with 5 min intervals. Thermodynamic parameters for thermal unfolding of rMaBGA were calculated according to Ding et al. [25].

4.2.4. Steady-State Kinetic of rMaBGA

The activity of rMaBGA was assayed with different concentrations of ONPG ranging from 0.25 to 5 mM to analyze the steady-state kinetic of the enzyme. The kinetic parameters were calculated by nonlinear fitting of the Michaelis–Menten Equation (1):

$$v = V_{max} \, [S]/(K_m + [S]) \tag{1}$$

where K_m and [S] are Michaelis constants and concentration of ONPG, respectively.

4.3. Synthesis of Galactooligosaccharides

4.3.1. Thin-Layer Chromatography Analysis

The transglycosylation reaction was conducted at 40 °C for 5 h by adding 3.5 U rMaBGA to 50 mM PBS buffer (pH 7.0) containing 480 mM lactose. Subsequently, the enzyme was inactivated by boiling for 2 min. The denatured enzyme was removed by centrifugation at 10,000× g for 15 min and the supernatant was used for thin-layer chromatography analysis. A solvent mixture consisting of 50% n-butanol, 20% ethanol, and 30% water was employed to develop the TLC plate in a developing chamber. The visualization reagents contained 0.5% 3,5-dihydroxytoluene and 20% H_2SO_4.

4.3.2. Characterization of the Products of Transglycosylation

The supernatant prepared as described above was concentrated by rotary evaporation and dissolved by 50% ethanol, which was then subjected to a prepacked column filled with Sephadex LH-20 and eluted with 50% ethanol. The elute was collected by a fraction collector and was analyzed by TLC. Fractions containing transglycosylation product were combined and concentrated by rotary evaporation. The concentrate was dissolved by the appropriate amount of water and filtered through a 0.22 μm membrane. Subsequently, the concentrated products were separated by HPLC (LC-10AdvP,

Mar. Drugs **2018**, *16*, 415

SHIMADZU, Kyoto, Japan) equipped with a semi-preparation YMC-Pack NH2 column, with a flow rate of 3 mL min^{-1} and temperature of 30 °C. The elution peaks were concentrated by rotary evaporation, then dissolved by appropriate amount of water, and further characterized by MS and NMR.

5. Conclusions

In the present work, a thermostable β-1,3-galactosidase from *Marinomonas* sp. BSi20414 was successfully heterologously expressed in *Escherichia coli* BL21 (DE3), with optimized over-expression conditions. The recombinant enzyme was further purified to electrophoretic purity and characterized biochemically. Although rMaBGA showed similar profiles of optimum catalytic pH and temperature to those of its wild-type counterpart, these two-form enzymes, which share an identical primary structure, exhibited different thermal stability and steady-state kinetics. It is assumed that the stability and the steady-state kinetics of the enzyme were altered by heterologous expression with the absence of post-translational modifications such as glycosylation. Furthermore, owing to the soluble over-expression, thermal stability, and selectivity toward β-1,3 linkage, rMaBGA was proven to be a promising alternative for biosynthesis of 3′-galactosyl-lactose, a probiotic with better bifidogenic effect than GOS with β-1,4 linkage and β-1,6 linkages.

Author Contributions: Y.Y. and B.C. conceived and designed the experiments; L.Z. and Q.Z. performed the experiments; H.D., Y.Y., L.Z., and Q.Z. analyzed the data; Y.Y. and B.C. contributed reagents/materials/analysis tools; H.D., Y.Y., and B.C. wrote the paper.

Funding: This research was funded by National Key R&D Program of China (2018YFC1406704, 2018YFC1406701), Youth Innovation Fund of Polar Science (201602), and Open Fund of Key Laboratory of Biotechnology and Bioresources Utilization of Dalian Minzu University (KF2015009).

Acknowledgments: We gratefully acknowledge the reviewers and editors for their deep and careful work in helping to improve the manuscript.

Conflicts of Interest: The authors declare no conflict of interest.

References

1. Panesar, P.S.; Kaur, R.; Singh, R.S.; Kennedy, J.F. Biocatalytic strategies in the production of galacto-oligosaccharides and its global status. *Int. J. Biol. Macromol.* **2018**, *111*, 667–679. [CrossRef] [PubMed]

2. Holscher, H.D. Dietary fiber and prebiotics and the gastrointestinal microbiota. *Gut Microbes* **2017**, *8*, 172–184. [CrossRef] [PubMed]

3. So, S.S.; Wan, M.L.; El-Nezami, H. Probiotics-mediated suppression of cancer. *Curr. Opin. Oncol.* **2017**, *29*, 62–72. [CrossRef] [PubMed]

4. Intanon, M.; Arreola, S.L.; Pham, N.H.; Kneifel, W.; Haltrich, D.; Nguyen, T.H. Nature and biosynthesis of galacto-oligosaccharides related to oligosaccharides in human breast milk. *Fems. Microbiol. Lett.* **2014**, *353*, 89–97. [CrossRef] [PubMed]

5. Vera, C.; Cordova, A.; Aburto, C.; Guerrero, C.; Suarez, S.; Illanes, A. Synthesis and purification of galacto-oligosaccharides: State of the art. *World J. Microbiol. Biotechnol.* **2016**, *32*, 197. [CrossRef] [PubMed]

6. Park, A.R.; Oh, D.K. Galacto-oligosaccharide production using microbial beta-galactosidase: Current state and perspectives. *Appl. Microbiol. Biotechnol.* **2010**, *85*, 1279–1286. [CrossRef] [PubMed]

7. Rastall, R.A. Functional oligosaccharides: Application and manufacture. *Annu. Rev. Food Sci. Technol.* **2010**, *1*, 305–339. [CrossRef] [PubMed]

8. Saqib, S.; Akram, A.; Halim, S.A.; Tassaduq, R. Sources of beta-galactosidase and its applications in food industry. *Biotechnology* **2017**, *7*, 79.

9. Oliveira, C.; Guimaraes, P.M.; Domingues, L. Recombinant microbial systems for improved beta-galactosidase production and biotechnological applications. *Biotechnol. Adv.* **2011**, *29*, 600–609. [CrossRef] [PubMed]

10. Bras, N.F.; Fernandes, P.A.; Ramos, M.J. QM/MM Studies on the beta-Galactosidase Catalytic Mechanism: Hydrolysis and Transglycosylation Reactions. *J. Chem. Theory Comput.* **2010**, *6*, 421–433. [CrossRef] [PubMed]

11. Chanalia, P.; Gandhi, D.; Attri, P.; Dhanda, S. Purification and characterization of beta-galactosidase from probiotic Pediococcus acidilactici and its use in milk lactose hydrolysis and galactooligosaccharide synthesis. *Bioorg. Chem.* **2018**, *77*, 176–189. [CrossRef] [PubMed]

12. Yin, H.; Pijning, T.; Meng, X.; Dijkhuizen, L.; van Leeuwen, S.S. Biochemical Characterization of the Functional Roles of Residues in the Active Site of the beta-Galactosidase from Bacillus circulans ATCC 31382. *Biochemistry* **2017**, *56*, 3109–3118. [CrossRef] [PubMed]

13. Carneiro, L.; Yu, L.; Dupree, P.; Ward, R.J. Characterization of a beta-galactosidase from Bacillus subtilis with transgalactosylation activity. *Int. J. Biol. Macromol.* **2018**, *120*, 279–287. [CrossRef] [PubMed]

14. Ding, H.; Zeng, Q.; Zhou, L.; Yu, Y.; Chen, B. Biochemical and Structural Insights into a Novel Thermostable beta-1,3-Galactosidase from *Marinomonas* sp. BSi20414. *Mar. Drugs* **2017**, *15*, 13. [CrossRef] [PubMed]

15. Jayaprakash, N.G.; Surolia, A. Role of glycosylation in nucleating protein folding and stability. *Biochem. J.* **2017**, *474*, 2333–2347. [CrossRef] [PubMed]

16. Nishi, H.; Shaytan, A.; Panchenko, A.R. Physicochemical mechanisms of protein regulation by phosphorylation. *Front. Genet.* **2014**, *5*, 270. [CrossRef] [PubMed]

17. Murn, J.; Shi, Y. The winding path of protein methylation research: Milestones and new frontiers. *Nat. Rev. Mol. Cell Biol.* **2017**, *18*, 517–527. [CrossRef] [PubMed]

18. Shental-Bechor, D.; Levy, Y. Effect of glycosylation on protein folding: A close look at thermodynamic stabilization. *Proc. Natl. Acad. Sci. USA* **2008**, *105*, 8256–8261. [CrossRef] [PubMed]

19. Rodriguez-Colinas, B.; Fernandez-Arrojo, L.; Ballesteros, A.O.; Plou, F.J. Galactooligosaccharides formation during enzymatic hydrolysis of lactose: Towards a prebiotic-enriched milk. *Food Chem.* **2014**, *145*, 388–394. [CrossRef] [PubMed]

20. Otieno, D.O. Synthesis of β-Galactooligosaccharides from Lactose Using Microbial β-Galactosidases. *Compr. Rev. Food Sci. Food Saf.* **2010**, *9*, 471–482. [CrossRef]

21. Depeint, F.; Tzortzis, G.; Vulevic, J.; I'Anson, K.; Gibson, G.R. Prebiotic evaluation of a novel galactooligosaccharide mixture produced by the enzymatic activity of Bifidobacterium bifidum NCIMB 41171, in healthy humans: A randomized, double-blind, crossover, placebo-controlled intervention study. *Am. J. Clin. Nutr.* **2008**, *87*, 785–791. [CrossRef] [PubMed]

22. Zeng, Q.; Wang, Y.; Sun, K.; Yu, Y.; Chen, B. Preliminary studies on the screening, identification and optimum fermentative conditions of a strain *Marinomonas* sp. BSi20414 isolated from arctic sea ice producing β-galactosidase. *J. Polar Res.* **2011**, 108–114.

23. Bradford, M.M. A rapid and sensitive method for the quantitation of microgram quantities of protein utilizing the principle of protein-dye binding. *Anal. Biochem.* **1976**, *72*, 248–254. [CrossRef]

24. Laemmli, U.K. Cleavage of structural proteins during the assembly of the head of bacteriophage T4. *Nature* **1970**, *227*, 680–685. [CrossRef] [PubMed]

25. Ding, H.; Gao, F.; Liu, D.; Li, Z.; Xu, X.; Wu, M.; Zhao, Y. Significant improvement of thermal stability of glucose 1-dehydrogenase by introducing disulfide bonds at the tetramer interface. *Enzym. Microb. Technol.* **2013**, *53*, 365–372. [CrossRef] [PubMed]

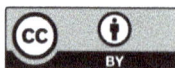

marine drugs

MDPI

Article

Extensive Tandem Duplication Events Drive the Expansion of the C1q-Domain-Containing Gene Family in Bivalves

Marco Gerdol [1,*] ⓘ, **Samuele Greco** [1] ⓘ and **Alberto Pallavicini** [1,2]

1 Department of Life Sciences, University of Trieste, 34127 Trieste, Italy;
   SAMUELE.GRECO@phd.units.it (S.G.); pallavic@units.it (A.P.)
2 National Institute of Oceanography and Applied Geophysics, 34151 Trieste, Italy
* Correspondence: mgerdol@units.it; Tel.: +39-040-5588676

Received: 30 August 2019; Accepted: 12 October 2019; Published: 14 October 2019

✓ check for updates

Abstract: C1q-domain-containing (C1qDC) proteins are rapidly emerging as key players in the innate immune response of bivalve mollusks. Growing experimental evidence suggests that these highly abundant secretory proteins are involved in the recognition of microbe-associated molecular patterns, serving as lectin-like molecules in the bivalve proto-complement system. While a large amount of functional data concerning the binding specificity of the globular head C1q domain and on the regulation of these molecules in response to infection are quickly accumulating, the genetic mechanisms that have led to the extraordinary lineage-specific expansion of the C1qDC gene family in bivalves are still largely unknown. The analysis of the chromosome-scale genome assembly of the Eastern oyster *Crassostrea virginica* revealed that the 476 oyster C1qDC genes, far from being uniformly distributed along the genome, are located in large clusters of tandemly duplicated paralogs, mostly found on chromosomes 7 and 8. Our observations point out that the evolutionary process behind the development of a large arsenal of C1qDC lectin-like molecules in marine bivalves is still ongoing and likely based on an unequal crossing over.

Keywords: innate immunity; lectins; complement system; C1q; bivalve mollusks; tandem duplication; pattern recognition receptors

---

1. Introduction

A growing body of evidence supports the idea that a proto-complement system, composed of C3, factor B and complement receptors, has an ancient origin in the animal tree of life [1]. Although several lineage-specific gene losses and acquisitions are likely to have reshaped the organization of the proto-complement system during its evolution, leading to its complete loss in some major extant taxa (e.g., insects), the activation of this primary defense system often relies on the recognition of microbe-associated molecular patterns (MAMPs) by different types of soluble lectin-like molecules. In vertebrate animals, two different types of pattern recognition receptors (PRRs) are involved in the lectin pathway of the complement system: mannan-binding lectins (MBLs) and ficolins. These proteins can recognize carbohydrate moieties associated with pathogens, triggering the activation of the complement proteolytic cascade, and eventually leading to the opsonization and killing of invading microbes.

The vertebrate complement component C1q is a connecting link between innate and adaptive immunity, as it enables complement activation through the recognition of antigen-complexed immunoglobulins, in the second arm of the complement system—the so-called classical pathway. Due to the absence of immunoglobulins, a proper classical pathway does not exist in invertebrates, making the activation of the complement system only possible in response to MAMP recognition by lectins, to the spontaneous hydrolysis of C3 (i.e., the alternative pathway), or to the direct binding of MAMPs by C1q, which is also observed in vertebrates [2]. In addition to the three monomeric units of the vertebrate C1q complex, the globular head C1q domain is also found in a number of different proteins with non-complement related functions, such as cerebellin, adiponectin, emilin, multimerin and others [3], defining the C1q-domain-containing (C1qDC) protein family and highlighting the high versatility of this structural scaffold [2].

In spite of the absence of an adaptive immune system, a large number of C1qDC proteins are encoded by the genomes of numerous metazoans which lack an adaptive immune system [4]. Due to the presence of several hundred C1qDC genes, bivalve mollusks most certainly emerge as the prime example of an animal group in which C1qDC proteins have met significant evolutionary success. For example, in stark contrast with most other protostomes, including gastropod and cephalopod mollusks, which only produce less than a dozen different C1qDC proteins [5,6], the genome of the Pacific oyster *Crassostrea gigas* harbors 337 C1qDC genes. Multiple transcriptome [7,8] and genome sequencing efforts have confirmed that C1qDC genes contribute to 0.5–1.5% of the entire repertoire of protein-coding genes of most bivalve species (e.g., 296 genes in *Pinctada fucata* [9], 445 in *Modiolus philippinarum* [10], 554 in *Saccostrea glomerata* [11] and over 1200 in *Ruditapes philipinarum* [12]). Curiously, this massive gene family expansion has been inferred to have occurred quite recently in bivalve evolution, since it only targeted all Pteriomorphia and Heterodonta, regardless of the environmental niche, but not the two remaining basal classes of Palaeoheterodonta and Protobranchia [13].

While it is still unclear whether all bivalve C1qDC proteins are involved in immune recognition [13], functional studies indicate that many of them play an important role as lectin-like molecules. The binding properties of the C1q domain enable the recognition of a broad range of MAMPs, such as peptidoglycan (PGN) and lipopolysaccharide (LPS)—the major components of Gram-positive and negative bacterial cell walls respectively—but also of other sugars associated with invading microbes, such as mannan [14,15], beta-1-3-glucan and yeast-glucan [16–18]. The impressive molecular diversification of bivalve C1qDC proteins has been hypothesized to be linked with a parallel functional specialization [16], which may further extend the range of potentially recognized MAMPs [19,20].

Bivalve C1qDC proteins are expressed in different tissues [13] and, upon secretion in the extracellular environment, they might be released in the hemolymph [7], in the extrapallial fluid [21] or in the mucus that covers the gills [13], offering a first line of defense against invading microorganisms in different body districts. The recognition of MAMPs by bivalve C1qDC proteins, which is probably aided by additional humoral factors, promotes the agglutination of bacterial cells [15,22], also triggering the migration and phagocytic activity of hemocytes [22–24], which clearly indicate an opsin-like function for these important soluble PRRs.

In vertebrates, the activation of the complement proteolytic cascade by C1q is effected by the presence a collagen tail, which also enables trimerization and the formation of a typical bouquet structure and defines the C1q-like type I domain architecture [20]. However, collagen tails are extremely rare in bivalves, which seem to either rely on a functionally analogous coiled-coil region for the assembly of oligomeric complexes (C1q-like type II proteins) and often completely lack N-terminal extensions (sghC1q proteins) [13].

Although several functional aspects remain to be fully investigated, the past decade has witnessed significant progress in the study of bivalve C1qDC proteins. Although these reports have contributed to a better elucidation of their functional significance in the context of immune response, the unavailability of high-quality genome assemblies has so far prevented the study of the genetic and molecular mechanisms that have led to the generation of several hundred C1qDC genes in this class of aquatic filter-feeding metazoans. Here, through the analysis of a high-quality chromosome-scale genome assembly [25], we investigate the genomic organization of the 476 C1qDC genes found in the Eastern oyster *Crassostrea virginica*, revealing a highly inhomogeneous distribution across chromosomes and a still-ongoing gene family expansion process which is mostly based on tandem gene duplication and episodic positive selection acting on newly generated gene copies. This process may have a significant impact of the functional diversification of these lectin-like molecules, resulting in the extension of the range of recognized MAMPs.

2. Results

2.1. The Repertoire of the Eastern Oyster C1qDC Genes

In total, 476 C1qDC genes were identified in the genome of *C. virginica* (detailed in Supplementary File 1). This number is in line with the previous report of 337 C1qDC genes in the congeneric species *C. gigas* [13], whose genome is slightly smaller (558 Mb vs. 685 Mb) [26], and similar to other Pteriomorphia [9–11].

Following the classification scheme previously proposed in another publication [13], oyster C1qDC proteins were labeled as follows: (i) sghC1qDC proteins, i.e., proteins containing a signal peptide, immediately followed by the C1q domain; (ii) sC1q-like type I proteins, i.e., secreted proteins containing a collagen tail before the C1q domain; (iii) sC1q-like type II proteins, i.e., secreted proteins containing a coiled-coil tail before the C1q domain; (iv) smultiC1q, i.e., secreted proteins containing multiple C1q domains; (v) other/uncertain, i.e., proteins with different domain architectures, or those resulting from likely incomplete annotation.

As in the case of the Pacific oyster, the majority of the C1qDCgenes (262, 55%) belonged to the sC1q-like type II category. SghC1q proteins were the second most abundant type, with 111 genes (23%); 21 genes encoded proteins with multiple C1q domains (three in most cases), which may or may not include a coiled-coil region (Table 1). No C1q-like type I protein was found in the Eastern oyster, confirming the observation that the association between the C1q domain and *N*-terminal collagen regions, typical of vertebrates, rarely occurs in bivalves [7,13].

Table 1. Details about the number and type of C1qDC genes found in the *Crassostrea virginica* genome.

	chr1	chr2	chr3	chr4	chr5	chr6	chr7	chr8	chr9	chr10	Total
Chromosome size (Mb)	65.67	61.72	77.06	59.69	98.70	51.26	57.83	75.94	104.16	32.65	684.68
Number of C1qDC genes	45	17	18	12	17	36	123	123	73	12	476
C1qDC density (genes/Mb)	0.67	0.28	0.23	0.28	0.17	0.70	2.13	1.63	0.70	0.37	0.70
sghC1q genes	8	0	4	3	1	2	18	63	12	0	111
sC1q-like type II genes	27	6	10	7	12	26	81	36	48	9	262
smultiC1q genes	3	1	0	2	1	0	1	14	0	0	21
sSUEL/C1q	0	10	0	0	0	0	6	0	0	0	16
Other C1qDc genes	7	0	4	0	3	8	17	10	13	3	63

A total of 79 genes were classified in the "other/uncertain" category. While in part these may correspond to truncated genes resulting from incorrect computational prediction (as previously shown for many C1qDC genes in *C. gigas* [13]), some may correspond to bona fide cytosolic or membrane-bound C1qDC proteins, which have been previously identified in other bivalve species [7,13]. An interesting subgroup of unusual C1qDC proteins was found to contain a D-galactoside/L-rhamnose-binding SUEL domain (acronym for sea urchin egg lectin), which is typically found in a number of lectins produced by marine echinoderms [27–29]. Although three sSUEL/C1q genes had been previously reported in the Pacific oyster, their number in the Eastern oyster (16) largely exceeds that of the congeneric species [13].

2.2. Chromosomal Distribution of Oyster C1qDC Genes

Far from being uniformly split among chromosomes, oyster C1qDC genes displayed a highly skewed distribution, with more than 50% genes being located on chromosomes 7 and 8. Indeed, while these two chromosomes contained 123 C1qDC genes each, others encoded as few as 12 C1qDC genes (i.e., chromosomes 4 and 10). This reflected a very uneven C1qDC gene density, ranging from 0.17 genes/Mb (chromosome 5) to 2.13 genes/Mb (chromosome 7), with the average genomic C1qDC gene density standing at 0.70 genes/Mb (Figure 1).

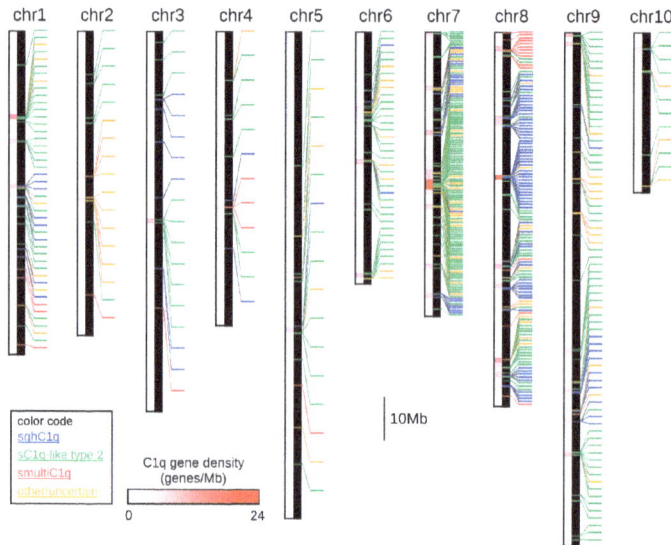

Figure 1. Chromosomal distribution of C1qDC genes in the *Crassostrea virginica* genome. The three main types of C1qDC genes (sghC1q, sC1q-like type 2, and smultiC1q) are indicated with different colors. C1qDC genes encoding proteins with a diverse domain organization, or of uncertain classification, were placed in the "other/uncertain" category. Chromosomes are drawn in scale.

C1qDC gene density was also largely non-homogeneous along chromosomes, as the genes were often placed in packed clusters, which often included more than a dozen units. This resulted in local peaks of very high gene density (i.e., >20 C1qDC genes/Mb in some regions of chromosome 7 and 8), as opposed to very large regions (>10 Mb) completely devoid of C1qDC genes (e.g., chromosome 3, 5 and 10) (Figure 1). Overall, 1.38% of the genes encoded by the *C. virginica* genome pertain to the C1qDC gene family. The relative abundance of C1qDC genes was however much higher for the two aforementioned chromosomes, standing at 4.78% and 3.16% for chromosome 7 and 8, respectively.

At the same time, a complete view of the localization of C1qDC genes in the genome (Figure 1) clearly shows that the different types of C1qDC genes were not evenly distributed. Type II C1q-like genes were the most abundant in all chromosomes, with the exception of chromosome 8, where the sghC1q type was the predominant one (Table 1). The high abundance of sghC1qDC genes in chromosome 8 was particularly notable, as 63 out of the 111 C1qDC genes of this type (57%) were found in this chromosome. Similarly, the majority of smultiC1qDC genes (14 out of 21) were found on chromosome 8, located in a dense cluster (Figure 1). On the other hand, most sSUELC1q genes (10 out of 16) were located on chromosome 2.

2.3. Most Oyster C1qDC Genes Are Tandemly Duplicated

The organization of oyster C1qDC genes in monotypic gene clusters (Figure 1) clearly suggest that these sequences are paralogous, which may have been generated by tandem gene duplication. We analyzed this evolutionary aspect in more depth by (i) inspecting the pairwise sequence similarity of the encoded proteins, and (ii) investigating their relative position. The clustering approach evidenced that 421 C1qDC proteins (88.44%) were grouped in clusters of at least two putative paralogs, and that 172 genes (36.13%) were grouped in large clusters (i.e., including ≥10 putative paralogous genes).

The C1qDC genes included in such large clusters were, for the most part, both evolutionarily closely related and spatially close to each other, as exemplified by one of the largest clusters identified in chromosome 7 (Figure 2a), which included 34 C1qDC genes, mostly of the C1q-like type II group. The phylogenetic analysis revealed that, of all C1qDC genes encoded by chromosome 7, these 34 genes created a well-supported monophyletic group (97% posterior probability), and they were organized in two distinct gene subclusters, containing 6 and 28 genes, respectively. The two subclusters were found to be separated by ~1.8 Mb sequence (Figure 2a) and, for the most part, included tandemly duplicated genes encoded on the same strand.

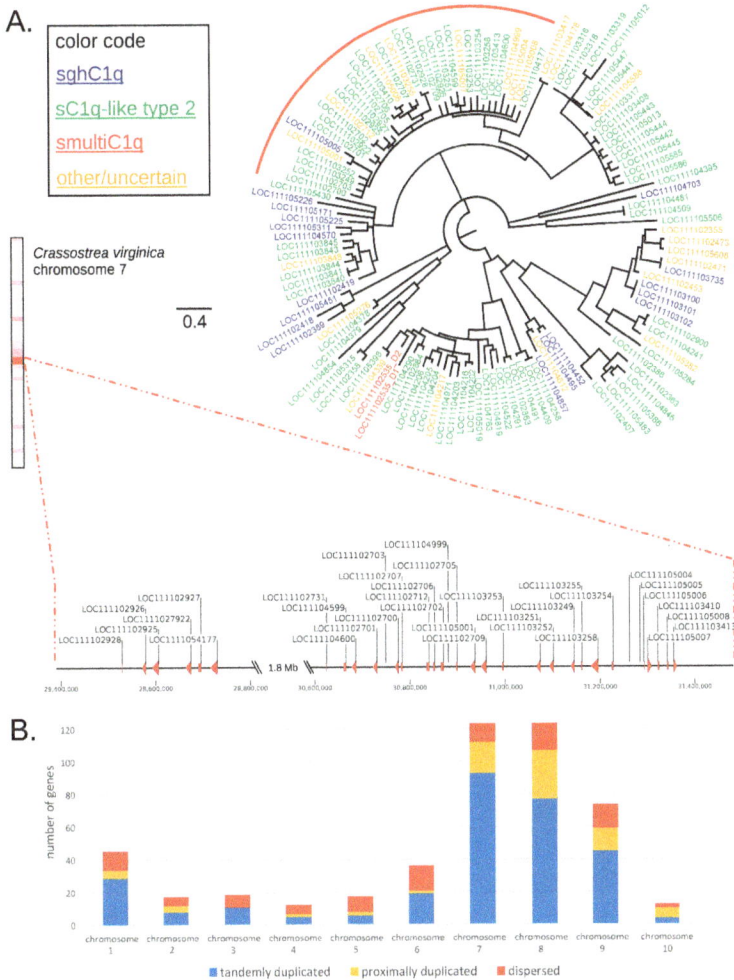

Figure 2. (**A**) Bayesian phylogenetic tree of the C1qDC proteins encoded by *Crassostrea virginica* chromosome 7. The three main types of C1qDC genes (sghC1q, sC1q-like type 2 and smultiC1q) are indicated with different colors. The location of the C1qDC genes pertaining to the monophyletic group indicated with a red circle is shown in detail in the zoomed-in chromosomal region. Nodes supported by posterior probability values <50% were collapsed. (**B**) Number of tandemly duplicated, proximally duplicated and dispersed C1qDC genes in each *C. virginica* chromosome.

The investigation carried out at the whole-genome scale confirmed the widespread occurrence of tandem duplications, which impacted 297 C1qDC genes (62.39%). In total, 84 genes (17.65%) were proximally duplicated (i.e., they were not directly flanked by C1qDC genes, but placed within 100 Kb distance from the closest one), and thus were the likely product of similar unequal crossing over processes [30] (Figure 2b). As previously mentioned, only a tiny fraction of the Eastern oyster C1qDC genes (i.e., <12%) were single-copy (i.e., they encoded proteins sharing <50% sequence similarity with other C1qDC proteins) and, in accordance with this observation, the occurrence of dispersed C1qDC genes (95 genes, 19.96%) was only slightly higher, showing the low prevalence of gene duplications driven by the activity of transposable elements. Chromosomes 7 and 8—i.e., the two chromosomes with the highest C1qDC gene density—were also those containing the highest proportion of tandemly or proximally duplicated genes (91.06% and 86.99%, respectively), confirming the fundamental importance of these processes in the bivalve C1qDC gene family expansion.

2.4. The Gene Duplication Process Is Still Ongoing and Is Paired with Diversifying Selection

Multiple lines of evidence suggest that the development of a very large repertoire of C1qDC genes in the Eastern oyster is the product of an evolutionary process that is still presently ongoing. Evidence in support of the very recent origin of paralogous C1qDC gene copies by tandem duplication is provided, for example, by the existence of eight nearly-identical genes, which encode proteins sharing 100% sequence identity at the amino acid level. In particular, three paralogous sghC1qDC genes located on chromosome 7 (i.e., LOC111103100, LOC111103101 and LOC111103102) share 100% sequence identity at the nucleotide level within the coding sequence, and only display small intronic indels due to the presence of microsatellites. A total of 65 C1qDC genes (13.63%) encode proteins with >95% sequence identity with the closest paralog, and this number rises to 89 genes (18.66%) for a sequence similarity threshold equal to 90%.

An additional example of this evolutionary process is given by a group of six highly similar paralogous sC1q-like type 2 genes found in chromosome 8 (i.e., LOC111105959, LOC111105960, LOC111105962, LOC111106427, LOC111106428 and LOC111109313), which all encode proteins of very similar length (249–251 aa) and share >90% sequence identity (Figure 3a). The six genes retain the same gene architecture, with conserved splicing donor and acceptor sites. Similarly, they display a nearly identical size of exons (with the only two exceptions of a 3nt-long in-frame deletion in LOC111105962 exon 1, and a 1nt-long deletion at the end of the coding sequence of LOC1111105960, which resulted in the acquisition of an additional codon at the 3′ end of the ORF). As expected, the intron was subject to more relaxed selective constraints compared with the two exons, displaying a higher evolutionary rate, as evidenced by the higher number of indels and SNPs (Figure 3a).

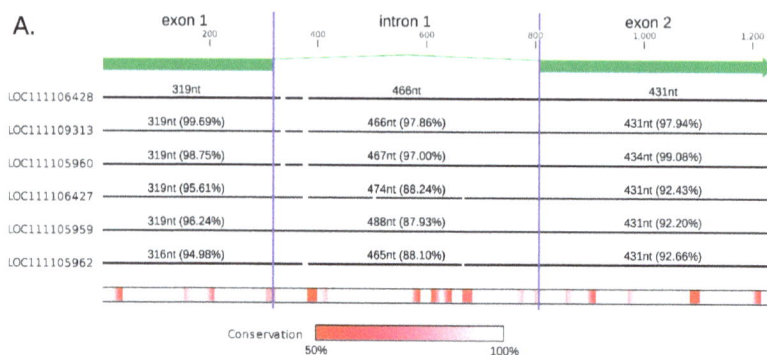

Figure 3. *Cont.*

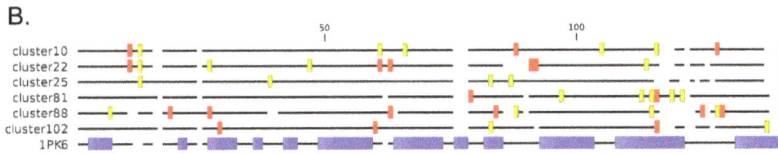

Figure 3. (A) Sequence comparison among the six sC1q-like type 2 paralogous genes LOC111105959, LOC111105960, LOC111105962, LOC111106427, LOC111106428 and LOC111109313, all found in chromosome 8. Identity percentages are shown for exon1, intron 1 and exon 2 separately, using the LOC111106428 sequence as a reference. Sequence conservation is shown with a heat map and indels are shown as line breaks. **(B)** Position of sites subject to positive selection in the six largest clusters of paralogous C1qDC genes identified in *C. virginica*. Strongly supported sites (i.e., detected with at least 2 different prediction methods) are shown in red. Sites with moderate support (i.e., detected with just one prediction method) are shown in yellow. The position of the beta strands in the human C1q chain A (PDB: 1PK6) are indicated by blue blocks.

BUSTED revealed strong evidence (*p*-value < 0.05) of episodic positive selection in the six largest clusters of paralogous C1qDC genes identified with a genome-wide analysis, suggesting that the gene duplication process is rapidly followed by molecular (and possibly functional) diversification through positive selection acting on a limited number of specific sites. In contrast with these hypervariable sites, the vast majority of the sites included in the globular C1q domain were found to evolve under negative selection, likely due to selective constraints linked with the maintenance of the typical 10-strand jelly-roll fold structure of the C1q domain itself, as well as of the contact surfaces between subunits required for oligomerization. The number of sites subject to significant diversifying selection, and their statistical support, largely varied from one cluster to the other. The four clusters that included C1q-like type 2 genes (i.e., cluster 10: 18 genes, cluster 22: 26 genes, cluster 81: 15 genes, and cluster 88: 19 genes) displayed between seven and 11 positively selected sites; i.e., roughly 5–10% of the sites included in the globular C1q head. The two clusters comprising sequences of different types (i.e., cluster 25: 16 sSUELC1q genes; cluster 102: 21 sghC1q genes) displayed a somewhat lower number of positively selected sites compared to the four aforementioned cases (four and five, respectively) (Figure 3b).

3. Discussion

In eukaryotes, small-scale gene duplication (i.e., independent from whole-genome duplication) can occur through a number of different mechanisms [31], which may or may not include the activity of transposable elements. Tandem gene duplications result in the creation of two adjacent paralogous genes, which are usually separated by a few Kb of intergenic sequence. Proximal gene duplications similarly result in the creation of two paralogous genes, which are placed at slightly longer distances compared with tandem duplications, and usually separated from each other by one or more genes. Both types of duplication are generally thought to arise from an unequal crossing over; i.e., from the misalignment of homologous regions of sister chromatids during meiosis [30]. An alternative process behind the creation of paralogous gene copies depends on the activity of transposable elements (TEs), such as DNA transposons [32] or retrotransposons [33]. In this case, new gene copies may either retain the original exon/intron architecture and regulatory features (DNA transposons), or completely lack introns, being detached from the promoter region of the original paralogous copy (retrotransposons). Even though the activity of TEs is sometimes spatially localized [34], in most cases, the new gene copies are dispersed; i.e., they are placed in genomic regions distant from their paralogs, often in different chromosomes.

Our investigation demonstrates that the predominant evolutionary process behind the massive expansion of the C1qDC gene family in bivalves is tandem gene duplication. This conclusion is supported by the observation that 62.39% of paralogous C1qDC genes are tandemly duplicated and that an additional 17.65% are proximally duplicated (Figure 2b). Hence, the widespread presence of C1qDC gene clusters in the Eastern oyster genome suggests that an unequal crossing over might be considered as the primary driving force behind this gene family expansion event. Our study further suggests that this process is still actively ongoing, since numerous identical or nearly-identical gene copies, inferred to have a very recent evolutionary origin, are present in dense gene clusters, which shows a highly inhomogeneous distribution along the genome.

However, this remarkable gene family expansion, with the extensive retention of newly generated gene copies, requires some additional explanation, as it seemingly contradicts the observation that the majority of duplicated genes with redundant function evolve under more relaxed selective constrains, being more prone to loss-of-function mutations, pseudogenization and consequent loss [35,36]. Over the years, multiple and partially overlapping theoretical models have been proposed to explain the fixation of duplicated genes in populations, which depend on a complex combination between the evolutionary dynamics of a given gene family and functional properties of the encoded proteins [37,38]. The retention of hundreds of C1qDc genes in the Eastern oyster, as well as in other bivalve species [5,7,13], most certainly indicates that the generation of tandemly and—in a minor way—proximally duplicated C1qDC genes represents an important evolutionary advantage in these filter-feeding organisms. Based on the functional information collected so far in oysters, scallops, mussels, clams and other bivalves, this advantage could arise from the neofunctionalization or subfunctionalization of new gene copies [39], which may acquire the ability to recognize additional MAMPs, extending the range of pathogenic microorganisms recognized, through the mutation of key sites involved in glycan recognition [16].

One key aspect that remained to be investigated was whether such molecular diversification is the result of relaxed selective constraints on redundant gene copies, or of positive selection acting on selected sites potentially involved in MAMP-binding, which could significantly affect the lectin-like function of oyster C1qDC proteins. The analysis of the six largest clusters of paralogous genes found in the *C. virginica* genome revealed highly supported traces of episodic positive selection, suggesting that duplicated gene copies undergo rapid molecular, and possibly functional, diversification. This process only seemed to act on a limited number of localized residues (4–11 per cluster, Figure 3b), which were in part shared by the different clusters and displayed a higher frequency in the hypervariable and gap-rich C-terminal part of the C1q domain (Figure 3b). On the other hand, the vast majority of the sites included in the C1q domain was subject to strong purifying selection, likely due to structural constraints. Our current knowledge of the sites involved in MAMP recognition in bivalve C1qDC proteins is virtually non-existent, and most of the information available concerning the residues involved in C1q ligand binding derives from very distantly related model organisms, such as mouse and human [40,41]. Consequently, the possibility to infer whether the position of positively selected sites in the 3D structure of the globular head C1q domain is paired with a functional specialization and to the acquisition of the ability to recognize novel ligands in tandemly duplicated C1qDC genes falls beyond our current reach.

Another interesting aspect revealed by this study was the complete lack of C1q-like type I proteins in *C. virginica*. In light of the recent report of the presence of this domain architecture in early-branching metazoans [42], its absence in the Eastern oyster suggests that bivalves do not necessarily require collagen tails for the activation of the proto-complement system. The presence of a very few non-orthologous C1q-like type I genes in other bivalve species [7,13] further reinforces the idea that alternative N-terminal structures (i.e., coiled-coil regions) are the predominant structure used for C1qDC protein oligomerization and the subsequent activation of the complement proteolytic cascade. The finding that 16 sSUEL/C1q genes were present in the Eastern oyster genome was another relevant result, since this domain combination, unique to Bivalvia, is highly reminiscent of the recently reported case of C1q-related proteins (QREPs) found in a few Caenogastropoda and Heterobranchia gastropod species [42]. As with sSUEL/C1q, these unusual proteins combine the C-terminal globular C1q domain with N-terminal domains with marked binding properties (i.e., two immunoglobulin-like domains). Altogether, these findings stimulate further research towards the functional characterization of these potentially multifunctional lectin-like proteins.

In summary, this study provides, for the first time, evidence supporting the important role of tandem gene duplication and an unequal crossing over in the expansion and molecular evolution of the C1qDC gene family in bivalves. Based on preliminary results, this rapid and still-ongoing process is likely paired with episodic diversifying selection, which only acts on a limited number of spatially localized residues, whose functional significance in MAMP binding should be investigated in depth in the future. Evolutionary processes analogous to those we have described for the Eastern oyster C1qDC genes may have targeted several other gene families involved in immune response, either as receptors or as effectors, that have similarly reportedly undergone massive lineage-specific expansion and molecular diversification [5,43,44].

4. Materials and Methods

4.1. Identification of C1qDC Genes

The annotated chromosome-scale nuclear genome assembly v.3.0 of *Crassostrea virginica* (Gmelin, 1791) [25] was downloaded from the GenBank repository (GCA_002022765.4). Protein-coding genes were virtually translated and the resulting amino acid sequences were screened for the presence of one or more C1q domains with HMMER v.3.2.1 [45], based on a 0.05 e-value threshold, using the PFAM profile of the C1q domain (PF00386) as a query. Positive hits were further refined by removing sequences with partial domains, taking into account the possibility of incorrect annotations.

All C1qDC proteins were further characterized as follows: the presence of *N*-terminal signal peptides and transmembrane regions was inspected with Phobius [46]; additional conserved protein domains were predicted with InterProScan v.5 [47] and coiled-coil regions were predicted with COILS [48], with a window length of 14, 21 and 28 amino acids, based on a probability threshold > 0.5. Protein nomenclature followed the scheme proposed in a previous publication [13] (see Section 2.1 for details).

4.2. Sequence Analysis of C1qDC Genes

The coordinates of each C1qDC gene were obtained from the genome GFF (General Feature Format) annotation file, and their positions were indicated on chromosomes, drawn to scale. The four gene categories indicated in Section 4.1 (with the exception of type I C1q-like genes, as no sequence of this type was identified) were indicated with different colors. The C1qDC gene density per Mb of genomic DNA sequence was computed using a 1 Mb sequence window length, and represented as a heat map on the side of each chromosome.

The amino acid sequences were clustered by similarity using CD-HIT v.4.8.1 [49], with different sequence identity thresholds to identify the products of putative gene duplication events. Sequences sharing > 50% pairwise identify were considered to be part of paralogous gene clusters and further classified as (i) tandemly duplicated genes, if they were flanked by at least one paralogous C1qDC genes, either at the 5′ or 3′ side; (ii) proximally duplicated genes, if the flanking genes were not pertaining to the C1qDC family, but the closest paralogous C1qDC was located within 100 Kb of distance; and (iii) dispersed genes, if the closest C1qDC gene was not located within 100 Kb of distance.

The evolutionary history of the C1qDC genes encoded by chromosome 7 (i.e., the oyster chromosome displaying the highest C1qDC gene density) was further investigated by generating a multiple sequence alignment (MSA) of all the encoded amino acid sequences. The MSA file, obtained with MUSCLE v.6.0 [50], was trimmed to only include the C1q domain; i.e., the region shared by all proteins. For smultiC1q proteins, each domain was separately added to the MSA. ModelTest-NG v.0.1.5 [51] estimated the WAG (Whelan And Goldman) model of molecular evolution [52], with a proportion of invariable sites and a gamma-shaped rate of variation across sites (WAG+G+I), as the best-fitting for the dataset analyzed. Phylogenetic inference was carried out with

MrBayes v.3.2.7a [53], running two parallel MCMC analyses with four chains each. The convergence of all estimated parameters was assessed with Tracer v.1.7.1 [54], based on the reaching of an effective sample size > 200; i.e., with 400,000 generations. The resulting phylogenetic tree was represented as a 50% majority rule consensus tree (i.e., nodes supported by posterior probability values <50% were collapsed).

4.3. Positive Selection Analysis

The six largest clusters of paralogous C1qDC genes, identified as described in Section 2.2, all containing 15 genes or more, were analyzed to detect the signatures of positive and negative selection as follows. First, the nucleotide sequences of the open reading frames were aligned with MEGA X [55], using MUSCLE [50], preserving the integrity of codon triplets. The obtained MSA files were trimmed to remove positions containing gaps in the alignment, as well as regions not included in the globular C1q domain. The resulting processed MSA files were processed with BUSTED [56] to detect domain-wise signatures of episodic positive selection, based on a *p*-value threshold < 0.05. The position of sites subject to positive selection was predicted with FUBAR, SLAC, FEL and MEME [57–59], based on a *p*-value threshold < 0.05 (or posterior probability > 0.95). All these tools were implemented with the use of the online Datamonkey 2.0 platform (https://datamonkey.org) [60]. Sites evolving under positive selection were categorized either as strongly supported (i.e., detected with at least two different methods) or as moderately supported (i.e., detected with just one method). Sites subject to positive selection were graphically represented in the alignment between the consensus sequences of the six selected clusters, using the experimentally determined structure of the chain A of the human C1q (PDB: 1PK6) [19] as a reference. The multiple sequence alignment was implemented with structural information using Expresso [61].

Supplementary Materials: The following are available online at http://www.mdpi.com/1660-3397/17/10/583/s1, Table S1: list of C1qDC genes identified in the *Crassostrea virginica* genome.

Author Contributions: Conceptualization, M.G. and A.P.; methodology, M.G. and S.G.; formal analysis, M.G. and S.G.; writing—original draft preparation, M.G.; writing—review and editing, M.G., S.G. and A.P.; visualization, M.G. and S.G.; supervision, A.P.; funding acquisition, A.P.

Funding: This project has received funding from the European Union's Horizon 2020 research and innovation programme under grant agreement No. 678589. Samuele Greco is supported by a grant from the Italian National Program for Antarctic Research, project PNRA16_00099.

Acknowledgments: We thank Davide Fracarossi for bioinformatics assistance.

Conflicts of Interest: The authors declare no conflict of interest. The funders had no role in the design of the study; in the collection, analyses, or interpretation of data; in the writing of the manuscript, or in the decision to publish the results.

References

1. Gorbushin, A.M. Immune repertoire in the transcriptome of Littorina littorea reveals new trends in lophotrochozoan proto-complement evolution. *Dev. Comp. Immunol.* **2018**, *84*, 250–263. [CrossRef] [PubMed]
2. Nayak, A.; Pednekar, L.; Reid, K.B.M.; Kishore, U. Complement and non-complement activating functions of C1q: A prototypical innate immune molecule. *Innate Immun.* **2012**, *18*, 350–363. [CrossRef] [PubMed]
3. Tom Tang, Y.; Hu, T.; Arterburn, M.; Boyle, B.; Bright, J.M.; Palencia, S.; Emtage, P.C.; Funk, W.D. The complete complement of C1q-domain-containing proteins in Homo sapiens. *Genomics* **2005**, *86*, 100–111. [CrossRef] [PubMed]
4. Carland, T.M.; Gerwick, L. The C1q domain containing proteins: Where do they come from and what do they do? *Dev. Comp. Immunol.* **2010**, *34*, 785–790. [CrossRef] [PubMed]
5. Zhang, L.; Li, L.; Guo, X.; Litman, G.W.; Dishaw, L.J.; Zhang, G. Massive expansion and functional divergence of innate immune genes in a protostome. *Sci. Rep.* **2015**, *5*, 8693. [CrossRef]
6. Gerdol, M.; Luo, Y.-J.; Satoh, N.; Pallavicini, A. Genetic and molecular basis of the immune system in the brachiopod *Lingula anatina*. *Dev. Comp. Immunol.* **2018**, *82*, 7–30. [CrossRef]

7. Gerdol, M.; Manfrin, C.; De Moro, G.; Figueras, A.; Novoa, B.; Venier, P.; Pallavicini, A. The C1q domain containing proteins of the Mediterranean mussel *Mytilus galloprovincialis*: A widespread and diverse family of immune-related molecules. *Dev. Comp. Immunol.* **2011**, *35*, 635–643. [CrossRef]
8. Zhang, L.; Li, L.; Zhu, Y.; Zhang, G.; Guo, X. Transcriptome analysis reveals a rich gene set related to innate immunity in the Eastern oyster (*Crassostrea virginica*). *Mar. Biotechnol.* **2014**, *16*, 17–33. [CrossRef]
9. Takeuchi, T.; Koyanagi, R.; Gyoja, F.; Kanda, M.; Hisata, K.; Fujie, M.; Goto, H.; Yamasaki, S.; Nagai, K.; Morino, Y.; et al. Bivalve-specific gene expansion in the pearl oyster genome: Implications of adaptation to a sessile lifestyle. *Zool. Lett.* **2016**, *2*, 3. [CrossRef]
10. Sun, J.; Zhang, Y.; Xu, T.; Zhang, Y.; Mu, H.; Zhang, Y.; Lan, Y.; Fields, C.J.; Hui, J.H.L.; Zhang, W.; et al. Adaptation to deep-sea chemosynthetic environments as revealed by mussel genomes. *Nat. Ecol. Evol.* **2017**, *1*, 0121. [CrossRef]
11. Powell, D.; Subramanian, S.; Suwansa-Ard, S.; Zhao, M.; O'Connor, W.; Raftos, D.; Elizur, A. The genome of the oyster Saccostrea offers insight into the environmental resilience of bivalves. *DNA Res. Int. J. Rapid Publ. Rep. Genes. Genomes* **2018**, *25*, 655–665. [CrossRef] [PubMed]
12. Mun, S.; Kim, Y.-J.; Markkandan, K.; Shin, W.; Oh, S.; Woo, J.; Yoo, J.; An, H.; Han, K. The Whole-Genome and Transcriptome of the Manila Clam (*Ruditapes philippinarum*). *Genome Biol. Evol.* **2017**, *9*, 1487–1498. [CrossRef]
13. Gerdol, M.; Venier, P.; Pallavicini, A. The genome of the Pacific oyster *Crassostrea gigas* brings new insights on the massive expansion of the C1q gene family in Bivalvia. *Dev. Comp. Immunol.* **2015**, *49*, 59–71. [CrossRef] [PubMed]
14. Zong, Y.; Liu, Z.; Wu, Z.; Han, Z.; Wang, L.; Song, L. A novel globular C1q domain containing protein (C1qDC-7) from *Crassostrea gigas* acts as pattern recognition receptor with broad recognition spectrum. *Fish. Shellfish. Immunol.* **2019**, *84*, 920–926. [CrossRef] [PubMed]
15. Cui, Y.; Wei, Z.; Shen, Y.; Li, C.; Shao, Y.; Zhang, W.; Zhao, X. A novel C1q-domain-containing protein from razor clam *Sinonovacula* constricta mediates G-bacterial agglutination as a pattern recognition receptor. *Dev. Comp. Immunol.* **2018**, *79*, 166–174. [CrossRef] [PubMed]
16. Wang, L.; Zhang, H.; Wang, M.; Zhou, Z.; Wang, W.; Liu, R.; Huang, M.; Yang, C.; Qiu, L.; Song, L. The transcriptomic expression of pattern recognition receptors: Insight into molecular recognition of various invading pathogens in Oyster *Crassostrea gigas*. *Dev. Comp. Immunol.* **2019**, *91*, 1–7. [CrossRef] [PubMed]
17. Wang, L.; Wang, L.; Kong, P.; Yang, J.; Zhang, H.; Wang, M.; Zhou, Z.; Qiu, L.; Song, L. A novel C1qDC protein acting as pattern recognition receptor in scallop *Argopecten irradians*. *Fish. Shellfish. Immunol.* **2012**, *33*, 427–435. [CrossRef]
18. Wang, L.; Wang, L.; Zhang, D.; Jiang, Q.; Sun, R.; Wang, H.; Zhang, H.; Song, L. A novel multi-domain C1qDC protein from Zhikong scallop Chlamys farreri provides new insights into the function of invertebrate C1qDC proteins. *Dev. Comp. Immunol.* **2015**, *52*, 202–214. [CrossRef]
19. Gaboriaud, C.; Juanhuix, J.; Gruez, A.; Lacroix, M.; Darnault, C.; Pignol, D.; Verger, D.; Fontecilla-Camps, J.C.; Arlaud, G.J. The Crystal Structure of the Globular Head of Complement Protein C1q Provides a Basis for Its Versatile Recognition Properties. *J. Biol. Chem.* **2003**, *278*, 46974–46982. [CrossRef]
20. Reid, K.B.M. Complement Component C1q: Historical Perspective of a Functionally Versatile, and Structurally Unusual, Serum Protein. *Front. Immunol.* **2018**, *9*, 764. [CrossRef]
21. Yin, Y.; Huang, J.; Paine, M.L.; Reinhold, V.N.; Chasteen, N.D. Structural characterization of the major extrapallial fluid protein of the mollusc *Mytilus edulis*: Implications for function. *Biochemistry* **2005**, *44*, 10720–10731. [CrossRef] [PubMed]
22. Li, S.; Ruan, Z.; Yang, X.; Li, M.; Yang, D. Immune recognition, antimicrobial and opsonic activities mediated by a sialic acid binding lectin from *Ruditapes philippinarum*. *Fish. Shellfish. Immunol.* **2019**, *93*, 66–72. [CrossRef] [PubMed]
23. Jiang, S.; Li, H.; Zhang, D.; Zhang, H.; Wang, L.; Sun, J.; Song, L. A C1q domain containing protein from *Crassostrea gigas* serves as pattern recognition receptor and opsonin with high binding affinity to LPS. *Fish. Shellfish. Immunol.* **2015**, *45*, 583–591. [CrossRef] [PubMed]
24. Li, H.; Kong, N.; Sun, J.; Wang, W.; Li, M.; Gong, C.; Dong, M.; Wang, M.; Wang, L.; Song, L. A C1qDC (CgC1qDC-6) with a collagen-like domain mediates hemocyte phagocytosis and migration in oysters. *Dev. Comp. Immunol.* **2019**, *98*, 157–165. [CrossRef]

25. Gómez-Chiarri, M.; Warren, W.C.; Guo, X.; Proestou, D. Developing tools for the study of molluscan immunity: The sequencing of the genome of the eastern oyster, *Crassostrea virginica*. *Fish. Shellfish. Immunol.* **2015**, *46*, 2–4. [CrossRef]

26. Zhang, G.; Fang, X.; Guo, X.; Li, L.; Luo, R.; Xu, F.; Yang, P.; Zhang, L.; Wang, X.; Qi, H.; et al. The oyster genome reveals stress adaptation and complexity of shell formation. *Nature* **2012**, *490*, 49–54. [CrossRef]

27. Hatakeyama, T.; Ichise, A.; Unno, H.; Goda, S.; Oda, T.; Tateno, H.; Hirabayashi, J.; Sakai, H.; Nakagawa, H. Carbohydrate recognition by the rhamnose-binding lectin SUL-I with a novel three-domain structure isolated from the venom of globiferous pedicellariae of the flower sea urchin Toxopneustes pileolus. *Protein Sci. Publ. Protein Soc.* **2017**, *26*, 1574–1583. [CrossRef]

28. Ozeki, Y.; Matsui, T.; Suzuki, M.; Titani, K. Amino acid sequence and molecular characterization of a D-galactoside-specific lectin purified from sea urchin (*Anthocidaris crassispina*) eggs. *Biochemistry* **1991**, *30*, 2391–2394. [CrossRef]

29. Carneiro, R.F.; Teixeira, C.S.; de Melo, A.A.; de Almeida, A.S.; Cavada, B.S.; de Sousa, O.V.; da Rocha, B.A.M.; Nagano, C.S.; Sampaio, A.H. L-Rhamnose-binding lectin from eggs of the *Echinometra lucunter*: Amino acid sequence and molecular modeling. *Int. J. Biol. Macromol.* **2015**, *78*, 180–188. [CrossRef]

30. Freeling, M. Bias in plant gene content following different sorts of duplication: Tandem, whole-genome, segmental, or by transposition. *Annu. Rev. Plant Biol.* **2009**, *60*, 433–453. [CrossRef]

31. Maere, S.; De Bodt, S.; Raes, J.; Casneuf, T.; Van Montagu, M.; Kuiper, M.; Van de Peer, Y. Modeling gene and genome duplications in eukaryotes. *Proc. Natl. Acad. Sci. USA.* **2005**, *102*, 5454–5459. [CrossRef] [PubMed]

32. Cusack, B.P.; Wolfe, K.H. Not born equal: Increased rate asymmetry in relocated and retrotransposed rodent gene duplicates. *Mol. Biol. Evol.* **2007**, *24*, 679–686. [CrossRef] [PubMed]

33. Kaessmann, H.; Vinckenbosch, N.; Long, M. RNA-based gene duplication: Mechanistic and evolutionary insights. *Nat. Rev. Genet.* **2009**, *10*, 19–31. [CrossRef] [PubMed]

34. Zhang, J.; Zuo, T.; Peterson, T. Generation of tandem direct duplications by reversed-ends transposition of maize ac elements. *PLoS Genet.* **2013**, *9*, e1003691. [CrossRef]

35. Wagner, A. The fate of duplicated genes: Loss or new function? *BioEssays News Rev. Mol. Cell. Dev. Biol.* **1998**, *20*, 785–788. [CrossRef]

36. Lynch, M.; Conery, J.S. The evolutionary fate and consequences of duplicate genes. *Science* **2000**, *290*, 1151–1155. [CrossRef]

37. Innan, H.; Kondrashov, F. The evolution of gene duplications: Classifying and distinguishing between models. *Nat. Rev. Genet.* **2010**, *11*, 97–108. [CrossRef]

38. Hahn, M.W. Distinguishing among evolutionary models for the maintenance of gene duplicates. *J. Hered.* **2009**, *100*, 605–617. [CrossRef]

39. Rastogi, S.; Liberles, D.A. Subfunctionalization of duplicated genes as a transition state to neofunctionalization. *BMC Evol. Biol.* **2005**, *5*, 28. [CrossRef]

40. Gaboriaud, C.; Frachet, P.; Thielens, N.M.; Arlaud, G.J. The Human C1q Globular Domain: Structure and Recognition of Non-Immune Self Ligands. *Front. Immunol.* **2012**, *2*, 92. [CrossRef]

41. Agrawal, A.; Shrive, A.K.; Greenhough, T.J.; Volanakis, J.E. Topology and structure of the C1q-binding site on C-reactive protein. *J. Immunol. Baltim. MD 1950* **2001**, *166*, 3998–4004. [CrossRef] [PubMed]

42. Gorbushin, A.M. Derivatives of the lectin complement pathway in Lophotrochozoa. *Dev. Comp. Immunol.* **2019**, *94*, 35–58. [CrossRef] [PubMed]

43. McDowell, I.C.; Modak, T.H.; Lane, C.E.; Gomez-Chiarri, M. Multi-species protein similarity clustering reveals novel expanded immune gene families in the eastern oyster Crassostrea virginica. *Fish. Shellfish. Immunol.* **2016**, *53*, 13–23. [CrossRef] [PubMed]

44. Gerdol, M.; Moreira, R.; Cruz, F.; Gómez-Garrido, J.; Vlasova, A.; Rosani, U.; Venier, P.; Naranjo-Ortiz, M.A.; Murgarella, M.; Balseiro, P.; et al. Massive gene presence/absence variation in the mussel genome as an adaptive strategy: First evidence of a pan-genome in Metazoa. *BioRxiv* **2019**, 781377. [CrossRef]

45. Finn, R.D.; Clements, J.; Eddy, S.R. HMMER web server: Interactive sequence similarity searching. *Nucleic Acids Res.* **2011**, *39*, W29–W37. [CrossRef]

46. Käll, L.; Krogh, A.; Sonnhammer, E.L.L. Advantages of combined transmembrane topology and signal peptide prediction—The Phobius web server. *Nucleic Acids Res.* **2007**, *35*, W429–W432. [CrossRef]

47. Finn, R.D.; Attwood, T.K.; Babbitt, P.C.; Bateman, A.; Bork, P.; Bridge, A.J.; Chang, H.-Y.; Dosztányi, Z.; El-Gebali, S.; Fraser, M.; et al. InterPro in 2017—beyond protein family and domain annotations. *Nucleic Acids Res.* **2017**, *45*, D190–D199. [CrossRef]

48. Lupas, A.; Van Dyke, M.; Stock, J. Predicting coiled coils from protein sequences. *Science* **1991**, *252*, 1162–1164. [CrossRef]

49. Li, W.; Godzik, A. Cd-hit: A fast program for clustering and comparing large sets of protein or nucleotide sequences. *Bioinformatics* **2006**, *22*, 1658–1659. [CrossRef]

50. Edgar, R.C. MUSCLE: Multiple sequence alignment with high accuracy and high throughput. *Nucleic Acids Res.* **2004**, *32*, 1792–1797. [CrossRef]

51. Darriba, D.; Posada, D.; Kozlov, A.M.; Stamatakis, A.; Morel, B.; Flouri, T. ModelTest-NG: A new and scalable tool for the selection of DNA and protein evolutionary models. *BioRxiv* **2019**, 612903. [CrossRef] [PubMed]

52. Whelan, S.; Goldman, N. A General Empirical Model of Protein Evolution Derived from Multiple Protein Families Using a Maximum-Likelihood Approach. *Mol. Biol. Evol.* **2001**, *18*, 691–699. [CrossRef] [PubMed]

53. Huelsenbeck, J.P.; Ronquist, F. MRBAYES: Bayesian inference of phylogenetic trees. *Bioinf. Oxf. Engl.* **2001**, *17*, 754–755. [CrossRef] [PubMed]

54. Rambaut, A.; Drummond, A.J.; Xie, D.; Baele, G.; Suchard, M.A. Posterior Summarization in Bayesian Phylogenetics Using Tracer 1.7. *Syst. Biol.* **2018**, *67*, 901–904. [CrossRef] [PubMed]

55. Kumar, S.; Stecher, G.; Li, M.; Knyaz, C.; Tamura, K. MEGA X: Molecular Evolutionary Genetics Analysis across Computing Platforms. *Mol. Biol. Evol.* **2018**, *35*, 1547–1549. [CrossRef] [PubMed]

56. Murrell, B.; Weaver, S.; Smith, M.D.; Wertheim, J.O.; Murrell, S.; Aylward, A.; Eren, K.; Pollner, T.; Martin, D.P.; Smith, D.M.; et al. Gene-wide identification of episodic selection. *Mol. Biol. Evol.* **2015**, *32*, 1365–1371. [CrossRef] [PubMed]

57. Kosakovsky Pond, S.L.; Frost, S.D.W. Not so different after all: A comparison of methods for detecting amino acid sites under selection. *Mol. Biol. Evol.* **2005**, *22*, 1208–1222. [CrossRef]

58. Murrell, B.; Wertheim, J.O.; Moola, S.; Weighill, T.; Scheffler, K.; Kosakovsky Pond, S.L. Detecting individual sites subject to episodic diversifying selection. *PLoS Genet.* **2012**, *8*, e1002764. [CrossRef]

59. Murrell, B.; Moola, S.; Mabona, A.; Weighill, T.; Sheward, D.; Kosakovsky Pond, S.L.; Scheffler, K. FUBAR: A fast, unconstrained bayesian approximation for inferring selection. *Mol. Biol. Evol.* **2013**, *30*, 1196–1205. [CrossRef]

60. Weaver, S.; Shank, S.D.; Spielman, S.J.; Li, M.; Muse, S.V.; Kosakovsky Pond, S.L. Datamonkey 2.0: A modern web application for characterizing selective and other evolutionary processes. *Mol. Biol. Evol.* **2018**, *35*, 773–777. [CrossRef]

61. Armougom, F.; Moretti, S.; Poirot, O.; Audic, S.; Dumas, P.; Schaeli, B.; Keduas, V.; Notredame, C. Expresso: Automatic incorporation of structural information in multiple sequence alignments using 3D-Coffee. *Nucleic Acids Res.* **2006**, *34*, W604–W608. [CrossRef] [PubMed]

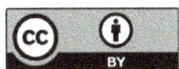

marine drugs

MDPI

Article

Tachypleus tridentatus Lectin Enhances Oncolytic Vaccinia Virus Replication to Suppress In Vivo Hepatocellular Carcinoma Growth

Gongchu Li *, Jianhong Cheng, Shengsheng Mei, Tao Wu and Ting Ye *

College of Life Sciences, Zhejiang Sci-Tech University, Hangzhou 310018, China;
cjh15067149909@163.com (J.C.); mss1053280369@163.com (S.M.); wutao0920@163.com (T.W.)
* Correspondence: lgc@zstu.edu.cn (G.L.); yeting@zstu.edu.cn (T.Y.);
   Tel.: +86-571-8684-3186 (G.L.); +86-571-8684-3199 (T.Y.)

Received: 20 May 2018; Accepted: 5 June 2018; Published: 7 June 2018

check for
updates

Abstract: Lectins play diverse roles in physiological processes as biological recognition molecules. In this report, a gene encoding *Tachypleus tridentatus* Lectin (TTL) was inserted into an oncolytic vaccinia virus (oncoVV) vector to form oncoVV-TTL, which showed significant antitumor activity in a hepatocellular carcinoma mouse model. Furthermore, TTL enhanced oncoVV replication through suppressing antiviral factors expression such as interferon-inducible protein 16 (IFI16), mitochondrial antiviral signaling protein (MAVS) and interferon-beta (IFN-β). Further investigations revealed that oncoVV-TTL replication was highly dependent on ERK activity. This study might provide insights into a novel way of the utilization of TTL in oncolytic viral therapies.

Keywords: TTL; oncolytic vaccinia virus; viral replication; ERK

1. Introduction

The horseshoe crab, as a "living fossil", has survived for more than 500 million years [1]. It can live solely on its hemolymph that contains granular hemocytes comprising 99% of the total hemocytes. The granules store many soluble defense molecules, such as lectins, clotting factors, clottable protein coagulogens, and C-reactive proteins [2,3]. Among those, Lectins, which are multivalent carbohydrate-binding proteins recognizing and binding with conserved pathogen associated molecular patterns (PAMPs) [4,5], agglutinate Gram-negative and Gram-positive bacteria by recognizing the structures of lipopolysaccharide (LPS) and lipoteichoic acid (LTA).

Lectins play diverse roles in physiological processes [6,7], including mediating interactions between cells during development and differentiation [8], and recognizing foreign molecules during immune responses [9]. Several lectins with a broad range of specificity have been identified in horseshoe crab [10]. In the Japanese horseshoe crab, there are six types of lectins, Tachylectin-1 (TL-1), Tachylectin-2 (TL-2), Tachylectin-3 (TL-3), Tachylectin-4 (TL-4) from hemocytes, and Tachylectin-5A (TL-5A) and Tachylectin-5B (TL-5B) from plasma. In the Taiwanese horseshoe crab, two types of lectins, *Tachypleus* plasma lectin 1 (TPL1) and *Tachypleus* plasma lectin 2 (TPL2), have been isolated and characterized as novel hemolymph proteins in the plasma of *Tachypleus tridentatus* [11]. TPL2, also named as *Tachypleus tridentatus* lectin (TTL), shows an 80% sequence identity with TL-3, and both TTL and TL-3 show ligand specificity toward lipopolysaccharides (LPSs), particularly O-antigen [12]. It has been reported that TTL directly interacted with L-rhamnose but not interact with D-galactose as demonstrated by a glycan array and Magnetic Reduction (MR) assay, implying that TTL might perform biological functions through recognizing rhamnose-containing molecules [12,13].

Oncolytic viruses are therapeutically useful viruses that preferentially replicate in cancer cells to elicit the killing effect [14]. A number of viruses including adenovirus, coxackie virus, vesicular stomatitis virus, measles virus, newcastle disease virus, parvovirus, poliovirus, reovirus, and vaccinia virus have now been clinically tested as oncolytic agents [15–18]. Vaccinia virus (VV) became famous as the most successful live biotherapeutic agent in the worldwide smallpox eradication program. VV replication occurs in the cytosol independent from the host cell nucleus [19,20]. Therefore, there is no possibility of chromosomal integration in contrast to other vector systems. Due to its unique features, VV is exploited as a therapeutic agent for the treatment of cancer. VV can be used for cancer therapy as cancer vaccines to stimulate antitumor immunity, or as a replicating virus vector sometimes harboring therapeutic genes to directly lyse tumor cells [21]. Arakawa et al. used an attenuated vaccinia virus to cure patients with metastatic lung and kidney cancer [22]. Kawa and Arakawa treated a multiple myeloma patient with the same attenuated vaccinia virus strain [23]. These studies indicated that oncolytic vaccinia virus had significant anticancer efficacy in various types of cancer. In previous studies, *Haliotis discus discus* sialic acid binding lectin (HddSBL), *Dicentrarchus labrax* fucose-binding lectin (DlFBL), and *Strongylocentrotus purpuratus* rhamnose-binding lectin (SpRBL) exogenously expressed through adenovirus vector showed suppressive effect on a variety of cancer cells in vitro [24,25]. Lectin from *Mytilus galloprovincialis* (MytiLec) was shown to be cytotoxic to diverse cancer cells through eliciting autophagy or apoptosis [26–28]. These data suggested that marine lectins may provide a distinct source of cancer therapeutic agents. Furthermore, our previous studies showed that oncolytic adenovirus vector harboring mannose binding lectin *Pinellia pedatisecta* agglutinin (PPA) showed an antileukemia effect in a mouse model [29], suggesting that harboring lectin genes may enhance the therapeutic effect of oncolytic viruses. In this study, marine lectin TTL was inserted to an oncolytic vaccinia virus (oncoVV) vector, which is deficient of thymidine kinase for cancer specific replication [30], to generate recombinant virus oncoVV-TTL. The antitumor effect of oncoVV-TTL and the underlying mechanisms were analyzed.

2. Results

2.1. oncoVV-TTL Suppressed Liver Cancer Cell Growth In Vivo

The FLAG tagged TTL was detected through Western blot with an antibody against FLAG in oncoVV-TTL treated cancer cells, but not in cells treated with PBS or oncoVV (Figure 1a), indicating that TTL is able to be expressed in cancer cells. To assess the efficacy of oncoVV-TTL against liver cancer in vivo, Balb/c nude mice were subcutaneously engrafted with MHCC97-H liver cancer cells stably expressing fire fly luciferase to establish a tumor-bearing mouse model [31]. The mice then received two injections of oncoVV-TTL or oncoVV for 1×10^7 plaque forming unit (PFU) each. PBS served as the negative control. As shown in Figure 1b, both oncoVV-TTL and oncoVV elicited antitumor efficacy. However, treatment with oncoVV-TTL resulted in a superior antitumor efficacy as compared to both oncoVV and PBS controls. Furthermore, bioluminescence was also monitored for the cancer cell burden in mice. Results confirm the antitumor effect of oncoVV-TTL as compared to oncoVV and PBS (Figure 1c). The significant suppressive effect of oncoVV-TTL compared with PBS and oncoVV was determined by statistical analysis (Figure 1d). Our data demonstrated the antitumor efficacy of oncoVV-TTL.

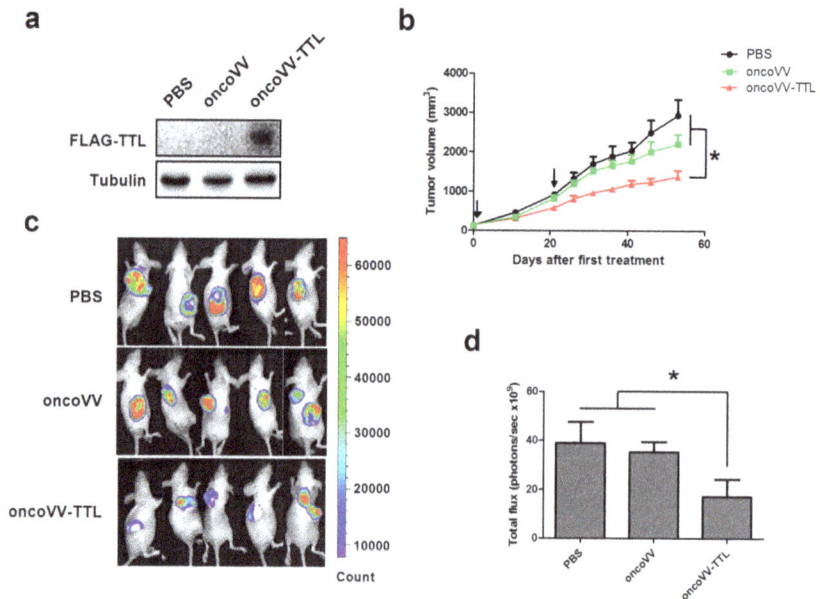

Figure 1. Intracellular expression of *Tachypleus tridentatus* lectin (TTL) in oncoVV-TTL infected cancer cells and the efficacy of oncoVV-TTL against hepatocellular carcinoma in vivo. (**a**) The expression of FLAG tagged TTL was determined by Western blot with an antibody against FLAG. Tubulin served as the loading control. (**b**) MHCC97-H cells were injected into the Balb/c nude mice. Mice were injected with PBS, oncoVV, or oncoVV-TTL after tumor size reached 120 mm^3. Arrows indicate two injections. Values are displayed as mean tumor size ±SEM. Statistically significant differences between treatments were represented by asterisks (* $p < 0.05$). Tumor growth curve of MHCC97-H tumors treated by different injections. (**c**) Representative MHCC97-H tumors 44 days after first treatment. Mice were imaged using the IVIS imaging system. (**d**) Quantification of fluorescence intensity of the MHCC97-H tumors 44 days after first treatment.

2.2. Oncolytic Vaccinia Virus Replication Improved by TTL

We then investigated the underlying mechanism of the antitumor effect of oncoVV-TTL. The viral replication was examined for oncoVV and oncoVV-TTL in liver cancer cell lines MHCC97-H and BEL-7404. As shown, oncoVV-TTL replicated significantly faster than oncoVV in MHCC97-H (Figure 2a), which was further confirmed in BEL-7404 cell line (Figure 2b). Thus, our data demonstrated that arming oncolytic vaccinia virus with TTL improved viral replication.

Intracellular signaling elements related to viral infection and replication were then analyzed. As reported previously, extracellular signal-regulated kinase (ERK) is required for vaccinia virus replication [32,33]. Interferon-inducible protein 16 (IFI16) senses viral DNA in the cytoplasm as well as the nucleus to initiate innate immune responses [34], and plays an important role in the initial steps of the inflammatory processes that precede the onset of autoimmune syndromes [35]. Mitochondrial antiviral signaling protein (MAVS) acts as an important factor in the induction of antiviral and inflammatory responses [36,37]. We then analyzed the phosphorylation level of ERK as well as the expression of IFI16 and MAVS through Western blotting. As shown in Figure 3a,b, oncoVV infection induced ERK phosphorylation in both MHCC97-H and BEL-7404 cell lines. Interestingly, oncoVV-TTL led to a significantly higher level of ERK phosphorylation as compared to oncoVV. We then investigated the effect of oncoVV-TTL on cellular levels of MAVS and IFI16. In MHCC97-H cells, oncoVV but not oncoVV-TTL induced the expression of MAVS and IFI16 (Figure 3a). In BEL-7404 cells, oncoVV triggered the expression of IFI16. On the contrary, oncoVV-TTL did not induce the IFI16 expression (Figure 3b). Our data demonstrated that TTL facilitated vaccinia virus replication in cancer cells through regulating intracellular signaling elements related to viral infection and replication.

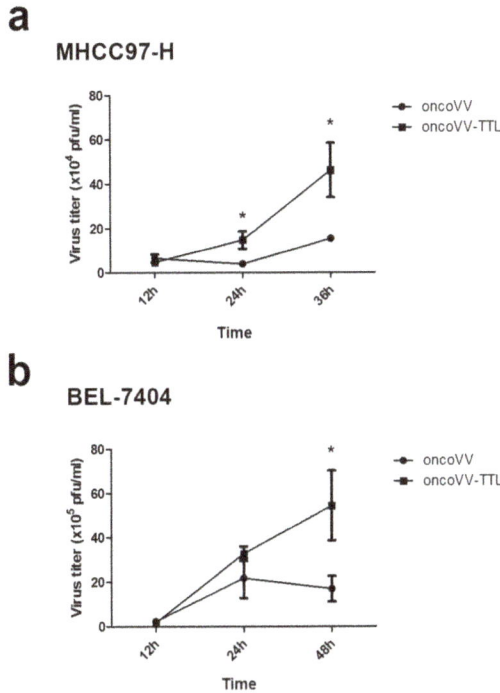

Figure 2. Replication of oncoVV-TTL in hepatocellular carcinoma cell lines. Replication of oncoVV and oncoVV-TTL in MHCC97-H cells (**a**) and BEL-7404 cells (**b**). Mean viral replication was determined by TCID$_{50}$ assay on MHCC97-H cells. Statistical analysis was carried out using a Students unpaired *t* test at each time point. (* $p < 0.05$).

Interferon-beta (IFN-β) regulates a wide range of genes, most of which are involved in the antiviral immune response, playing an important role in inducing non-specific resistance against a broad range of viral infections [38,39]. To determine the effect of oncoVV-TTL infection on IFN-β induction, IFN-β reporter assay was performed in MHCC97-H cells. Results showed that oncoVV induced the upregulation of IFN-β transcription, which was significantly suppressed through TTL harboring (Figure 3c). Taken together, our results indicated that TTL favors oncolytic vaccinia virus replication through suppressing the antiviral response of cancer cells.

2.3. The Role of ERK Activity on oncoVV-TTL Replication

The role of ERK activity in oncoVV-TTL replication was further analyzed. U0126, an inhibitor of mitogen-activated protein kinase kinase (MEK) 1/2-mediated phosphorylation of ERK1/2 [40,41], was used to treat liver cancer cell lines in combination with oncoVV or oncoVV-TTL. Results showed that in MHCC97-H cells the virus titers of oncoVV-TTL but not oncoVV were markedly reduced with the combination of U0126 (Figure 4a). In BEL-7404 cell lines, the effect of U0126 on oncoVV-TTL and oncoVV replication yielded essentially similar results as in MHCC97-H (Figure 4b). Our results indicated that oncoVV-TTL replication was highly dependent on ERK activity.

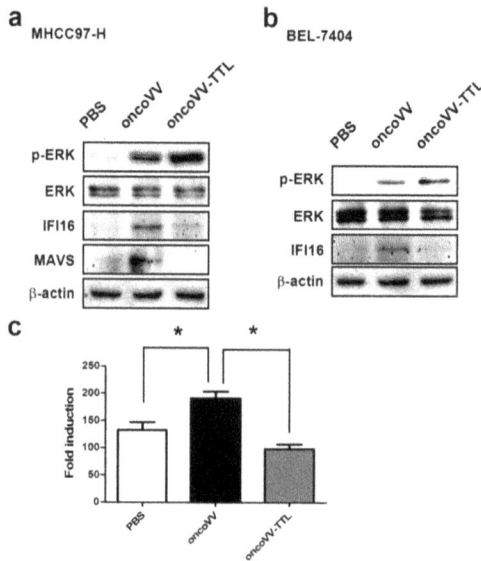

Figure 3. Intracellular signaling elements regulated by oncoVV-TTL. MHCC97-H cells (**a**) or BEL-7404 cells (**b**) were treated with 5MOI of oncoVV-TTL or oncoVV for 24 h, and cells were also treated with PBS as a negative control. Western blot was performed with antibodies against phosphor-extracellular signal-regulated kinase (ERK), ERK, interferon-inducible protein 16 (IFI16), mitochondrial antiviral signaling protein (MAVS) and β-actin. β-actin served as the loading control. (**c**) Activity of interferon-beta (IFN-β) promoter was analyzed through a duo-luciferase reporter assay kit. Statistically significant differences between treatments were represented by asterisks (* $p < 0.05$).

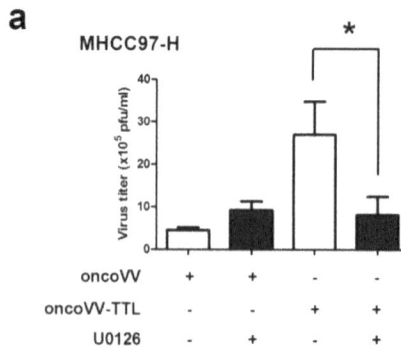

Figure 4. *Cont.*

b

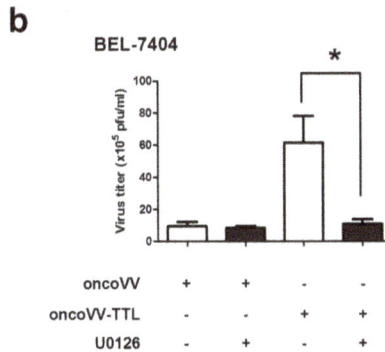

Figure 4. Virus replication was dependent on ERK activity. MHCC97-H cells (**a**) or in BEL-7404 cells (**b**) were infected with oncoVV, oncoVV-TTL respectively with or without the combination of ERK inhibitor U0126. Virus titers were then measured through $TCID_{50}$ aasay. Statistically significant differences between treatments were represented by asterisks (* $p < 0.05$).

3. Discussion

The utilization of lectins in antitumor therapies are greatly limited by their in vivo immunogenicity and toxicity. Vaccinia viruses provide promising vectors for oncolytic therapies and have been developed to be valuable agents for preclinical and clinical evaluations due to their safety and effect [42–45]. In the work presented, A *Tachypleus tridentatus* plasma lectin TTL was genetically inserted into an oncoVV vector and the antitumor activity was evaluated. We showed that TTL enhanced the antitumor activity of oncoVV due to its ability to promote virus replication in liver cancer cells. Further studies showed that the TTL harboring significantly suppressed the oncoVV induced antiviral factors, and the replication of oncoVV-TTL was highly dependent on ERK activation. Importantly, our study did not find obvious toxicity of oncoVV-TTL in this hepatocellular carcinoma mouse model. Therefore, our studies suggest that harboring lectin genes in oncolytic viral vectors could be an important novel direction to overcome the in vivo toxicity of lectins for further development of lectin based antitumor agents.

Viruses need to overcome host antiviral responses for effective replication and spreading. Human cells have evolved a series of viral restriction factors that directly inhibit various steps of viral replication [46,47]. Nucleus associated IFI16 protein, as an innate DNA sensor, regulates inflammatory cytokines and type I interferon (IFN) production [48]. In addition, Mitochondrial antiviral signaling protein (MAVS) acts as an important factor in the induction of antiviral and inflammatory responses [49]. In this study, TTL upregulated the oncoVV induced ERK phosphorylation and suppressed the antiviral factors such as IFN-β, IFI16 and MAVS induced by oncoVV. Therefore, the relationship between ERK activity and antiviral factors still remains unclear pending further investigations.

4. Materials and Methods

4.1. Cell Culture and Transfection

The human embryonic kidney cell line 293A, hepatocellular carcinoma cell lines MHCC97-H and BEL-7404 were provided by American Type Culture Collection (Rockville, MD, USA). Cells were incubated in Dulbecco's modified Eagle's medium supplemented with 1% penicillin/streptomycin solution, 1% L-Glutamine and 10% fetal bovine serum, maintained at 37 °C in a humidified 5% CO_2. Appropriate amounts of plasmids were transfected into cells by using Thermo Scientific

TurboFect Transfection Reagent (Thermo Fisher Scientific Inc., Waltham, MA, USA) following the manufacturer's instruction.

4.2. Plasmid Construction

The plasmid pEGFP-Flag-TTL encoding TTL (GenBank accession no. AF264068) gene was purchased from Shanghai Generay Biotech Co., Ltd., Shanghai, China. For recombinant expression in cell lines MHCC97-H and BEL-7404, the Flag-TTL gene was cloned into the pCB plasmid using primers 5'-GA*AGATCT*ATGGATTACAAGGATGACGACGATAAGGGAATTTTCAAAGTGT-3' (forward) with a *Bgl*II site (italic) and 5'-GC*TCTAGA*TTACTTAATTATTATAATAGGTCCA-3' (reverse) with a *Xba*I site (italic). The sequence was confirmed by Shanghai Generay Biotech Company.

4.3. Vaccinia Virus Construction

The vaccinia virus was generated in our laboratory previously. After HEK-293A cells infected with wild type vaccinia virus about 2–4 h, pCB-Flag-TTL were transfected into 293A cells. Mycophenolic acid, dioxopurine, and hypoxanthine were added to screen effective oncoVV-TTL. Recombinant viruses were gathered from cell culture medium, and purified through CsCl gradient centrifugation. The virus titers were determined by $TCID_{50}$ (median tissue culture infective dose).

4.4. Infectious Progeny Production

To determine virus progeny production, 5×10^4 cells (MHCC97-H, BEL-7404) were plated in 24-well plates. Cells were infected with 5MOI (multiplicity of infection) of the Vaccinia virus oncoVV-TTL or oncoVV. After 24 h, 36 h and 48 h, cells were collected and washed twice with PBS. After three freeze/thaw cycles in $-80\ ^\circ$C and 37 $^\circ$C, the production was determined by $TCID_{50}$ assay on 293A cells.

4.5. Animal Experiments

Balb/c nude mice of 4–5 weeks age were used for hepatocellular carcinoma tumor-bearing mouse model. MHCC97-H at 2.5×10^6 cells/mouse were injected subcutaneously into the mice on the back. Mice were randomly grouped and in situ injected with two injections of oncolytic vaccinia virus for 1×10^7 plaque-forming units (PFU) each. Then we measured the volume of tumor every five days. The tumor volume was calculated using the formula: length (mm) $\times$ width (mm)^2 $\times$ 0.5. After injection of D-luciferin into mice, bioluminescence was measured through the Caliber IVIS kinetics (Caliper life sciences, Hopkinton, MA, USA). Regions of interest were measured through the IVIS software.

All animal studies were approved by the Institutional Animal Care and Use Committee (IACUC) of Zhejiang Sci-Tech University (2017-1), Hangzhou, Zhejiang, China.

4.6. Reporter Assay

IFN-β firefly luciferase reporter plasmid was constructed previously. Reporter assay was performed using a duo-luciferase assay kit (GeneCopoeia, Inc., Rockville, MD, USA) according to the manufacturer's instructions. Briefly, MHCC97-H or BEL-7404 cells were co-transfected with Renilla luciferase control plasmid and IFN-β luciferase reporter plasmid, followed by treatment with PBS, 5 MOI of oncoVV or oncoVV-TTL for 24 h. Then cells were lysed and IFN-β luciferase activity was normalized to Renilla luciferase activity.

4.7. Western Blotting Analysis

The cell extracts were separated in SDS-PAGE gel and transferred onto nitrocellulose membranes. The membranes were then immersed in Tris-buffered saline and Tween-20 containing 5% of bovine serum albumin at room temperature for 1 h. Subsequently, the membrane was incubated with the primary antibody, followed by incubation with secondary antibodies for 1 h at room temperature. After washing with Tris-buffered saline, the bands were detected under a Tanon 5500 chemiluminescence image system (Tanon Inc., Shanghai, China).

Goat anti-MAVS, IFI16 antibodies were purchased from Santa Cruz Biotechnology Inc. (Dallas, TX, USA). Rabbit anti-ERK1/2 and phospho-ERK1/2 antibodies were purchased from Cell Signaling Technology Inc. (Danvers, MA, USA). Rabbit anti-β-actin was purchased from Bioss Antibodies (Beijing, China). The HRP conjugated goat anti-rabbit and goat anti-mouse antibodies were purchased from MultiSciences (Lianke) Biotech Co., Ltd. (Hangzhou, China).

4.8. Statistical Analysis

Differences among the different treatment groups were determined by student's *t*-test. $p < 0.05$ was considered significant.

5. Conclusions

Our studies showed that oncoVV-TTL elicited significant antitumor activity in a hepatocellular carcinoma mouse model. TTL enhanced viral replication through inhibiting the antiviral immune response in hepatocellular carcinoma cells. Furthermore, oncoVV-TTL replication was demonstrated to be depended on ERK activity. Our studies might provide insights into the utilization of marine lectin genes such as TTL in oncolytic viral therapies. However, the underlying mechanism of the TTL functions in cancer cells still remains unclear pending further investigations.

Author Contributions: G.L. conceived and designed the experiments; G.L., J.C., S.M., and T.W. performed the experiments; G.L. analyzed the data; T.Y. wrote the paper; G.L. revised the paper.

Acknowledgments: This work was supported by Zhejiang Provincial Natural Science Foundation grant LZ16D060002, National Natural Science Foundation of China grant 81572986, Guangzhou Shiyao Biotechnology Co., Ltd., and Zhejiang Provincial Top Key Discipline of Biology.

Conflicts of Interest: The authors declare no conflict of interest.

References

1. Xia, X. Phylogenetic relationship among horseshoe crab species: Effect of substitution models on phylogenetic analyses. *Syst. Biol.* **2000**, *49*, 87–100. [CrossRef] [PubMed]
2. Iwanaga, S. The molecular basis of innate immunity in the horseshoe crab. *Curr. Opin. Immunol.* **2002**, *14*, 87–95. [CrossRef]
3. Kurata, S.; Ariki, S.; Kawabata, S. Recognition of pathogens and activation of immune responses in drosophila and horseshoe crab innate immunity. *Immunobiology* **2006**, *211*, 237–249. [CrossRef] [PubMed]
4. Loris, R. Principles of structures of animal and plant lectins. *Biochim. Biophys. Acta* **2002**, *1572*, 198–208. [CrossRef]
5. Richardson, M.B.; Williams, S.J. MCL and mincle: C-type lectin receptors that sense damaged self and pathogen-associated molecular patterns. *Front. Immunol.* **2014**, *5*, 288–288. [CrossRef] [PubMed]
6. Elola, M.T.; Blidner, A.G.; Ferragut, F.; Bracalente, C.; Rabinovich, G.A. Assembly, organization and regulation of cell-surface receptors by lectin-glycan complexes. *Biochem. J.* **2015**, *469*, 1–16. [CrossRef] [PubMed]
7. Lambert, A.A.; Gilbert, C.; Richard, M.; Beaulieu, A.D.; Tremblay, M.J. The C-type lectin surface receptor DCIR acts as a new attachment factor for HIV-1 in dendritic cells and contributes to trans- and cis-infection pathways. *Blood* **2008**, *112*, 1299–1307. [CrossRef] [PubMed]
8. Mikkola, M.; Toivonen, S.; Tamminen, K.; Alfthan, K.; Tuuri, T.; Satomaa, T.; Natunen, J.; Saarinen, J.; Tiittanen, M.; Lampinen, M. Lectin from *Erythrina cristagalli* supports undifferentiated growth and differentiation of human pluripotent stem cells. *Stem Cells Dev.* **2013**, *22*, 707–716. [CrossRef] [PubMed]
9. Kawabata, S.; Koshiba, T.; Shibata, T. The lipopolysaccharide-activated innate immune response network of the horseshoe crab. *Invert. Surviv. J.* **2009**, *6*, 59–77.
10. Kawabata, S.I.; Iwanaga, S. Role of lectins in the innate immunity of horseshoe crab. *Dev. Comp Immunol.* **1999**, *23*, 391–400. [CrossRef]
11. Kuo, T.H.; Chuang, S.C.; Chang, S.Y.; Liang, P.H. Ligand specificities and structural requirements of two *Tachypleus* plasma lectins for bacterial trapping. *Biochem. J.* **2006**, *393*, 757–766. [CrossRef] [PubMed]

12. Chen, S.C.; Yen, C.H.; Yeh, M.S.; Huang, C.J.; Liu, T.Y. Biochemical properties and cDNa cloning of two new lectins from the plasma of *Tachypleus tridentatus*: *Tachypleus* plasma lectin 1 and 2$^+$. *J. Biol. Chem.* **2001**, *276*, 9631–9639. [CrossRef] [PubMed]
13. Ng, S.-K.; Huang, Y.-T.; Lee, Y.-C.; Low, E.-L.; Chiu, C.-H.; Chen, S.-L.; Mao, L.-C.; Chang, D.T. A recombinant horseshoe crab plasma lectin recognizes specific pathogen-associated molecular patterns of bacteria through Rhamnose. *PLoS ONE* **2014**, *9*, e115296. [CrossRef] [PubMed]
14. Russell, S.J.; Peng, K.W.; Bell, J.C. Oncolytic virotherapy. *Nat. Biotechnol.* **2012**, *30*, 658–670. [CrossRef] [PubMed]
15. Guo, Z.S.; Thorne, S.H.; Bartlett, D.L. Oncolytic virotherapy: Molecular targets in tumor-selective replication and carrier cell-mediated delivery of oncolytic viruses. *Biochim. Biophys. Acta* **2008**, *1785*, 217–231. [CrossRef] [PubMed]
16. Chernajovsky, Y.; Layward, L.; Lemoine, N. Controversy: Fighting cancer with oncolytic viruses. *Br. Med. J.* **2006**, *332*, 170–172. [CrossRef] [PubMed]
17. Jacobsen, K.A. Analysis of a mathematical model for tumor therapy with a fusogenic oncolytic virus. *Math. Biosci.* **2015**, *270*, 169–182. [CrossRef] [PubMed]
18. Saha, D.; Ahmed, S.S.; Rabkin, S.D. Exploring the antitumor effect of virus in malignant glioma. *Drug Future* **2015**, *40*, 739–749.
19. Carroll, M.W.; Kovacs, G.R. Virus-based vectors for gene expression in mammalian cells: Vaccinia virus. *New Compr. Biochem.* **2003**, *38*, 125–136.
20. Mallardo, M.; Leithe, E.; Schleich, S.; Roos, N.; Doglio, L.; Krijnse, L.J. Relationship between vaccinia virus intracellular cores, early mRNAs, and DNA replication sites. *J. Virol.* **2002**, *76*, 5167–5183. [CrossRef] [PubMed]
21. Guse, K.; Cerullo, V.; Hemminki, A. Oncolytic vaccinia virus for the treatment of cancer. *Expert Opin. Biol. Ther.* **2011**, *11*, 595–608. [CrossRef] [PubMed]
22. Arakawa, S.; Hamami, G.; Umezu, K.; Kamidono, S.; Ishigami, J.; Arakawa, S. Clinical trial of attenuated vaccinia virus as strain in the treatment of advanced adenocarcinoma. *J. Cancer Res. Clin.* **1987**, *113*, 95–98. [CrossRef]
23. Kawa, A.; Arakawa, S. The effect of attenuated vaccinia virus AS strain on multiple myeloma: A case report. *J. Exp. Med.* **1987**, *57*, 79–81.
24. Wu, B.; Mei, S.; Cui, L.; Zhao, Z.; Chen, J.; Wu, T.; Li, G. Marine lectins DLFBL and HddSBL fused with soluble coxsackie-adenovirus receptor facilitate adenovirus infection in cancer cells but have different effects on cell survival. *Mar. Drugs* **2017**, *15*, 73. [CrossRef] [PubMed]
25. Wu, L.; Yang, X.; Duan, X.; Cui, L.; Li, G. Exogenous expression of marine lectins DLFBL and SpRBL induces cancer cell apoptosis possibly through PRMT5-E2F-1 pathway. *Sci. Rep.* **2014**, *4*, 4505. [CrossRef] [PubMed]
26. Terada, D.; Kawai, F.; Noguchi, H.; Unzai, S.; Hasan, I.; Fujii, Y.; Park, S.Y.; Ozeki, Y.; Tame, J.R. Crystal structure of Mytilec, a galactose-binding lectin from the mussel *Mytilus galloprovincialis* with cytotoxicity against certain cancer cell types. *Sci. Rep.* **2016**, *6*, 28344. [CrossRef] [PubMed]
27. Hasan, I.; Sugawara, S.; Fujii, Y.; Koide, Y.; Terada, D.; Iimura, N.; Fujiwara, T.; Takahashi, K.G.; Kojima, N.; Rajia, S.; et al. Mytilec, a mussel R-type lectin, interacts with surface glycan Gb3 on burkitt's lymphoma cells to trigger apoptosis through multiple pathways. *Mar. Drugs* **2015**, *13*, 7377–7389. [CrossRef] [PubMed]
28. Fujii, Y.; Dohmae, N.; Takio, K.; Kawsar, S.M.; Matsumoto, R.; Hasan, I.; Koide, Y.; Kanaly, R.A.; Yasumitsu, H.; Ogawa, Y.; et al. A lectin from the mussel *Mytilus galloprovincialis* has a highly novel primary structure and induces glycan-mediated cytotoxicity of globotriaosylceramide-expressing lymphoma cells. *J. Biol. Chem.* **2012**, *287*, 44772–44783. [CrossRef] [PubMed]
29. Li, G.; Li, X.; Wu, H.; Yang, X.; Zhang, Y.; Chen, L.; Wu, X.; Cui, L.; Wu, L.; Luo, J.; et al. Cd123 targeting oncolytic adenoviruses suppress acute myeloid leukemia cell proliferation in vitro and in vivo. *Blood Cancer J.* **2014**, *4*, e194. [CrossRef] [PubMed]
30. Mccart, J.A.; Ward, J.M.; Lee, J.; Hu, Y.; Alexander, H.R.; Libutti, S.K.; Moss, B.; Bartlett, D.L. Systemic cancer therapy with a tumor-selective vaccinia virus mutant lacking thymidine kinase and vaccinia growth factor genes. *Cancer Res.* **2001**, *61*, 8751–8757. [PubMed]
31. Gnant, M.F.; Noll, L.A.; Irvine, K.R.; Puhlmann, M.; Terrill, R.E.; Jr, A.H.; Bartlett, D.L. Tumor-specific gene delivery using recombinant vaccinia virus in a rabbit model of liver metastases. *J. Natl. Cancer Inst.* **1999**, *91*, 1744–1750. [CrossRef] [PubMed]
32. Andrade, A.A.; Silva, P.N.; Pereira, A.C.; De Sousa, L.P.; Ferreira, P.C.; Gazzinelli, R.T.; Kroon, E.G.; Ropert, C.; Bonjardim, C.A. The vaccinia virus-stimulated mitogen-activated protein kinase (MAPK) pathway is required for virus multiplication. *Biochem. J.* **2004**, *381*, 437–446. [CrossRef] [PubMed]

33. Kim, Y.; Lee, C. Extracellular signal-regulated kinase (ERK) activation is required for porcine epidemic diarrhea virus replication. *Virology* **2015**, *484*, 181–193. [CrossRef] [PubMed]

34. Unterholzner, L.; Keating, S.M.; Horan, K.A.; Jensen, S.B.; Sharma, S.; Sirois, C.M.; Jin, T.; Latz, E.; Xiao, T.S.; Fitzgerald, K.A. IFI16 is an innate immune sensor for intracellular DNA. *Nat. Immunol.* **2010**, *11*, 997–1004. [CrossRef] [PubMed]

35. Mondini, M.; Vidali, M.; Airò, P.; De, A.M.; Riboldi, P.; Meroni, P.L.; Gariglio, M.; Landolfo, S. Role of the interferon-inducible gene IFI16 in the etiopathogenesis of systemic autoimmune disorders. *Ann. N. Y. Acad. Sci.* **2007**, *1110*, 47–56. [CrossRef] [PubMed]

36. Li, X.D.; Sun, L.; Chen, Z.J. Hepatitis C virus protease NS3/4A cleaves mitochondrial antiviral signaling protein off the mitochondria to evade innate immunity. *Proc. Nat. Acad. Sci. USA* **2005**, *102*, 17717–17722. [CrossRef] [PubMed]

37. Li, X.D.; Chiu, Y.H.; Ismail, A.S.; Behrendt, C.L.; Wightcarter, M.; Hooper, L.V.; Chen, Z.J. Mitochondrial antiviral signaling protein (MAVS) monitors commensal bacteria and induces an immune response that prevents experimental colitis. *Proc. Nat. Acad. Sci. USA* **2011**, *108*, 17390–17395. [CrossRef] [PubMed]

38. Petersen, T.; Møller-Larsen, A.; Ellermanneriksen, S.; Thiel, S.; Christensen, T. Effects of interferon-beta therapy on elements in the antiviral immune response towards the human herpesviruses EBV, HSV, and VZV, and to the human endogenous retroviruses HERV-H and HERV-W in multiple sclerosis. *J. Neuroimmunol.* **2012**, *249*, 105–108. [CrossRef] [PubMed]

39. Dewitteorr, S.J.; Mehta, D.R.; Collins, S.E.; Suthar, M.S.; Gale, M., Jr.; Mossman, K.L. Long double-stranded RNA induces an antiviral response independent of IFN regulatory factor 3, IFN-beta promoter stimulator 1, and IFN. *J. Immunol.* **2009**, *183*, 6545–6553. [CrossRef] [PubMed]

40. Satoh, T.; Nakatsuka, D.; Watanabe, Y.; Nagata, I.; Kikuchi, H.; Namura, S. Neuroprotection by MAPK/ERK kinase inhibition with u0126 against oxidative stress in a mouse neuronal cell line and rat primary cultured cortical neurons. *Neurosci. Lett.* **2000**, *288*, 163–166. [CrossRef]

41. Kennedy, R.A.; Kemp, T.J.; Sugden, P.H.; Clerk, A. Using u0126 to dissect the role of the extracellular signal-regulated kinase 1/2 (ERK1/2) cascade in the regulation of gene expression by endothelin-1 in cardiac myocytes. *J. Mol. Cell. Cardiol.* **2006**, *41*, 236–247. [CrossRef] [PubMed]

42. Advani, S.J.; Buckel, L.; Chen, N.G.; Scanderbeg, D.J.; Geissinger, U.; Zhang, Q.; Yu, Y.A.; Aguilar, R.J.; Mundt, A.J.; Szalay, A.A. Preferential Replication of Systemically Delivered Oncolytic Vaccinia Virus in Focally Irradiated Glioma Xenografts. *Clin. Cancer Res.* **2012**, *18*, 2579–2590. [CrossRef] [PubMed]

43. Breitbach, C.J.; Burke, J.; Jonker, D.; Stephenson, J.; Haas, A.R.; Chow, L.Q.M.; Nieva, J.; Hwang, T.H.; Moon, A.; Patt, R. Intravenous delivery of a multi-mechanistic cancer-targeted oncolytic poxvirus in humans. *Nature* **2011**, *477*, 99–102. [CrossRef] [PubMed]

44. Hwang, T.H.; Moon, A.; Burke, J.; Ribas, A.; Stephenson, J.; Breitbach, C.J.; Daneshmand, M.; Silva, N.D.; Parato, K.; Diallo, J.S. A Mechanistic Proof-of-concept Clinical Trial with JX-594, a Targeted Multi-mechanistic Oncolytic Poxvirus, in Patients with Metastatic Melanoma. *Mol. Ther.* **2011**, *19*, 1913–1922. [CrossRef] [PubMed]

45. Chard, L.S.; Maniati, E.; Wang, P.; Zhang, Z.; Gao, D.; Wang, J.; Cao, F.; Ahmed, J.; El, K.M.; Hughes, J. A vaccinia virus armed with interleukin-10 is a promising therapeutic agent for treatment of murine pancreatic cancer. *Clin. Cancer Res.* **2015**, *21*, 405–416. [CrossRef] [PubMed]

46. García-Sastre, A. Induction and evasion of type I interferon responses by influenza viruses. *Virus Res.* **2011**, *162*, 12–18. [CrossRef] [PubMed]

47. Duggal, N.K.; Emerman, M. Evolutionary conflicts between viruses and restriction factors shape immunity. *Nat. Rev. Immunol.* **2012**, *12*, 687–695. [CrossRef] [PubMed]

48. Goubau, D.; Deddouche, S.; Reis, E.S.C. Cytosolic sensing of viruses. *Immunity* **2013**, *38*, 855–869. [CrossRef] [PubMed]

49. Belgnaoui, S.M.; Paz, S.; Hiscott, J. Orchestrating the interferon antiviral response through the mitochondrial antiviral signaling (MAVS) adapter. *Curr. Opin. Immunol.* **2011**, *23*, 564–572. [CrossRef] [PubMed]

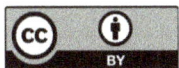

marine drugs

MDPI

Article

Haliotis discus discus Sialic Acid-Binding Lectin Reduces the Oncolytic Vaccinia Virus Induced Toxicity in a Glioblastoma Mouse Model

Gongchu Li *, Shengsheng Mei, Jianhong Cheng, Tao Wu and Jingjing Luo *

College of Life Sciences, Zhejiang Sci-Tech University, Hangzhou 310018, China; mss1053280369@163.com (S.M.); cjh15067149909@163.com (J.C.); wutao0920@163.com (T.W.)
* Correspondence: lgc@zstu.edu.cn (G.L.); deepstoh@163.com (J.L.); Tel.: +86-571-8684-3186 (G.L. & J.L.)

Received: 4 April 2018; Accepted: 25 April 2018; Published: 26 April 2018

check for updates

Abstract: Although oncolytic viruses provide attractive vehicles for cancer treatment, their adverse effects are largely ignored. In this work, rat C6 glioblastoma cells were subcutaneously xenografted into mice, and a thymidine kinase-deficient oncolytic vaccinia virus (oncoVV) induced severe toxicity in this model. However, oncoVV-HddSBL, in which a gene encoding *Haliotis discus discus* sialic acid-binding lectin (HddSBL) was inserted into oncoVV, significantly prolonged the survival of mice as compared to the control virus. HddSBL reduced the tumor secreted serum rat IL-2 level upregulated by oncoVV, promoted viral replication, as well as inhibited the expression of antiviral factors in C6 glioblastoma cell line. Furthermore, HddSBL downregulated the expression levels of histone H3 and H4, and upregulated histone H3R8 and H4R3 asymmetric dimethylation, confirming the effect of HddSBL on chromatin structure suggested by the transcriptome data. Our results might provide insights into the utilization of HddSBL in counteracting the adverse effects of oncolytic vaccinia virus.

Keywords: HddSBL; oncolytic vaccinia virus; glioblastoma; adverse effects

1. Introduction

Glioblastoma is the most common primary brain tumor and shows poor prognosis. The 2-year overall survival of glioblastoma patients is approximately 25% after current standard radiation and chemotherapy [1,2]. The failure of effective treatment for glioblastoma is at least partly due to the restricted permeation of drugs across the blood–brain barrier (BBB) [3,4]. Therefore, novel technologies for safer and effective clinical application are essential.

Oncolytic virotherapy is a promising treatment modality that selectively targets cancerous tissues without harming normal tissues [5]. In this strategy, virus vectors are usually designed by deleting genes important for viral replication in normal cells and inserting therapeutic genes. Through specifically infecting cancer cells, viruses amplify in the tumor and infect more cancer cells [6]. Several viruses, including measles virus (MV) [7], myxoma virus (MYXV) [8], adenovirus (Ad) [9,10], herpes simplex virus (HSV) [11–13], and vaccinia virus (VV) [14] have been utilized in glioblastoma treatment. Compared with other viral vectors, vaccinia virus offers several advantages, including large packing capacity of exogenous genes, the ability of overcoming BBB for effective tumor treatment, and rapid replication in cytoplasm, instead of integration into the host genome [15]. Oncolytic vaccinia viruses (oncoVV) have been used in clinical trials, including GLV-1h68 [16] and JX-594 [17–20]. JX-594 has a deletion of the thymidine kinase gene, and expression of human granulocyte-macrophage colony stimulating factor (GM-CSF) and β-galactosidase (β-gal) proteins, and has showed enhanced cytotoxicity in mouse GL261 glioma cells, compared with reovirus or VSVΔM51. However, the adverse effects of oncolytic viruses have been largely ignored.

Lectins, distributed ubiquitously in plants, animals, and fungi, are highly diverse carbohydrate-binding proteins, which selectively recognize and bind distinct sugar-containing receptors on cellular surfaces [21,22]. Regarding their biochemical properties, lectins hold not only potential for cancer diagnosis and prognosis, but also show great potential for application in cancer therapy, through activating apoptotic- or autophagic-related signaling pathways. Previous studies have showed the anticancer potential of various lectins, including galectin [23,24], mistletoe lectin [25], concanavalin A [26], and MytiLec [27–30]. In our previous work, we have demonstrated the anticancer efficiency of adenovirus-mediated lectin expression, including mannose-binding lectin from *Pinellia pedatisecta* agglutinin (PPA) [31], *Ulva pertusa* lectin 1 [32], *Strongylocentrotus purpuratus* rhamnose binding lectin (SpRBL), *Dicentrarchus labrax* fucose binding lectin (DlFBL) [33], and *Haliotis discus discus* sialic acid-binding lectin (HddSBL), which elicited significant in vitro and in vivo suppressive effects on a variety of tumor cells. HddSBL exogenously expressed from adenovirus vectors has shown significant growth inhibition on hepatocellular carcinoma Hep3B cells, colon carcinoma SW480 cells, and lung cancer cell lines A549 and H1299 [34].

Here, we show that an oncoVV with the deletion of thymidine kinase gene was toxic to mice subcutaneously xenografted with rat C6 glioblastoma cells. Interestingly, the survival of C6 glioblastoma xenograft mice was prolonged by oncoVV harboring HddSBL (oncoVV-HddSBL) as compared to the control oncoVV virus. We further showed that HddSBL downregulated serum rat interleukin-2 (IL-2) levels, inhibited the production of intracellular antiviral factors, promoted viral replication, and influenced histone methylation.

2. Results

2.1. HddSBL Reduced the Toxicity of OncoVV in a Subcutaneous C6 Glioblastoma Xenograft Mouse Model

We first assessed the efficacy of oncoVV and oncoVV-HddSBL in a subcutaneous glioblastoma xenograft model. Rat C6 glioblastoma xenografts were grown in the right flank of athymic BALB/c nude mice. The xenograft model was established by day 10 and the tumor volume reached about 100 mm^3, followed by intraperitoneal injection of PBS, oncoVV, or oncoVV-HddSBL. As shown in Figure 1a, oncoVV exhibited severe toxicity. However, the survival of the oncoVV-HddSBL group was significantly prolonged as compared to the oncoVV group. Our unpublished data have demonstrated the safety of this control oncoVV virus to several other tumor-bearing mouse models, indicating that the toxicity of oncoVV shown here was induced through acting on C6 tumors. Therefore, we further investigated the effect of oncoVV-HddSBL on C6 xenografts, as well as C6 tumor cells.

2.2. OncoVV-HddSBL Reduced Tumor Secretion of Rat IL-2

We then investigated the potential mechanisms underlying prolonged survival of mice by oncoVV-HddSBL. After 15 days of the first injection of VV, secretion of rat IL-2 in the xenograft tumors was measured by ELISA assay (Figure 1b). Compared to the PBS control, the oncoVV enhanced the secretion of IL-2 ($p < 0.05$), while the oncoVV-HddSBL significantly reduced the secretion of IL-2 compared to the oncoVV group ($p < 0.05$). The transcription levels of rat IL-2 in vitro were investigated by RT-PCR analysis after C6 cells were infected with 5 multiplicity of infection (MOI) of VVs (Figure 1c), which was consistent with ELISA assay results. Furthermore, the activity of inflammation related transcription factors nuclear factor-κB (NF-κB) and activator protein-1 (AP-1) was upregulated in oncoVV-HddSBL-treated C6 cells, as compared to PBS and oncoVV controls (Figure 2). Taken together, our data suggested that the prolonged survival of C6 mice by oncoVV-HddSBL might be due to the significant reduction of IL-2 secretion from tumor cells, whereas the activation of inflammatory transcription factors NF-κB and AP-1 limited this effect.

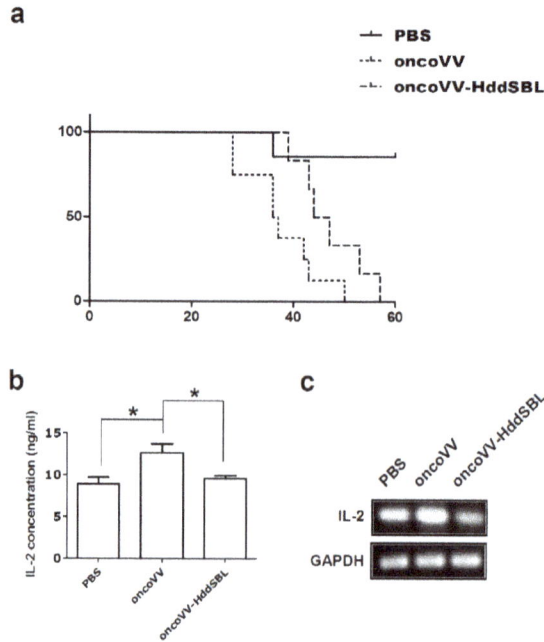

Figure 1. The oncolytic vaccinia virus (oncoVV)-*Haliotis discus discus* sialic acid-binding lectin (HddSBL) reduced toxicity and prolonged survival of mice compared to the oncoVV. (**a**) Kaplan–Meier survival curves of C6 glioblastoma xenograft mouse model. (**b**) ELISA assay of IL-2 secretion. (**c**) Reverse transcriptase-polymerase chain reaction (RT-PCR) analysis of rat IL-2 at mRNA levels.

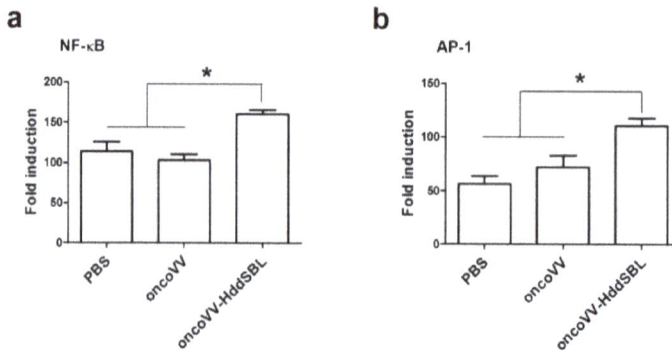

Figure 2. The effects of oncoVV and oncoVV-HddSBL on (**a**) NF-κB and (**b**) AP-1 activation in C6 glioblastoma cells using NF-κB or AP-1 reporter assay. * $p < 0.05$.

2.3. Virus Replication in Rat C6 Glioblastoma Cells

After rat C6 glioblastoma cells were infected with 5 MOI oncoVV or oncoVV-HddSBL for 36 h, total RNA was extracted from cells, differentially expressed genes were screened, and transcriptome sequencing analysis was carried out. The result of gene enrichment analysis is shown in Figure 3. Then, the representing differentially expressed genes were selected and shown in Figure 4, including several factors related to intracellular viral controlling. Therefore, C6 glioblastoma cells were then infected with 5 MOI oncoVV or oncoVV-HddSBL, and virus replication was investigated at 24 h and 36 h. The results showed that the oncoVV-HddSBL was nearly 2-fold higher at 24 h and 7-fold higher at 36 h than that of control oncoVV (Figure 5a). We then investigated the transcription levels of antiviral factors IFIT2 (interferon-induced protein with tetratricopeptide repeats 2), IFIT3, and DDX58 (DEAD-box helicase 58) by RT-PCR. The transcription of IFIT2, IFIT3, and DDX58 was upregulated in oncoVV group, while the oncoVV-HddSBL dramatically decreased their levels as compared to oncoVV treatment (Figure 5b), which was consistent with the transcriptome data shown in Figure 4.

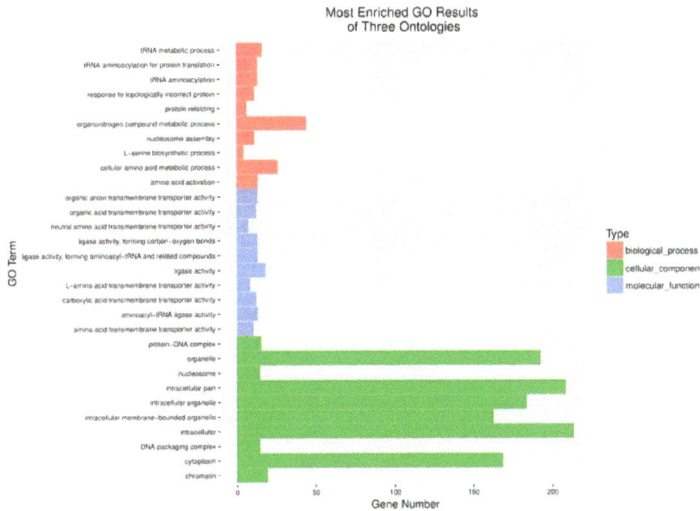

Figure 3. Functional categorization of up-regulated genes based on gene ontology (GO) annotations between oncoVV and oncoVV-HddSBL treatments.

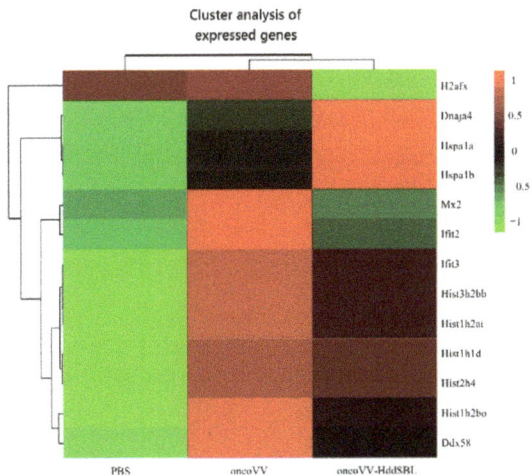

Figure 4. Screening and functional analysis of differentially expressed genes after treatment of C6 glioblastoma cells with PBS, oncoVV (5 MOI), and oncoVV-HddSBL (5 MOI) for 36 h. Scale bar is in log10.

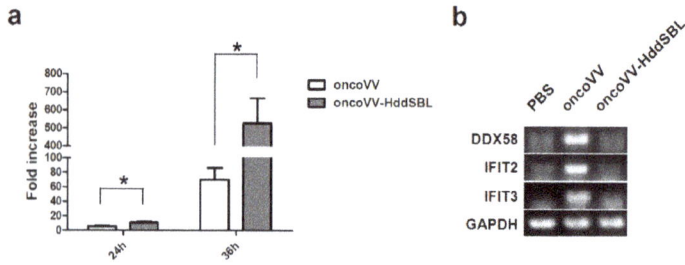

Figure 5. HddSBL promoted viral replication and inhibited antiviral factors in C6 glioblastoma cells. (**a**) Viral replication in C6 glioblastoma cells; (**b**) RT-PCR for mRNA levels of antiviral genes. * $p < 0.05$.

2.4. The Effect of HddSBL on Histone Modification

As shown in our transcriptome data, among the most significant categories, we found terms related to chromatin structure such as "nucleosome", "protein–DNA complex", "DNA packaging complex", and "chromatin". We then verified the effect of HddSBL on chromatin structure regulation. The oncoVV-HddSBL treatment showed significant downregulation of histone H3 and histone H4, and upregulation of histone H3 Arg8 asymmetric methylation (H3R8me2a), and histone H4 Arg3 asymmetric methylation (H4R3me2a) in C6 glioblastoma cells (Figure 6). Our results indicated that HddSBL influenced histone modification, which was consistent with the result of transcriptome data. Furthermore, the expression of FLAG-tagged HddSBL was also verified by Western blot with an antibody against FLAG.

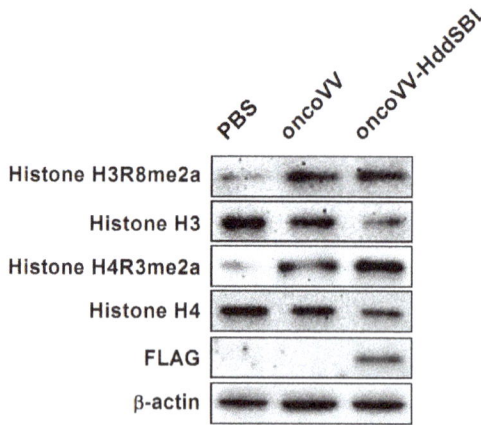

Figure 6. The effect of oncoVV-HddSBL on histone modification. C6 glioblastoma cells were treated with PBS, 5 MOI of oncoVV or oncoVV-HddSBL, and histone H3, H4, H3R8, and H4R3 asymmetric dimethylation levels, as well as the expression of FLAG-tagged HddSBL were analyzed by Western blot.

3. Discussion

Oncolytic viruses provide an alternative tool for cancer treatment. The transgenes can be integrated into recombinant vectors to form tumor-selective, multi-mechanistic antitumor agents. Deletion of viral genes that are necessary for replication in normal cells greatly enhances cancer cell-specific replication of oncolytic viruses [35]. Their oncolytic effects can be enhanced through the insertion of foreign antitumor genes [36,37]. Due to the large packing capacity of exogenous genes, VV is particularly attractive as a potential therapeutic agent for the treatment of malignant tumors. However, the adverse effects of

VV have been ignored in many studies. In this work, we demonstrated the potential for lectin HddSBL carried by oncoVV for reducing the oncoVV-induced severe toxicity in treatment of glioblastoma.

The interferons (IFNs) induced protein with tetratricopeptide repeats (IFITs) family participates in diverse processes in response to viral infection [38]. IFIT2 is located in microtubules, and plays an important role in cell proliferation and microtubule dynamics. IFIT3 is located in the cytoplasm and mitochondria, and is also recognized as an antiviral protein. Our study showed that HddSBL inhibits the oncoVV-induced antiviral factors, which favored oncoVV replication in C6 cells. In addition, previous studies have demonstrated that a high dose of IL-2 led to substantial acute toxicity [39,40]. In our study, a decrease in IL-2 secretion was shown to be associated with prolonged survival of oncoVV-HddSBL-treated mice. Thus, our results have suggested that HddSBL affected multiple signaling pathways related to immune responses induced by oncoVV. Therefore, further investigations into the underlying mechanism may help to develop oncoVV-HddSBL into an agent for controlling oncoVV toxicity.

4. Materials and Methods

4.1. Cell Culture and Production of oncoVV-HddSBL

Rat C6 glioblastoma cells and human embryonic kidney cells HEK293A were obtained from American Type Culture Collection (Rockville, MD, USA) and were cultured in DMEM medium (Gibco, Thermo Fisher Scientific, Waltham, MA, USA) with 10% fetal bovine serum (FBS, Gibco). The gene encoding *Haliotis discus discus* sialic acid-binding lectin (HddSBL, GenBank accession No. EF103404) was integrated into the plasmid pCB with a thymidine kinase (TK) gene deletion to form pCB-HddSBL. The plasmid was cotransfected into HEK293A cells using Effectene Transfection Reagent (Qiagen, Hilden, Germany) with WR vaccinia virus to generate oncoVV-HddSBL through homologous recombination. OncoVV without transgene has been constructed previously as control virus. The viruses were amplified in HEK293A cells and purified by sucrose-gradient ultracentrifugation.

4.2. Subcutaneous C6 Glioblastoma Xenograft Mouse Model

Mice were cared for in accordance with the Guide for the Care and Use of Laboratory Animals. Xenograft tumors (rat C6 glioblastoma) were established by injecting 1×10^5 cells in 100 μL PBS subcutaneously into the right flank of 4–5 weeks old female BALB/c nude mice (Shanghai Slack Animal Laboratory, China), with each group consisting of 7 mice. Treatment started when tumor size reached about 100 mm^3. OncoVV or oncoVV-HddSBL was injected intraperitoneally at 1×10^7 plaque-forming units (pfu) in 100 μL PBS twice. Control animals received intraperitoneal injections of PBS. The survival of mice was monitored every day.

4.3. ELISA Assay for IL-2 Secretion

The secretion of IL-2 in tumors was determined by ELISA assay using the Rat IL-2 ELISA Kit (Multi Science, CA, USA) according to the manufacturer's instructions. Briefly, mice serum samples were obtained from tumor veins after 15 days of the first injection of VVs. Serum samples were incubated with anti-Rat IL-2 antibody in ELISA plate for 1.5 h at room temperature. Then, the samples were washed 6 times with washing buffer and incubated with streptavidin-HRP for 0.5 h at room temperature. After washing three times in washing buffer, samples were incubated with substrate solution for 30 min at room temperature. The absorbance of the sample at 450 nm was read on an absorption spectrophotometer after the addition of stop solution.

4.4. Screening and Functional Analysis of Differentially Expressed Genes and Analysis of Gene Enrichment

Rat C6 glioblastoma cells were plated at 5×10^6 in 10 cm dishes ($n = 3$). After culture overnight, cells were infected at a multiplicity of infection (MOI) of 5 with oncoVV or oncoVV-HddSBL for 36 h. PBS served as the negative control. Total RNA was extracted from cells using TRIzol reagent (Invitrogen, Waltham,

MA, USA). Differentially expressed genes were screened, and the transcriptome sequencing and analysis was carried out by Vazyme Biotech Co., Ltd. (Nanjing, China).

4.5. Virus Replication Assay

To determine the viral replication capacity of VVs in C6 glioblastoma cells, cells were plated on 24-well plates at 1×10^5 cells per well one day before treatment with viruses. Then, cells were infected with oncoVV or oncoVV-HddSBL at a MOI of 2 for 2 h, 24 h, and 36 h. Cells and culture medium were collected and lysed with three cycles of freeze-thawing at the time interval indicated. Then, the supernatants were collected by centrifugation, and viral titers were measured through tissue culture infectious dose (TCID50) assay.

4.6. Semi-Quantitative Reverse Transcription Polymerase Chain Reaction (RT-PCR) Analysis

C6 glioblastoma cells were seeded at a density of 8×10^4 cells per well on the 24 well plate. MOI of 5 oncoVV or oncoVV-HddSBL were added, respectively, the next day. Total RNA was extracted from cells using TRIzol reagent (Invitrogen) according to the manufacturer's instructions. The total RNA was then reverse transcribed into cDNA using reverse transcription kit (TOYOBO). Primer sequences for GAPDH used were 5′-ATGGTGAAGGTCGGTGTGAAC-3′ (sense) and 5′-ATGGGTTTCCCGTTGATGAC-3′ (antisense). The PCR primers for rat IL-2 were 5′-ATGTACAGCATGCAGCTCGC-3′ (sense) and 5′-GATATTTCAATTCTGTGGCC-3′ (antisense). The PCR primers for IFIT3 were 5′-CCATTGCCATGTACCGCCTA-3′ (sense) and 5′-GCATCTTCAACCAACCGCTC-3′ (antisense). The PCR primers for IFIT2 were 5′-ATGCCACTTCACCTGGAACC-3′ (sense) and 5′-CTTCGGCTTCCCCTAAGCAT-3′ (antisense). The PCR primers for DDX58 were 5′-TGCAAGGCGCTCTTTCTGTA-3′ (sense) and 5′-CAAAGCCTTCAAACCTCCGC-3′ (antisense).

4.7. Western Blot Analysis

Cells were plated at 1×10^6 in 60 mm dishes. After infected with MOI of 5 oncoVV or oncoVV-HddSBL respectively, cells were harvested in ice-cold cell lysis buffer (Beyotime Institute of Biotechnology, Shanghai, China). The extracts were then subjected to SDS-PAGE and transferred to nitrocellulose membranes. The membranes were subsequently blocked with 5% bovine serum albumin for 2 h at room temperature and incubated at 4 °C overnight with corresponding antibodies. After washing with TBST buffer (0.01 M Tris-buffered saline with 0.1% Tween-20), the membrane was incubated with HRP-conjugated secondary antibodies for 1 h at room temperature. After washing with TBS buffer, membranes were exposed to the Tanon 5500 chemiluminescence image system (Tanon Inc., Shanghai, China). Anti-histone H3, anti-histone H4, anti-flag, and anti-β-actin antibodies were obtained from Cell Signaling Technology Inc. (Danvers, MA, USA). Histone H3 dimethyl Arg8 asymmetric and Histone H4 dimethyl Arg3 asymmetric antibodies were purchased from Active Motif (Carlsbad, CA, USA).

4.8. Reporter Assay

To determine the impact of viruses on NF-κB and AP-1 activation, we co-transfected rat C6 glioblastoma cells with the *Renilla* luciferase control plasmid together with reporter plasmids coding for firefly luciferase gene downstream of NF-κB or AP-1 binding sites, followed by treatment of C6 glioblastoma cells with PBS, oncoVV (MOI 5), or oncoVV-HddSBL (MOI 5) for 24 h ($n = 3$). The ratio of firefly to *Renilla* luciferase activity was measured using a dual-luciferase assay system (GeneCopoeia, Inc., Rockville, MD, USA).

4.9. Statistical Analysis

Statistical significance was determined with Student's *t*-test. $p < 0.05$ was considered significant.

5. Conclusions

In this work, a subcutaneous C6 glioblastoma xenograft model was established, and oncoVV-HddSBL exhibited the ability to prolong the survival of tumor-bearing mice as compared to the control virus oncoVV. The tumor secreted serum IL-2 level was downregulated in the oncoVV-HddSBL group compared to the oncoVV group. Furthermore, oncoVV-HddSBL exhibited higher viral replication capability, and intracellular antiviral factors, including DDX58, IFIT2, and IFIT3, induced by oncoVV, were dramatically decreased by HddSBL. HddSBL was also shown to modulate the histone modification and may influence the chromatin structure. Taken together, HddSBL reduced the oncoVV induced toxicity in a C6 glioblastoma mouse model by affecting multiple signaling pathways.

Author Contributions: G.L. conceived and designed the experiments; G.L., S.M., J.C., and T.W. performed the experiments; G.L. analyzed the data; G.L. and J.L. wrote the paper.

Funding: This work was supported by National Natural Science Foundation of China grant 81572986, Zhejiang Provincial Natural Science Foundation grant LZ16D060002, and Zhejiang Provincial Top Key Discipline of Biology.

Conflicts of Interest: The authors declare no conflict of interest.

References

1. Van Tellingen, O.; Yetkin-Arik, B.; de Gooijer, M.C.; Wesseling, P.; Wurdinger, T.; de Vries, H.E. Overcoming the blood-brain tumor barrier for effective glioblastoma treatment. *Drug Resist. Update* **2015**, *19*, 1–12. [CrossRef] [PubMed]
2. Tanaka, S.; Louis, D.N.; Curry, W.T.; Batchelor, T.T.; Dietrich, J. Diagnostic and therapeutic avenues for glioblastoma: No longer a dead end? *Nat. Rev. Clin. Oncol.* **2013**, *10*, 14–26. [CrossRef] [PubMed]
3. Kim, S.S.; Harford, J.B.; Pirollo, K.F.; Chang, E.H. Effective treatment of glioblastoma requires crossing the blood-brain barrier and targeting tumors including cancer stem cells: The promise of nanomedicine. *Biochem. Biophys. Res. Commun.* **2015**, *468*, 485–489. [CrossRef] [PubMed]
4. Jue, T.R.; McDonald, K.L. The challenges associated with molecular targeted therapies for glioblastoma. *J. Neuro-Oncol.* **2016**, *127*, 427–434. [CrossRef] [PubMed]
5. Russell, S.J.; Peng, K.W.; Bell, J.C. Oncolytic virotherapy. *Nat. Biotechnol.* **2012**, *30*, 658–670. [CrossRef] [PubMed]
6. Fukuhara, H.; Ino, Y.; Todo, T. Oncolytic virus therapy: A new era of cancer treatment at dawn. *Cancer Sci.* **2016**, *107*, 1373–1379. [CrossRef] [PubMed]
7. Allen, C.; Opyrchal, M.; Aderca, I.; Schroeder, M.A.; Sarkaria, J.N.; Domingo, E.; Federspiel, M.J.; Galanis, E. Oncolytic measles virus strains have significant antitumor activity against glioma stem cells. *Gene Ther.* **2013**, *20*, 444–449. [CrossRef] [PubMed]
8. Zemp, F.J.; McKenzie, B.A.; Lun, X.; Reilly, K.M.; McFadden, G.; Yong, V.W.; Forsyth, P.A. Cellular factors promoting resistance to effective treatment of glioma with oncolytic myxoma virus. *Cancer Res.* **2014**, *74*, 7260–7273. [CrossRef] [PubMed]
9. Oh, E.; Hong, J.; Kwon, O.J.; Yun, C.O. A hypoxia- and telomerase-responsive oncolytic adenovirus expressing secretable trimeric TRAIL triggers tumour-specific apoptosis and promotes viral dispersion in TRAIL-resistant glioblastoma. *Sci. Rep.* **2018**, *8*, 1420. [CrossRef] [PubMed]
10. Shimazu, Y.; Kurozumi, K.; Ichikawa, T.; Fujii, K.; Onishi, M.; Ishida, J.; Oka, T.; Watanabe, M.; Nasu, Y.; Kumon, H.; et al. Integrin antagonist augments the therapeutic effect of adenovirus-mediated REIC/Dkk-3 gene therapy for malignant glioma. *Gene Ther.* **2015**, *22*, 146–154. [CrossRef] [PubMed]
11. Duebgen, M.; Martinez-Quintanilla, J.; Tamura, K.; Hingtgen, S.; Redjal, N.; Wakimoto, H.; Shah, K. Stem cells loaded with multimechanistic oncolytic herpes simplex virus variants for brain tumor therapy. *J. Natl. Cancer Inst.* **2014**, *106*, dju090. [CrossRef] [PubMed]
12. Alvarez-Breckenridge, C.A.; Choi, B.D.; Suryadevara, C.M.; Chiocca, A. Potentiating oncolytic viral therapy through an understanding of the initial immune responses to oncolytic viral infection. *Curr. Opin. Virol.* **2015**, *13*, 25–32. [CrossRef] [PubMed]
13. Meisen, W.H.; Wohleb, E.S.; Jaime-Ramirez, A.C.; Bolyard, C.; Yoo, J.Y.; Russell, L.; Hardcastle, J.; Dubin, S.; Muili, K.; Yu, J.H.; et al. The Impact of Macrophage- and Microglia-Secreted TNF alpha on Oncolytic HSV-1

Therapy in the Glioblastoma Tumor Microenvironment. *Clin. Cancer Res.* **2015**, *21*, 3274–3285. [CrossRef] [PubMed]

14. Kober, C.; Rohn, S.; Weibel, S.; Geissinger, U.; Chen, N.H.G.; Szalay, A.A. Microglia and astrocytes attenuate the replication of the oncolytic vaccinia virus LIVP 1.1.1 in murine GL261 gliomas by acting as vaccinia virus traps. *J. Transl. Med.* **2015**, *13*, 216. [CrossRef] [PubMed]

15. Advani, S.J.; Buckel, L.; Chen, N.G.; Scanderbeg, D.J.; Geissinger, U.; Zhang, Q.; Yu, Y.A.; Aguilar, R.J.; Mundt, A.J.; Szalay, A.A. Preferential Replication of Systemically Delivered Oncolytic Vaccinia Virus in Focally Irradiated Glioma Xenografts. *Clin. Cancer Res.* **2012**, *18*, 2579–2590. [CrossRef] [PubMed]

16. Mell, L.K.; Brumund, K.T.; Daniels, G.A.; Advani, S.J.; Zakeri, K.; Wright, M.E.; Onyeama, S.J.; Weisman, R.A.; Sanghvi, P.R.; Martin, P.J.; et al. Phase I Trial of Intravenous Oncolytic Vaccinia Virus (GL-ONC1) with Cisplatin and Radiotherapy in Patients with Locoregionally Advanced Head and Neck Carcinoma. *Clin. Cancer Res.* **2017**, *23*, 5696–5702. [CrossRef] [PubMed]

17. Breitbach, C.J.; Burke, J.; Jonker, D.; Stephenson, J.; Haas, A.R.; Chow, L.Q.M.; Nieva, J.; Hwang, T.H.; Moon, A.; Patt, R.; et al. Intravenous delivery of a multi-mechanistic cancer-targeted oncolytic poxvirus in humans. *Nature* **2011**, *477*, 99–102. [CrossRef] [PubMed]

18. Murphy, A.M.; Rabkin, S.D. Current status of gene therapy for brain tumors. *Transl. Res.* **2013**, *161*, 339–354. [CrossRef] [PubMed]

19. Hwang, T.H.; Moon, A.; Burke, J.; Ribas, A.; Stephenson, J.; Breitbach, C.J.; Daneshmand, M.; De Silva, N.; Parato, K.; Diallo, J.S.; et al. A Mechanistic Proof-of-concept Clinical Trial with JX-594, a Targeted Multi-mechanistic Oncolytic Poxvirus, in Patients with Metastatic Melanoma. *Mol. Ther.* **2011**, *19*, 1913–1922. [CrossRef] [PubMed]

20. Parato, K.A.; Breitbach, C.J.; Le Boeuf, F.; Wang, J.H.; Storbeck, C.; Ilkow, C.; Diallo, J.S.; Falls, T.; Burns, J.; Garcia, V.; et al. The Oncolytic Poxvirus JX-594 Selectively Replicates in and Destroys Cancer Cells Driven by Genetic Pathways Commonly Activated in Cancers. *Mol. Ther.* **2012**, *20*, 749–758. [CrossRef] [PubMed]

21. Jiang, Q.L.; Zhang, S.; Tian, M.; Zhang, S.Y.; Xie, T.; Chen, D.Y.; Chen, Y.J.; He, J.; Liu, J.; Ouyang, L.; et al. Plant lectins, from ancient sugar-binding proteins to emerging anti-cancer drugs in apoptosis and autophagy. *Cell Prolif.* **2015**, *48*, 17–28. [CrossRef] [PubMed]

22. Hyun, J.Y.; Park, C.W.; Liu, Y.; Kwon, D.; Park, S.H.; Park, S.; Pai, J.; Shin, I. Carbohydrate Analogue Microarrays for Identification of Lectin-Selective Ligands. *Chembiochem* **2017**, *18*, 1077–1082. [CrossRef] [PubMed]

23. Thijssen, V.L.; Heusschen, R.; Caers, J.; Griffioen, A.W. Galectin expression in cancer diagnosis and prognosis: A systematic review. *BBA-Rev. Cancer* **2015**, *1855*, 235–247. [CrossRef] [PubMed]

24. Yau, T.; Dan, X.L.; Ng, C.C.W.; Ng, T.B. Lectins with Potential for Anti-Cancer Therapy. *Molecules* **2015**, *20*, 3791–3810. [CrossRef] [PubMed]

25. Han, S.Y.; Hong, C.E.; Kim, H.G.; Lyu, S.Y. Anti-cancer effects of enteric-coated polymers containing mistletoe lectin in murine melanoma cells in vitro and in vivo. *Mol. Cell. Biochem.* **2015**, *408*, 73–87. [CrossRef] [PubMed]

26. Chang, C.P.; Yang, M.C.; Liu, H.S.; Lin, Y.S.; Lei, H.Y. Concanavalin A induces autophagy in hepatoma cells and has a therapeutic effect in a murine in situ hepatoma model. *Hepatology* **2007**, *45*, 286–296. [CrossRef] [PubMed]

27. Terada, D.; Kawai, F.; Noguchi, H.; Unzai, S.; Hasan, I.; Fujii, Y.; Park, S.Y.; Ozeki, Y.; Tame, J.R.H. Crystal structure of MytiLec, a galactose-binding lectin from the mussel Mytilus galloprovincialis with cytotoxicity against certain cancer cell types. *Sci. Rep. UK* **2016**, *6*, 28344. [CrossRef] [PubMed]

28. Hasan, I.; Gerdol, M.; Fujii, Y.; Rajia, S.; Koide, Y.; Yamamoto, D.; Kawsar, S.M.A.; Ozeki, Y. cDNA and Gene Structure of MytiLec-1, A Bacteriostatic R-Type Lectin from the Mediterranean Mussel (*Mytilus galloprovincialis*). *Mar. Drugs* **2016**, *14*, 92. [CrossRef] [PubMed]

29. Hasan, I.; Sugawara, S.; Fujii, Y.; Koide, Y.; Terada, D.; Iimura, N.; Fujiwara, T.; Takahashi, K.G.; Kojima, N.; Rajia, S.; et al. MytiLec, a Mussel R-Type Lectin, Interacts with Surface Glycan Gb3 on Burkitt's Lymphoma Cells to Trigger Apoptosis through Multiple Pathways. *Mar. Drugs* **2015**, *13*, 7377–7389. [CrossRef] [PubMed]

30. Fujii, Y.; Dohmae, N.; Takio, K.; Kawsar, S.M.A.; Matsumoto, R.; Hasan, I.; Koide, Y.; Kanaly, R.A.; Yasumitsu, H.; Ogawa, Y.; et al. A Lectin from the Mussel Mytilus galloprovincialis Has a Highly Novel Primary Structure and Induces Glycan-mediated Cytotoxicity of Globotriaosylceramide-expressing Lymphoma Cells. *J. Biol. Chem.* **2012**, *287*, 44772–44783. [CrossRef] [PubMed]

31. Li, G.; Li, X.; Wu, H.; Yang, X.; Zhang, Y.; Chen, L.; Wu, X.; Cui, L.; Wu, L.; Luo, J.; et al. CD123 targeting oncolytic adenoviruses suppress acute myeloid leukemia cell proliferation in vitro and in vivo. *Blood Cancer J.* **2014**, *4*, e194. [CrossRef] [PubMed]

32. Li, G.C.; Zhao, Z.Z.; Wu, B.B.; Su, Q.S.; Wu, L.Q.; Yang, X.Y.; Chen, J. Ulva pertusa lectin 1 delivery through adenovirus vector affects multiple signaling pathways in cancer cells. *Glycoconj. J.* **2017**, *34*, 489–498. [CrossRef] [PubMed]

33. Wu, L.Q.; Yang, X.Y.; Duan, X.M.; Cui, L.Z.; Li, G.C. Exogenous expression of marine lectins DlFBL and SpRBL induces cancer cell apoptosis possibly through PRMT5-E2F-1 pathway. *Sci. Rep.* **2014**, *4*, 4505. [CrossRef] [PubMed]

34. Yang, X.Y.; Wu, L.Q.; Duan, X.M.; Cui, L.Z.; Luo, J.J.; Li, G.C. Adenovirus Carrying Gene Encoding Haliotis discus discus Sialic Acid Binding Lectin Induces Cancer Cell Apoptosis. *Mar. Drugs* **2014**, *12*, 3994–4004. [CrossRef] [PubMed]

35. Kirn, D.H.; Thorne, S.H. Targeted and armed oncolytic poxviruses: A novel multi-mechanistic therapeutic class for cancer. *Nat. Rev. Cancer* **2009**, *9*, 64–71. [CrossRef] [PubMed]

36. Bartlett, D.L.; Liu, Z.Q.; Sathaiah, M.; Ravindranathan, R.; Guo, Z.B.; He, Y.K.; Guo, Z.S. Oncolytic viruses as therapeutic cancer vaccines. *Mol. Cancer* **2013**, *12*, 103. [CrossRef] [PubMed]

37. Zhang, Q.; Yu, Y.A.; Wang, E.; Chen, N.; Dannel, R.L.; Munson, P.J.; Marincola, F.M.; Szalay, A.A. Eradication of solid human breast tumors in nude mice with an intravenously injected light-emitting oncolytic vaccinia virus. *Cancer Res.* **2007**, *67*, 10038–10046. [CrossRef] [PubMed]

38. Zhou, X.; Michal, J.J.; Zhang, L.F.; Ding, B.; Lunney, J.K.; Liu, B.; Jiang, Z.H. Interferon Induced IFIT Family Genes in Host Antiviral Defense. *Int. J. Biol. Sci.* **2013**, *9*, 200–208. [CrossRef] [PubMed]

39. Pachella, L.A.; Madsen, L.T.; Dains, J.E. The Toxicity and Benefit of Various Dosing Strategies for Interleukin-2 in Metastatic Melanoma and Renal Cell Carcinoma. *J. Adv. Pract. Oncol.* **2015**, *6*, 212–221. [PubMed]

40. Acquavella, N.; Kluger, H.; Rhee, J.; Farber, L.; Tara, H.; Ariyan, S.; Narayan, D.; Kelly, W.; Sznol, M. Toxicity and activity of a twice daily high-dose bolus interleukin 2 regimen in patients with metastatic melanoma and metastatic renal cell cancer. *J. Immunother.* **2008**, *31*, 569–576. [CrossRef] [PubMed]

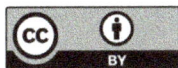

marine drugs

MDPI

Article

MytiLec-1 Shows Glycan-Dependent Toxicity against Brine Shrimp *Artemia* and Induces Apoptotic Death of Ehrlich Ascites Carcinoma Cells In Vivo

Imtiaj Hasan [1,*], A.K.M. Asaduzzaman [1], Rubaiya Rafique Swarna [1], Yuki Fujii [2], Yasuhiro Ozeki [3], Md. Belal Uddin [1] and Syed Rashel Kabir [1,*]

1   Department of Biochemistry and Molecular Biology, Faculty of Science, University of Rajshahi, Rajshahi-6205, Bangladesh
2   Department of Pharmacy, Faculty of Pharmaceutical Science, Nagasaki International University, 2825-7 Huis Ten Bosch, Sasebo, Nagasaki 859-3298, Japan
3   Department of Life and Environmental System Science, School of Sciences, Yokohama City University, 22-2 Seto, Kanazawa-ku, Yokohama 236-0027, Japan
*   Correspondence: hasanimtiaj@yahoo.co.uk (I.H.); rashelkabir@ru.ac.bd (S.R.K.); Tel.: +880-721-711109 (I.H.); +880-721-711506 (S.R.K.); Fax: +880-721-711114 (I.H.); +880-721-711114 (S.R.K.)

check for
updates

Received: 18 July 2019; Accepted: 23 August 2019; Published: 28 August 2019

Abstract: MytiLec-1, a 17 kDa lectin with β-trefoil folding that was isolated from the Mediterranean mussel (*Mytilus galloprovincialis*) bound to the disaccharide melibiose, Galα(1,6) Glc, and the trisaccharide globotriose, Galα(1,4) Galβ(1,4) Glc. Toxicity of the lectin was found to be low with an LC_{50} value of 384.53 μg/mL, determined using the *Artemia* nauplii lethality assay. A fluorescence assay was carried out to evaluate the glycan-dependent binding of MytiLec-1 to *Artemia* nauplii. The lectin strongly agglutinated Ehrlich ascites carcinoma (EAC) cells cultured in vivo in Swiss albino mice. When injected intraperitoneally to the mice at doses of 1.0 mg/kg/day and 2.0 mg/kg/day for five consecutive days, MytiLec-1 inhibited 27.62% and 48.57% of cancer cell growth, respectively. Antiproliferative activity of the lectin against U937 and HeLa cells was studied by 3-(4,5-dimethylthiazol-2-yl)-2,5-diphenyltetrazolium bromide (MTT) assay in vitro in RPMI-1640 medium. MytiLec-1 internalized into U937 cells and 50 μg/mL of the lectin inhibited their growth of to 62.70% whereas 53.59% cell growth inhibition was observed against EAC cells when incubated for 24 h. Cell morphological study and expression of apoptosis-related genes (p53, Bax, Bcl-X, and NF-κB) showed that the lectin possibly triggered apoptosis in these cells.

Keywords: apoptosis-related genes; Ehrlich ascites carcinoma; toxicity; lectin; MytiLec-1; *Mytilus galloprovincialis*

1. Introduction

Over time, well-organized defense mechanisms have been evolved in living systems for their survival. Lectins are a group of structurally diverse glycan-binding proteins that take part in the defense mechanism of invertebrates by specifically recognizing foreign particles and as effector molecules [1]. Lectins can bind to cell-surface glycoconjugates present in organisms that result in cell agglutination. They are also responsible for various intracellular and intercellular cell signaling and signal transduction. These proteins are present in diverse organisms, implicated in many essential cellular and molecular recognition processes and play a number of physiological roles including immunomodulatory [2], antitumor [3,4], antifungal [5,6], antibacterial [7,8], and antiviral [9] activities.

Over the last 30 years, lectins from marine organisms have received much attention from researchers. Though lectins from marine species are relatively new, researchers are trying to reveal their characteristics and biological applications in living organisms. They are present in more than 300 species and most of their structures, amino acid sequences, and carbohydrate specificities have been determined [10].

Lectins from marine organisms are classified into many families: C-type lectins, P-type lectins, F-type lectins, galectins, intelectins, rhamnose-binding lectins, and R-type lectins [1,11–13]. MytiLec (formerly MGL), which is an α-galactose-binding lectin, was first placed in the R-type lectin family, though it did not possess the additional toxic domain, a characteristic feature of R-type lectins [14]. Later, a new family known as 'mytilectin' was introduced [8]. At present, there are four members in the mytilectin family. Identification and elimination of microbial pathogens are the suggested physiological functions of the members of this family, whereas distinct antimicrobial activities are considered to be their hallmarks. As the first member of the mytilectin family, an α-D-galactose binding mussel lectin from *Crenomytilus grayanus* (CGL) interacted with gram positive and gram negative bacteria [15,16]. The third and fourth member of the mytilectin family, MCL (from *Mytilus californianus*) and MTL (from *Mytilus trossulus*) also showed growth suppressive activities against different bacteria and fungi [1,17].

The second member, MytiLec, a 17-kDa polypeptide, was isolated from the bivalve *Mytilus galloprovincialis* [14]. Based on the transcriptome analysis, three isoforms (MytiLec-1, -2, and -3) of this protein have been reported so far [8,14], whereas the aerolysin-like domain was present in MytiLec-2 and -3. Despite of not having that domain, MytiLec-1 could inhibit bacterial growth like its counterparts [8] and similar to CGL, interacted with Gb3-containing glycosphingolipid-enriched microdomains on Burkitt's lymphoma (Raji) cell surface to trigger apoptosis [18–20]. In this study, glycan-based cell regulatory activities of MytiLec-1 was observed using two different living systems, i.e., aquatic crustaceans (brine shrimp *Artemia* nauplii) and various cancer cells. Toxicity of MytiLec-1 was checked against brine shrimp with evidence to its ability to bind with glycans expressed on those. Previous reports on the anticancer activity of MytiLec-1 were based on in vitro studies. In this work, for the first time, in vivo antiproliferative activity of MytiLec-1 was checked against Ehrlich's ascites carcinoma cell lines using Swiss albino mice. An effort was also made to partially elucidate the apoptotic pathway of this anticancer activity. In addition, antitumor effect of the lectin against U937 and HeLa cell lines was investigated in vitro.

2. Results

2.1. Purification and Confirmation of the Molecular Mass of MytiLec-1

Purified MytiLec-1 showed strong hemagglutination activity as it agglutinated human erythrocytes at the minimum concentration of 12 μg/mL. It migrated on SDS-PAGE as a single band with a molecular mass of 17 kDa (Figure 1).

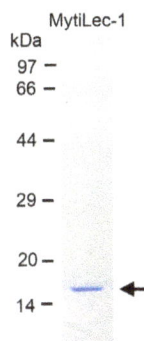

Figure 1. Purification of MytiLec-1 with a molecular weight of 17 kDa. Markers: Phosphorylase b (97 kDa), serum albumin (66 kDa), ovalbumin (44 kDa), carbonic anhydrase (29 kDa), trypsin inhibitor (20 kDa), and lysozyme (14 kDa).

2.2. Toxicity of MytiLec-1 against Brine Shrimp Artemia Nauplii

At the concentrations of 25–200 µg/mL of MytiLec-1, mortality rate of *Artemia* nauplii was 0% to 33%, and the rate increased to 50% when the concentration rose to 400 µg/mL and the LC_{50} value was determined to be 384.53 µg/mL (Figure 2).

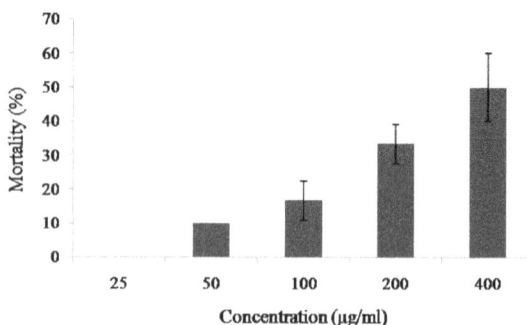

Figure 2. Percentage of mortality of brine shrimp nauplii treated with different concentrations of MytiLec-1. Data are expressed in mean ± S.D.

2.3. Binding of FITC-Labeled Lectins to Artemia Nauplii Detected by Fluorescence Microscopy

Binding of MytiLec-1 to *Artemia* nauplii was confirmed by fluorescence microscopy. Figure 3A and 3B showed the absence and presence of green color of Fluorescein isothiocyanate (FITC)-BSA and FITC-MytiLec-1 in their digestive tracts, respectively. This binding was affected by the presence of melibiose (ligand sugar of MytiLec-1), as intensity of the green color became diminished (Figure 3C).

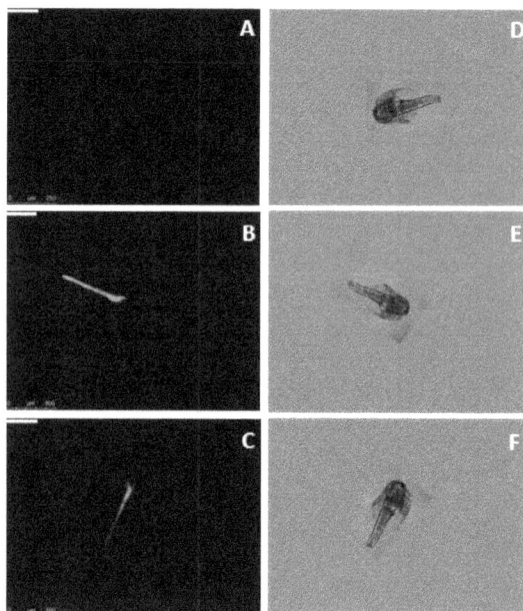

Figure 3. Binding of Fluorescein isothiocyanate (FITC)-labeled MytiLec-1 to *Artemia* nauplii detected by fluorescence and brightfield microscopy. Green color indicates the presence of FITC-labeled MytiLec-1 in the digestive tract of the animal. (**A,D**): FITC-BSA; (**B,E**): FITC-MytiLec-1; (**C,F**): FITC-MytiLec-1 with melibiose sugar.

2.4. Agglutination of Ehrlich Ascites Carcinoma Cells

MytiLec-1 strongly agglutinated Ehrlich ascites carcinoma (EAC) cells at concentrations of 50 and 100 µg/mL (Figure 4), whereas the minimum agglutination concentration was 16 µg/mL.

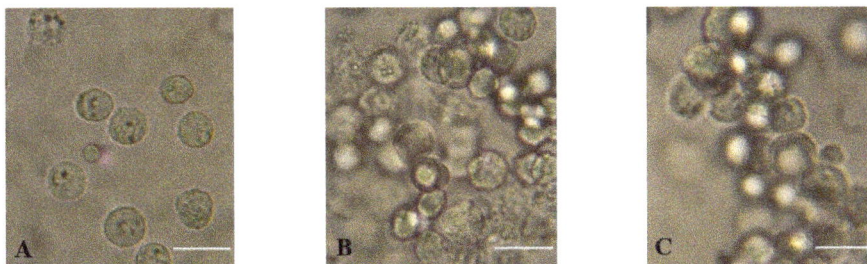

Figure 4. Agglutination of Ehrlich ascites carcinoma (EAC) cells by MytiLec-1. (**A**). Untreated control cells; (**B**). EAC cells treated with 50 µg/mLand (**C**). 100 µg/mL of MytiLec-1. Scale bar: 25 µm.

2.5. In Vivo Antitumor Activity of MytiLec-1

When treated with intraperitoneal injection of MytiLec-1 for five days, growth of EAC cells in tumor-bearing Swiss albino mice became reduced comparing to EAC cells in untreated (or control) mice. At the doses of 1 and 2 mg/kg/day of MytiLec-1, around 28% and 49% cell growth inhibition were found (Figure 5).

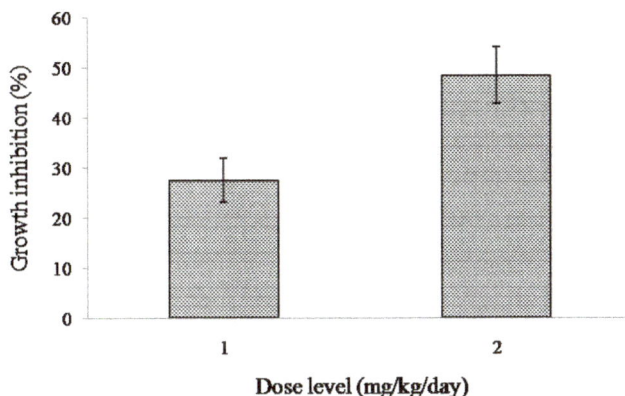

Figure 5. Inhibition of the growth of control and MytiLec-1 treated EAC cells. Data are expressed in mean ± S.D ($n = 6$).

2.6. Morphological Examination of Ehrlich Ascites CarcinomaCells

EAC nuclei from cells in the control group were found to be in round and normal shape (Figure 6A). Contrarily, MytiLec-1 treated cells showed characteristic morphological alterations (irregular shapes, nuclear condensation, and presence of apoptotic bodies) when observed by fluorescence (Figure 6B) and bright field microscopes (Figure 6C).

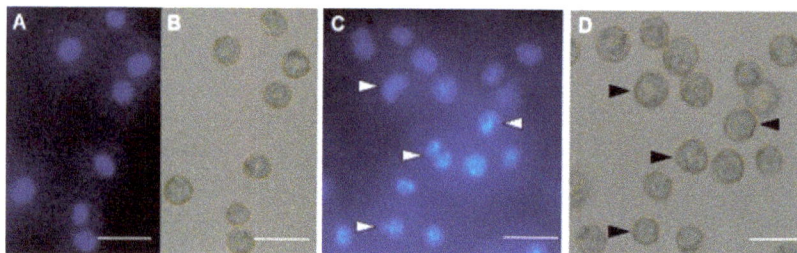

Figure 6. MytiLec-1 induces apoptotic morphological features in EAC cells. Cells were stained with Hoechst-33342 dye to be observed by fluorescence (**A,C**) and bright field microscopes (**B,D**). (**A,B**) Untreated control cells. (**C,D**) Cells treated with 50 mg/mL of MytiLec-1 for 24 h. Scale bar: 50 μm. White and black arrows represent cells undergoing apoptosis.

2.7. Expression of Apoptosis-Related Genes

The expression level of Bax was high in MytiLec-1 treated EAC cells although no expression was found in control EAC cells. Opposite results were found in case of Bcl-X and NF-κB genes. Expression of these genes became upregulated in control EAC cells and lectin-treated EAC cells showed no expression at all. Though it was very low, expression of p53 gene was observed in the lectin-treated cells. Expression of glyceraldehyde 3-phosphate dehydrogenase (GAPDH) was satisfactory to confirm the quality of mRNA from lectin-treated and control EAC cells (Figure 7).

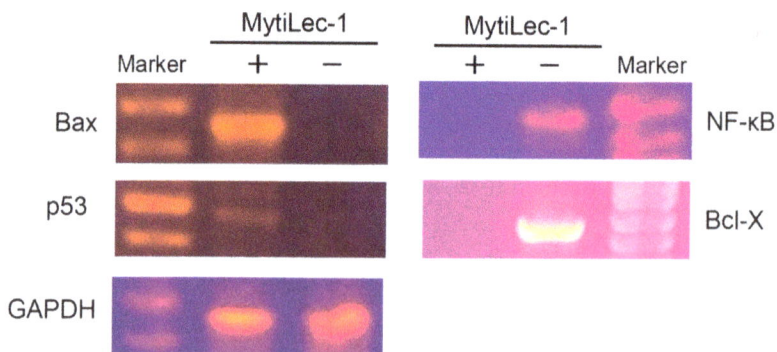

Figure 7. Amplification of apoptosis related genes. Total RNA was extracted from MytiLec-1 treated (+) and untreated (−) EAC cells and reverse transcription was performed. PCR reaction was carried out using primers specific for Bax, NF-κB, p53, Bcl-X, and GAPDH whereas products were separated on 1.5% agarose gel and stained with ethidium bromide.

2.8. Internalization of MytiLec-1 into U937 Cells

Not only binding with U937 cells, MytiLec-1 was observed to be internalized into those cells by fluorescence microscopy. Similar result had been found for Burkitt's lymphoma cells where the lectin induced morphological changes in cells [19]. In this case, changes in cell morphology were observed after 1 h of incubation with MytiLec-1 (Figure 8).

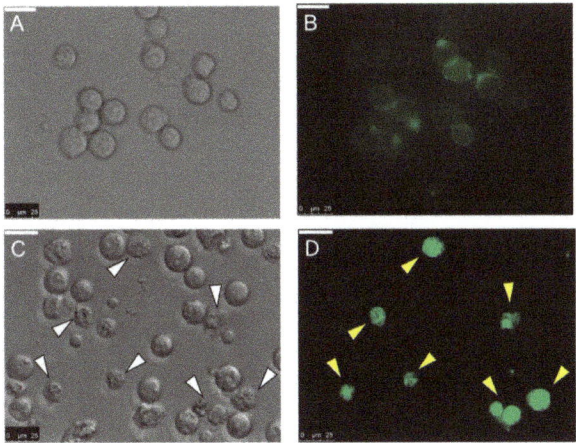

Figure 8. Internalization of MytiLec-1 into U937 cells. Cells were observed by phase contrast (**A,C**) and fluorescence microscopy (**B,D**). Incubation time: 5 min (**A,B**)and 1 h (**C,D**). Scale bar: 25 μm.

2.9. In Vitro Antiproliferative Activity of MytiLec-1 against U937 and HeLa Cell Lines

MTT assay showed a dose dependent effect of MytiLec-1 against U937 and HeLa cells. U937 cells were slightly more susceptible to MytiLec-1 comparing to HeLa cells. Around 36–63% of cell growth inhibition of U937 cells was found at the protein concentration of 12.5–50 μg/mL (Figure 9A), whereas against HeLa cells, 32–54% of cell growth inhibition was observed (Figure 9B).

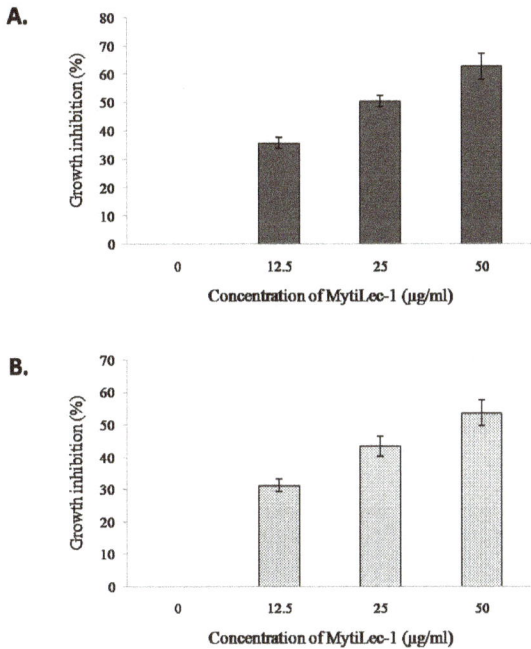

Figure 9. Growth inhibition of human cancer cells after treatment with MytiLec-1. Cell proliferation of U937 (**A**) and HeLa (**B**) cells was measured by an MTT assay ($n = 3$, mean ± S.D) after treating those with different doses of MytiLec-1.

3. Discussion

MytiLec-1 showed mild lethality with an LC_{50} value of 384.53 µg/mL (Figure 2). In a previous study, CvL-2, another galactose-binding trimeric lectin from *Cliona varians*, was reported to have lower lethality (LC_{50} value of 850.1 µg/mL) since the Sea cucumber (*Holothuria grisea*) lectin HGL was highly toxic (LC_{50} value of 9.5 µg/mL) against *Artemia* nauplii [21]. Two other lectins, H-1 and H-2, from a marine sponge *Haliclona caerulea*, showed higher toxicity (LC_{50} value of 6.4 and 142.1 µg/mL, respectively) than MytiLec-1, putting it in a category of mildly toxic lectins [22].

It became evident that the lectin bound to the digestive tract of *Artemia* nauplii (Figure 3B). Heavily glycosylated digestive tract of nauplii might contain α-galactoside sugars that became specifically recognized by MytiLec-1 as addition of 0.1M melibiose [Gal(α1-6)Glc] sugar reduced the binding of FITC-labeled MytiLec-1 (Figure 3C). This finding was in line with the properties of previously reported lectins from the genus *Canavalia* [23]. Though plant lectins are usually more toxic than animal lectins, this result suggested that animal lectins follow similar mechanisms to interrupt the functions of gut cells of *Artemia* or to destroy those cells [24,25].

A number of marine lectins, including MytiLec-1, have been reported to bind the outer sugar chains of glycoconjugates on cancer cell surface and induce anti-cancer effects [4]. Members from the Mytilidae lectin family are fairly distributed in nature and many of the structural and biological properties of MytiLec have already been elucidated. It is a lectin with β-trefoil fold and specific binding property to Gb3 (Galα1-4Galβ1-4Glc). Antitumor activities and mechanism of action of both forms, natural and artificial, of MytiLec-1 has been studied in vitro against Burkitt's lymphoma Raji cells [17,19,20,26]. As both animal studies and clinical studies are essential to check the possibility to utilize the lectin for chemotherapeutic treatment, this work attempted an in vivo study on Ehrlich's ascites carcinoma.

Ehrlich ascites carcinoma cells are the adapted ascites form of mammary adenocarcinoma cells. Many lectins agglutinated these cells in various concentrations and inhibited their growth [27–30]. It has long been established that cell membranes of EAC cells contain a family of α-D-galactosyl containing glycoproteins and glycolipids [31,32], which are ligand sugars of MytiLec-1. The lectin strongly agglutinated EAC cells (Figure 4) with a minimum concentration of 16 µg/mL. It had been reported that Jacalin, another α-D-galactosyl specific lectin from Jackfruit, agglutinated the same cells at a minimum concentration of 8 µg/mL [33].

After confirming the glycan-specific agglutination activity, the lectin was injected into Swiss albino mice to study its antiproliferative activity. At doses of 1 mg/kg/day and 2 mg/kg/day, MytiLec-1 showed around 28% and 49% of cell growth inhibition (Figure 5). A lectin from *Pisum sativum* exhibited growth inhibition rates of 63% and 44% against EAC cells at concentrations of 2.8 mg/kg/day and 1.4 mg/kg/day, respectively [34]. In the case of KRL-2 from *Kaempferia rotunda*, 41% and 59% of EAC cell growth inhibition was found at the doses of 3 mg/kg/day and 6 mg/kg/day [27]. At a fixed concentration of 100 µg/mL, plant extracts with lectin activity from *Ricinus communis* and *Amaranthus hybridus* led to 54 and 45% growth inhibition of EAC cells, respectively [35,36]. Considering these results, antiproliferative activity of MytiLec-1 to EAC cells is quite significant despite of its low toxicity to brine shrimp. In Figure 6, fluorescence and optical microscopy of EAC cells from the MytiLec-1 treated mice showed early-apoptotic morphological changes in shape and size along with membrane blebbing, cell shrinkage, nuclear condensation and formation of apoptotic bodies, comparing to round sized cells with regular nuclei from the control mice.

Apoptosis, a common type of programmed cell death, takes place in response to various cellular damages, stress, and molecular stimuli. This highly regulated process plays significant roles in the development and homeostasis of eukaryotic organisms. Induction of apoptosis by a lectin from *Kaempferia rotunda* has been reported to occur in EAC cells. Expression of Bax genes increased significantly with a marked decrease of Bcl-2 and Bcl-X genes [37]. Involvement of p53 genes had also become evident through its increased expression when two other plant lectins from *Geodorum densiflorum* and *Solanum tuberosum* inhibited the growth of EAC cells [28,30]. In p53-dependent mitochondrial pathways, p53 upregulates the transcription of pro-apoptotic genes, including Bax and Bak, and downregulates anti-apoptotic genes, including Bcl-2, Bcl-X, and Bcl-w, to augment apoptosis in many cancer cells [38]. In this study, a faint band of p53 was observed in MytiLec-1 treated cells, whereas the band for Bax was very prominent. Upon binding to Bcl-2 family proteins, p53 aids Bax to become available to transmit an apoptotic signal to mitochondria. Cytochrome c got released through the Bax-Bak oligomeric pores and switched on the caspase cascade, leading to apoptosis [39]. Figure 7 shows complete downregulation of the expression of anti-apoptotic gene Bcl-X and transcriptional factor NF-κB indicating a possible augmentation of the above process [40]. We also noticed the overexpression of Bax, which probably regulated the function of Bcl-X [28]. We should not rule out the possibility of a p53-independent pathway as Bax and Bak had been previously reported to trigger apoptosis in the absence of p53 [41–43] and both these pathways can run concurrently [39].

It had been reported that U937 and HeLa cells possess glycosphingolipids Gb3 as a cell surface receptor to bind with various molecules like lectins and toxins [44,45]. MytiLec-1 was previously reported to internalize into Burkitt's lymphoma cells to cause cytotoxicity [19]. In the present study, the lectin showed the same tendency to incorporate into U937 cells (Figure 8). Another marine lectin, HOL-18 from Japanese black sponge (*Halichondria okadai*) also went inside of a number of cancer cells including HeLa, MCF-7, and T47D to inhibit their growth but did not response to Caco-2 cells [46]. A lactose-binding fungal lectin showed the same behavior but did not cause cytotoxicity of HeLa cells [47]. Therefore, MytiLec-1 perhaps specifically interacted with Gb3 to reduce the growth of both U937 and HeLa cells. The MTT assay also showed that U937 cells were more susceptible (63%) to MytiLec-1 than HeLa cells (54%) at the concentration of 50 µg/mL (Figure 9). Being a lot more toxic in nature, ricin (first member of the lectin with β-trefoil folding) triggered cell death in U937 cells in a much lower concentration [48,49]. Many other lectins from animal and plant sources had been reported to exert dose-dependent growth inhibitory effects against U937 and HeLa cell lines, proceeding to apoptosis and cell death [50–53].

4. Experimental Design

4.1. Materials

Melibosyl-agarose column was prepared by packing agarose gel immobilized melibiose (Galα1-6Glc) (EY Laboratories Inc., San Mateo, CA, USA) in Poly-Prep chromatography column (Bio-Rad Laboratories, Irvine, CA, USA). RPMI-1640 medium, fetal calf serum, and Hoechst-33342 were purchased from Sigma Aldrich (St. Louis, MO, USA). Penicillin-streptomycin was bought from Roche Diagnostics. Standard protein markers for SDS-PAGE were purchased from Takara Bio Inc. (Kyoto, Japan). Poly-L-lysine-coated slides used in this study were from MilliporeSigma (Darmstadt, Germany). All other chemical/reagents, each of the highest purity grades were from Wako Pure Chemical Co. (Osaka, Japan) and Sigma Aldrich (St. Louis, MO, USA).

4.2. Purification of Protein

Mytilus galloprovincialis mussels were commercially purchased from the local market of Yokohama, Japan. Gills and mantles are homogenized with 2-amino-2-(hydroxymethyl)propane-1,3-diol;hydrochloride (Tris-HCl) buffer (pH 7.4). The crude supernatant was applied on a melibiosyl-agarose affinity column and MytiLec-1 was eluted by using Tris-HCl buffer containing 100 mM of melibiose sugar [14]. Eluted MytiLec-1 was dialyzed against Tris-HCl buffer to remove the sugar. Purity of the protein was checked by using SDS-PAGE (sodium dodecyl sulfate polyacrylamide gel electrophoresis) in 16% (w/v) polyacrylamide gel as described by Laemmli [54].

4.3. Brine Shrimp Nauplii Lethality Assay

Toxicity of MytiLec-1 was checked using brine shrimp nauplii (*Artemia salina*) lethality assay [55]. Shrimp nauplii were placed in six vials (ten in each vial) and MytiLec-1 was added to the vials at final concentrations of 0.0, 25.0, 50.0, 75.0, 100.0, and 200.0 µg/mL. The volume of each vial was adjusted by adding artificial sea water. Artificial sea water was prepared by dissolving 38 g of NaCl in 1 L of distilled water. To adjust the pH to 7.0, sodium tetraborate salt was added to it. The vials were kept at 30 °C for 24 h under a light source. Three replicates were used for each experiment. Percentage of mortality of the nauplii was calculated for each concentration and LC_{50} value of MytiLec-1 was determined using Probit analysis [56].

4.4. Preparation of Fluorescein Isothioycanate (FITC)-Labeled Proteins

FITC-labeled MytiLec-1 was prepared by conjugating purified MytiLec-1 (2 mg) with NH_2-reactive fluorescein isothioycanate (Dojindo Laboratories, Kumamoto, Japan) following the manufacturer's protocol. A washing buffer (PBS, i.e., phosphate-buffered saline: 0.01M sodium phosphate buffer, 0.027M KCl and 0.15M NaCl, pH 7.4) was prepared. FITC-lectin was passed through a Sephadex G-25 column to remove unconjugated FITC molecules. The FITC-labeled MytiLec-1 was then dialyzed for 12 h against distilled water. Similarly, Bovine serum albumin (BSA) protein was labeled to FITC, which produced FITC-BSA.

4.5. Fluorescence Microscopy of Artemia Nauplii

Artemia nauplii were incubated with FITC-MytiLec-1, FITC-BSA (50 µg/mL) and FITC-MytiLec-1 (with 0.1M melibiose sugar) and kept overnight. The shrimp were then washed thrice in PBS, placed on slides, and examined using an optical and fluorescence microscopy (Olympus IX71, Seoul, Korea). 498 nm lasers were used for the excitation of FITC.

4.6. Experimental Animals and Ethical Clearance

Swiss albino mice were collected from the ICDDR'B (International Center for Diarrheal Diseases Research, Dhaka, Bangladesh). This investigation was officially recognized by the Institutional Animal, Medical Ethics, Biosafety, and Biosecurity Committee (IAMEBBC) for Experimentations on Animals, Human, Microbes and Living Natural Sources (Memo No. 55/320/IAMEBBC/IBSc), Institute of Biological Sciences (IBSc), University of Rajshahi, Rajshahi, Bangladesh.

4.7. Ehrlich Ascites Carcinoma Cell Agglutination

In this next step, 50 µL of hemagglutination buffer was prepared and used to check the agglutination of EAC cells. The protein solution (50 µL) was serially diluted in a titer plate and then 50 µL of 2% EAC cells in saline were added. The plate was shaken for 7 min by a microshaker as well as incubated at 34 °C for 60 min.

4.8. Determination of Growth Inhibition of Ehrlich Ascites Carcinoma Cells

EAC cells were maintained through an intraperitoneal transformation into the Swiss albino mice in every two weeks. Development of ascites carcinoma in all mice was confirmed by the increase of their weight (data not shown). Cells were collected from a mouse bearing 1-week old ascites tumors and their concentration was adjusted to 4×10^6 cells/mL with 0.9% normal saline. After counting cells using a haemocytometer, their viability was verified by 0.4% trypan blue exclusion assay. Further, 0.1 mL of tumor cells (99% viable) were injected intraperitoneNaly into each Swiss albino mouse. The mice were divided into three groups with a minimum number of six mice in each group. One group was kept as the control group and after 24 h, the other two groups of mice were treated with an intraperitoneal injection of MytiLec-1 at the doses of 1.0 and 2.0 mg/kg/day. After five days treatment, mice in each group were slaughtered on the sixth day. EAC cells from each mouse was harvested in 0.9% saline by intraperitoneal injection and counted by a haemocytometer. The total number of viable cells in every mouse of the treated groups was compared with those of the control group. The percentage of inhibition was calculated by using the following formula:

$$\text{Percentage of inhibition} = 100 - \{(\text{cells from MytiLec-1 treated mice/cells from control mice}) \times 100\}$$

4.9. Examination of Morphological Alteration and Nuclear Damages of Ehrlich Ascites Carcinoma Cells by Hoechst Staining

Signs of apoptosis of EAC cells were morphologically observed without and with MytiLec-1 using an optical and fluorescence microscopy (Olympus IX71, Seoul, Korea). EAC cells were collected from the mice treated with and without MytiLec-1 (2.0 mg/kg/day) for five consecutive days and washed thrice with PBS. Cells were then stained with 0.1 μg/mL of Hoechst-33342 at 37 °C for 20 min in the dark and washed again with PBS to remove the unbound dye.

4.10. Isolation of RNA from Ehrlich Ascites Carcinoma Cells and Expression of Apoptosis-Related Genes

Tiangen Biotech reagent kit (Beijing, China) was used to isolate the total RNA from EAC cells collected from lectin-treated and lectin-untreated Swiss albino mice. Concentration and purity of the isolated RNAs were determined by a spectrophotometer at 260 and 280 nm. RNA quality was checked by 1.4% agarose gel electrophoresis as the gel was stained with 10 μg/mL of ethidium bromide and the bands were visualized with a gel documentation system (Cleaver Scientific Ltd., Rugby, UK). cDNA samples were prepared from the isolated RNA following the manufacturer's protocol (Applied Biosystems, Walthum, MA, USA). Primer sequences used in this study are shown in Table 1.

Table 1. List of primers.

Primer	Forward	Reverse
GAPDH	GTGGAAGGACTCATGACCACAG	CTGGTGCTCAGTGTAGCCCAG
Bax	CCTGCTTCTTTCTTCATCGG	AGGTGCCTGGACTCTTGGGT
Bcl-X	TTGGACAATGGACTGGTTGA	GTAGAGTGGATGGTCAGTG
NF-κB	AACAAAATGCCCCACGGTTA	GGGACGATGCAATGGACTGT
p53	GCGTCTTAGAGACAGTTGCCT	GGATAGGTCGGCGGTTCATGC

The program for amplification reactions was fixed at 95 °C for 3 min, 94 °C for 30 s, 55 °C 30 s, 72 °C for 50 s, and 72 °C for 10 min. Eventually, it was held at 20 °C in the thermal cycler (GeneAtlas, Tokyo, Japan). Expression of a housekeeping gene (GAPDH) was checked to confirm the quality of mRNA of the lectin-treated and untreated samples. All PCR reactions were analyzed by 1.4% agarose gel electrophoresis in the presence of a 100 bp DNA ladder (Sigma) as marker.

4.11. Cell Culture

HeLa (cervical cancer cells) and U937 (myeloid leukemia cells) were obtained from the Riken Cell Bank, Tsukuba, Japan and were cultured in RPMI-1640 medium with 10% fetal calf serum, and 1% (v/v) penicillin–streptomycin, in 25 cm² tissue culture flasks at a humidified atmosphere of 5% CO_2 at 37 °C. Cells were sub-cultured at regular intervals whenever the confluence reached to 70–80%.

4.12. Incubation of Fluorescein Isothiocyanate (FITC)-Conjugated MytiLec-1 with U937 Cells

Next, 2 mg of MytiLec-1 was conjugated with NH_2-reactive fluorescein Isothiocyanate (Dojindo Laboratories, Kumamoto, Japan) according to the manufacturer's instructions. U937 cells were cultured, taken on 18 mm round cover slips, and incubated with 100 μg/mL of FITC-MytiLec-1 from 5 min to 1 h. Cells were fixed with 4% paraformaldehyde for 15 min and observed using a Leica TCS SP5 confocal microscope (Wetzlar, Germany).

4.13. 3-(4,5-Dimethylthiazol-2-yl)-2,5-Diphenyl Tetrazolium Bromide (MTT) Colorimetric Assay of Different Cancer Cell Lines

MTT colorimetric assay was performed to determine the proliferation of U937 and HeLa cells according to a previous report [27]. Cells (2×10^4 in 150 µL RPMI 1640 media) were seeded in a 96-well flat bottom culture plate and incubated at 37 °C in a CO_2 incubator for 24 h. Cells were then incubated again for 48 h in the absence and presence of various concentrations (50–12.5 µg/mL) of MytiLec-1. Media containing only U937 and HeLa cells were used as positive controls. After carefully draining the aliquot, 10 mM of PBS (180 µL) and MTT (20 µL, 5 mg/mL MTT in PBS) were added and incubated for 8 h at 37 °C. The aliquot was removed again and 200 µL of acidic isopropanol was added to every well and incubated again at 37 °C for 30 min. The absorbance was recorded at 570 nm by a culture plate reader. Three wells were employed for each concentration and the following equation was followed to calculate the cell proliferation inhibition ratio:

$$\text{Proliferation inhibition ratio (\%)} = \{(A - B) \times 100\}/A$$

where A is the OD_{570} nm of the cellular homogenate (control) without MytiLec-1 and B is the OD_{570} nm of the cellular homogenate with MytiLec-1.

4.14. Statistical Analysis

For each of the studied parameters, experimental results were presented as mean ± standard error (SE) for three replicates. Data were subjected to one-way analysis of variance (ANOVA) followed by Dunnett's test, using the SPSS Statistics software package, v. 10 (IBM Corporation, Armonk, NY, USA). Differences with $p < 0.05$ were considered as statistically significant.

5. Conclusions

In this study, it became evident that MytiLec-1 was mildly cytotoxic, strictly glycan-dependent in its actions, and effectively inhibited the growth of different cancer cells in vivo and in vitro. The protein activated Bax/Bak genes eventually caused apoptosis, possibly through a p53-dependent pathway. MytiLec-1 can be considered significantly active against cancer cells, but further studies are necessary to resolve the explicit intrinsic molecular mechanism of action of MytiLec-1.

Author Contributions: I.H. did the majority of the study and wrote the A.K.M.A., and R.R.S. were involved in experimental works and data analysis. Y.F. supported purification of MytiLec-1. Y.O., M.B.U., and S.R.K. provided laboratory support, conducted the study and improved the manuscript through careful review and helpful suggestions.

Funding: This study was supported in part by JSPS KAKENHI under grant no. JP19K06239 (Y.O. and Y.F.) and JP18K07458 (Y.F.).

Acknowledgments: Authors would like to thank Ruhul Amin, Senior Scientific Officer, Bangladesh Council of Scientific and Industrial Research (BCSIR), Rajshahi, Bangladesh for providing laboratory support.

Conflicts of Interest: The authors declare no conflict of interest.

References

1. Garcia-Maldonado, E.; Cano-Sanchez, P.; Hernandez-Santoyo, A. Molecular and functional characterization of a glycosylated galactose-binding lectin from *Mytilus californianus*. *Fish Shellfish Immunol.* **2017**, *66*, 564–574. [CrossRef]
2. Rubinstein, N.; Ilarregui, J.M.; Toscano, M.A.; Rabinovich, G.A. The role of galectins in the initiation, amplification and resolution of the inflammatory response. *Tissue Antigens* **2004**, *64*, 1–12. [CrossRef] [PubMed]
3. Liu, B.; Bian, H.J.; Bao, J.K. Plant lectins: Potential antineoplastic drugs from bench to clinic. *Cancer Lett.* **2010**, *287*, 1–12. [CrossRef] [PubMed]

4. Yau, T.; Dan, X.; Ng, C.C.W.; Ng, T.B. Lectins with potential for anticancer therapy. *Molecules* **2015**, *20*, 3791–3810. [CrossRef] [PubMed]
5. Varrot, A.; Basheer, S.M.; Imberty, A. Fungal lectins: Structure, function and potential applications. *Curr. Opin. Struct. Biol.* **2013**, *23*, 678–685. [CrossRef] [PubMed]
6. Herre, J.; Willment, J.A.; Gordon, S.; Brown, G.D. The role of Dectin-1 in antifungal immunity. *Crit. Rev. Immunol.* **2004**, *24*, 193–203. [CrossRef] [PubMed]
7. Breitenbach, B.C.L.C.; Marcelino, D.S.S.P.; Felix, O.W.; de Moura, M.C.; Viana, P.E.; Soares, G.F.; Guedes, P.P.M.; Napoleao, T.H.; Dos, S.C.M.T. Lectins as antimicrobial agents. *J. Appl. Microbiol.* **2018**, *125*, 1238–1252. [CrossRef] [PubMed]
8. Hasan, I.; Gerdol, M.; Fujii, Y.; Rajia, S.; Koide, Y.; Yamamoto, D.; Kawsar, S.M.A.; Ozeki, Y. cDNA and Gene Structure of MytiLec-1, A Bacteriostatic R-Type Lectin from the Mediterranean Mussel (*Mytilus galloprovincialis*). *Mar. Drugs* **2016**, *14*, 92. [CrossRef]
9. Mitchell, C.A.; Ramessar, K.; O'Keefe, B.R. Antiviral lectins: Selective inhibitors of viral entry. *Antiviral. Res.* **2017**, *142*, 37–54. [CrossRef]
10. Cheung, R.C.F.; Wong, J.H.; Pan, W.; Chan, Y.S.; Yin, C.; Dan, X.; Ng, T.B. Marine lectins and their medicinal applications. *Appl. Microbiol. Biotechnol.* **2015**, *99*, 3755–3773. [CrossRef]
11. Kilpatrick, D.C. Animal lectins: A historical introduction and overview. *Biochim. Biophys. Acta.* **2002**, *1572*, 187–197. [CrossRef]
12. Vasta, G.R.; Ahmed, H.; Tasumi, S.; Odom, E.W.; Saito, K. Biological roles of lectins in innate immunity: Molecular and structural basis for diversity in self/nonself recognition. *Adv. Exp. Med. Biol.* **2007**, *598*, 389–406. [PubMed]
13. Varki, A.; Etzler, M.E.; Cummings, R.D.; Esko, J.D. *Discovery and Classification of Glycan-binding Proteins, In Essentials of Glycobiology*, 2nd ed.; Varki, A., Cummings, R.D., Esko, J.D., Freeze, H.H., Stanley, P., Bertozzi, C.R., Hart, G.W., Etzler, M.E., Eds.; Cold Spring Harbor Laboratory Press: New York, NY, USA, 2009; pp. 375–394.
14. Fujii, Y.; Dohmae, N.; Takio, K.; Kawsar, S.M.A.; Matsumoto, R.; Hasan, I.; Koide, Y.; Kanaly, R.A.; Yasumitsu, H.; Ogawa, Y.; et al. A lectin from the mussel *Mytilus galloprovincialis* has a highly novel primary structure and induces glycan-mediated cytotoxicity of globotriaosylceramide-expressing lymphoma cells. *J. Biol. Chem.* **2012**, *287*, 44772–44783. [CrossRef]
15. Belogortseva, N.I.; Molchanova, V.I.; Kurika, A.V.; Skobun, A.S.; Glazkova, V.E. Isolation and characterization of new GalNAc/Gal-specific lectin from the sea mussel *Crenomytilus grayanus*. *Comp. Biochem. Physiol. C Pharmacol. Toxicol. Endocrinol.* **1998**, *119*, 45–50. [CrossRef]
16. Kovalchuk, S.N.; Chikalovets, I.V.; Chernikov, O.V.; Molchanova, V.I.; Li, W.; Rasskazov, V.A.; Lukyanov, P.A. cDNA cloning and structural characterization of a lectin from the mussel *Crenomytilus grayanus* with a unique amino acid sequence and antibacterial activity. *Fish Shellfish Immunol.* **2013**, *35*, 1320–1324. [CrossRef] [PubMed]
17. Chikalovets, I.V.; Kondrashina, A.S.; Chernikov, O.V.; Molchanova, V.I.; Lukyanov, P.A. Isolation and general characteristics of lectin from the mussel *Mytilus trossulus*. *Chem. Nat. Comp.* **2013**, *48*, 1058–1061. [CrossRef]
18. Chernikov, O.; Kuzmich, A.; Chikalovets, I.; Molchanova, V.; Hua, K.F. Lectin CGL from the sea mussel *Crenomytilus grayanus* induces Burkitt's lymphoma cells death via interaction with surface glycan. *Int. J. Biol. Macromol.* **2017**, *104*, 508–514. [CrossRef]
19. Hasan, I.; Sugawara, S.; Fujii, Y.; Koide, Y.; Terada, D.; Iimura, N.; Fujiwara, T.; Takahashi, K.G.; Kojima, N.; Rajia, S.; et al. MytiLec, a Mussel R-Type Lectin, interacts with surface glycan Gb3 on Burkitt's lymphoma cells to trigger apoptosis through multiple pathways. *Mar. Drugs* **2015**, *13*, 7377–7389. [CrossRef]
20. Terada, D.; Kawai, F.; Noguchi, H.; Unzai, S.; Hasan, I.; Fujii, Y.; Park, S.; Ozeki, Y.; Tame, J.R.H. Crystal structure of MytiLec, a galactose-binding lectin from the mussel *Mytilus galloprovincialis* with cytotoxicity against certain cancer cell types. *Sci. Rep.* **2016**, *6*, 28344. [CrossRef]
21. Moura, R.M.; Melo, A.A.; Carneiro, R.F.; Rodrigues, C.R.; Delatorre, P.; Nascimento, K.S.; Saker-Sampaio, S.; Nagano, C.S.; Cavada, B.S.; Sampaio, A.H. Hemagglutinating/Hemolytic activities in extracts of marine invertebrates from the Brazilian coast and isolation of two lectins from the marine sponge *Cliona varians* and the sea cucumber *Holothuria grisea*. *An. Acad. Bras. Cienc.* **2015**, *87*, 973–984. [CrossRef]

22. Carneiro, R.F.; de Melo, A.A.; Nascimento, F.E.; Simplicio, C.A.; Nascimento, K.S.; Rocha, B.A.; Saker-Sampaio, S.; Moura, R.M.; Mota, S.S.; Cavada, B.S.; et al. Halilectin 1 (H-1) and Halilectin 2 (H-2): Two new lectins isolated from the marine sponge *Haliclona caerulea*. *J. Mol. Recognit.* **2013**, *26*, 51–58. [CrossRef] [PubMed]

23. Arruda, F.V.; Melo, A.A.; Vasconcelos, M.A.; Carneiro, R.F.; Barroso-Neto, I.L.; Silva, S.R.; Pereira-Junior, F.N.; Nagano, C.S.; Nascimento, K.S.; Teixeira, E.H.; et al. Toxicity and binding profile of lectins from the Genus *canavalia* on brine shrimp. *Biomed. Res. Int.* **2013**, *2013*, 154542. [CrossRef] [PubMed]

24. Pusztai, A.; Bardocz, S. Biological effects of plant lectins on the gastrointestinal tract: Metabolic consequences and applications. *Trends Glycosci. Glyc.* **1996**, *8*, 149–165. [CrossRef]

25. Miyake, K.; Tanaka, T.; McNeil, P.L. Lectin-based food poisoning: A new mechanism of protein toxicity. *PLoS ONE* **2007**, *2*, e687. [CrossRef] [PubMed]

26. Terada, D.; Voet, A.R.D.; Noguchi, H.; Kamata, K.; Ohki, M.; Addy, C.; Fujii, Y.; Yamamoto, D.; Ozeki, Y.; Tame, J.R.H.; et al. Computational design of a symmetrical beta-trefoil lectin with cancer cell binding activity. *Sci. Rep.* **2017**, *7*, 5943. [CrossRef] [PubMed]

27. Ahmed, F.R.S.; Amin, R.; Hasan, I.; Asaduzzaman, A.K.M.; Kabir, S.R. Antitumor properties of a methyl-β-D-galactopyranoside specific lectin from *Kaempferia rotunda* against Ehrlich ascites carcinoma cells. *Int. J. Biol. Macromol.* **2017**, *102*, 952–959. [CrossRef]

28. Kabir, K.M.A.; Amin, R.; Hasan, I.; Asaduzzaman, A.K.M.; Khatun, H.; Kabir, S.R. *Geodorum densiflorum* rhizome lectin inhibits Ehrlich ascites carcinoma cell growth by inducing apoptosis through the regulation of BAX, p53 and NF-κB genes expression. *Int. J. Biol. Macromol.* **2019**, *125*, 92–98. [CrossRef]

29. Hasan, I.; Islam, F.; Ozeki, Y.; Kabir, S.R. Antiproliferative activity of cytotoxic tuber lectins from *Solanum tuberosum* against experimentally induced Ehrlich ascites carcinoma in mice. *Afr. J. Biotechnol.* **2014**, *13*, 1679–1685.

30. Kabir, S.R.; Rahman, M.M.; Amin, R.; Karim, M.R.; Mahmud, Z.H.; Hossain, M.T. *Solanum tuberosum* lectin inhibits Ehrlich ascites carcinoma cells growth by inducing apoptosis and G2/M cell cycle arrest. *Tumour. Biol.* **2016**, *37*, 8437–8444. [CrossRef]

31. Eckhardt, A.E.; Goldstein, I.J. An α-D-galactopyranosyl-containing glycoprotein from Ehrlich ascites tumor cell plasma membranes. In *Glycoconjugate Research*, 1st ed.; Gregory, J.D., Jeanloz, R.W., Eds.; Academic Press Inc.: New York, NY, USA, 1979; pp. 1043–1045.

32. Sakakibara, F.; Kawauchi, H.; Takayanagi, G.; Ise, H. Egg lectin of *Rana japonica* and its receptor glycoprotein of Ehrlich tumor cells. *Cancer Res.* **1979**, *39*, 1347–1352.

33. Ahmed, H.; Chatterjee, B.P.; Debnath, A.K. Interaction and in vivo growth inhibition of Ehrlich ascites tumor cells by jacalin. *J. Biosci.* **1988**, *13*, 419–424. [CrossRef]

34. Kabir, S.R.; Nabi, M.M.; Haque, A.; Zaman, R.U.; Mahmud, Z.H.; Reza, M.A. Pea lectin inhibits growth of Ehrlich ascites carcinoma cells by inducing apoptosis and G2/M cell cycle arrest in vivo in mice. *Phytomedicine* **2013**, *20*, 1288–1296. [CrossRef] [PubMed]

35. Al-Mamun, M.A.; Akter, Z.; Uddin, M.J.; Ferdaus, K.M.K.B.; Hoque, K.M.F.; Ferdousi, Z.; Reza, M.A. Characterization and evaluation of antibacterial and antiproliferative activities of crude protein extracts isolated from the seeds of *Ricinus communis* in Bangladesh. *BMC Complement. Altern. Med.* **2016**, *16*, 211. [CrossRef] [PubMed]

36. Al-Mamun, M.A.; Husna, J.; Khatun, M.; Hasan, R.; Kamruzzaman, M.; Hoque, K.M.F.; Reza, M.A.; Ferdousi, Z. Assessment of antioxidant, anticancer and antimicrobial activity of two vegetable species of *Amaranthus* in Bangladesh. *BMC Complement. Altern. Med.* **2016**, *16*, 157. [CrossRef] [PubMed]

37. Reza, M.A.; Kabir, S.R. Antibacterial activity of *Kaempferia rotunda* rhizome lectin and its induction of apoptosis in Ehrlich ascites carcinoma cells. *Appl. Biochem. Biotechnol.* **2014**, *172*, 2866–2876.

38. Groc, L.; Bezin, L.; Jiang, H.; Jackson, T.S.; Levine, R.A. Bax, Bcl-2, and cyclin expression and apoptosis in rat substantia nigra during development. *Neurosci. Lett.* **2001**, *306*, 198–202. [CrossRef]

39. Li, F.; Chen, X.; Xu, B.; Zhou, H. Curcumin induces p53-independent necrosis in H1299 cells via a mitochondria-associated pathway. *Mol. Med. Rep.* **2015**, *12*, 7806–7814. [CrossRef]

40. Baichwal, V.R.; Baeuerle, P.A. Activate NF-kappa B or die? *Curr. Biol.* **1997**, *7*, R94–R96. [CrossRef]

41. Tong, Q.S.; Zheng, L.D.; Wang, L.; Liu, J.; Qian, W. BAK overexpression mediates p53-independent apoptosis inducing effects on human gastric cancer cells. *BMC Cancer* **2004**, *4*, 33. [CrossRef]

42. Degenhardt, K.; Chen, G.; Lindsten, T.; White, E. BAX and BAK mediate p53-independent suppression of tumorigenesis. *Cancer Cell.* **2002**, *2*, 193–203. [CrossRef]

43. Strobel, T.; Swanson, L.; Korsmeyer, S.; Cannistra, S.A. BAX enhances paclitaxel-induced apoptosis through a p53-independent pathway. *Proc. Natl. Acad. Sci. USA.* **1996**, *93*, 14094–14099. [CrossRef] [PubMed]

44. Mise, K.; Akifusa, S.; Watarai, S.; Ansai, T.; Nishihara, T.; Takehara, T. Involvement of ganglioside GM3 in G2/M cell cycle arrest of human monocytic cells induced by *Actinobacillus actinomycetemcomitans* cytolethal distending toxin. *Infect. Immun.* **2005**, *73*, 4846–4852. [CrossRef] [PubMed]

45. Matsushima-Hibiya, Y.; Watanabe, M.; Hidari, K.I.J.; Miyamoto, D.; Suzuki, Y.; Kasama, T.; Kanazawa, T.; Koyama, K.; Sugimura, T.; Wakabayashi, K. Identification of glycosphingolipid receptors for Pierisin-1, a guanine-specific ADP-ribosylaing toxin from the cabbage butterfly. *J. Biol. Chem.* **2003**, *278*, 9972–9978. [CrossRef] [PubMed]

46. Hasan, I.; Ozeki, Y. Histochemical localization of N-acetylhexosamine-binding lectin HOL-18 in Halichondria okadai (Japanese black sponge), and its antimicrobial and cytotoxic anticancer effects. *Int. J. Biol. Macromol.* **2019**, *124*, 819–827. [CrossRef] [PubMed]

47. Zurga, S.; Nanut, M.P.; Kos, J.; Sabotic, J. Fungal lectin MpL enables entry of protein drugs into cancer cells and their subcellular targeting. *Oncotarget* **2017**, *8*, 26896–26910. [CrossRef] [PubMed]

48. Oda, T.; Iwaoka, J.; Komatsu, N.; Muramatsu, T. Involvement of N-acetylcysteine-sensitive pathways in ricin-induced apoptotic cell death in U937 cells. *Biosci. Biotechnol. Biochem.* **1999**, *63*, 341–348. [CrossRef]

49. Hasegawa, N.; Kimura, Y.; Oda, T.; Komatsu, N.; Muramatsu, T. Isolated ricin B-chain-mediated apoptosis in U937 cells. *Biosci. Biotechnol. Biochem.* **2000**, *64*, 1422–1429. [CrossRef]

50. Koyama, Y.; Katsuno, Y.; Miyoshi, N.; Hayakawa, S.; Mita, T.; Muto, H.; Isemura, S.; Aoyagi, Y.; Isemura, M. Apoptosis induction by lectin isolated from the mushroom *Boletopsis leucomelas* in U937 cells. *Biosci. Biotechnol. Biochem.* **2002**, *66*, 784–789. [CrossRef]

51. Carvalho, F.C.; Soares, S.G.; Tamarozzi, M.B.; Rego, E.M.; Roque-Barreira, M.C. The recognition of N-glycans by the lectin ArtinM mediates cell death of a human myeloid leukemia cell line. *PLoS ONE* **2011**, *6*, e27892. [CrossRef]

52. Rabelo, L.; Monteiro, N.; Serquiz, R.; Santos, P.; Oliveira, R.; Oliveira, A.; Rocha, H.; Morais, A.H.; Uchoa, A.; Santos, E. A lactose-binding lectin from the marine sponge *Cinachyrella apion* (Cal) induces cell death in human cervical adenocarcinoma cells. *Mar. Drugs* **2012**, *10*, 727–743. [CrossRef]

53. Fujii, Y.; Fujiwara, T.; Koide, Y.; Hasan, I.; Sugawara, S.; Rajia, S.; Kawsar, S.M.A.; Yamamoto, D.; Araki, D.; Kanaly, R.A.; et al. Internalization of a novel, huge lectin from *Ibacus novemdentatus* (slipper lobster) induces apoptosis of mammalian cancer cells. *Glycoconj. J.* **2017**, *34*, 85–94. [CrossRef] [PubMed]

54. Laemmli, U.K. Cleavage of structural proteins during the assembly of the head of bacteriophage T4. *Nature* **1970**, *227*, 680–685. [CrossRef] [PubMed]

55. Kabir, S.R.; Zubair, M.A.; Nurujjaman, M.; Haque, M.A.; Hasan, I.; Islam, M.F.; Hossain, M.T.; Hossain, M.A.; Rakib, M.A.; Alam, M.T.; et al. Purification and characterization of a Ca^{2+} dependent novel lectin from *Nymphaea nouchali* Tuber with antiproliferative activities. *Biosci. Rep.* **2011**, *31*, 465–475. [CrossRef] [PubMed]

56. Finney, D.J. *Probit Analysis*, 3rd ed.; Cambridge University Press: London, UK, 1971; p. 333.

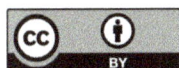

MDPI

St. Alban-Anlage 66

4052 Basel

Switzerland

Tel. +41 61 683 77 34

Fax +41 61 302 89 18

www.mdpi.com

Marine Drugs Editorial Office

E-mail: marinedrugs@mdpi.com

www.mdpi.com/journal/marinedrugs